AF480107

Essentials of
Herbal Options

Essentials of
Herbal Options

Prof (Dr.) Tapan Kumar Chatterjee

M. Pharm. (J.U), Ph.D (J.U.), FIC (Cal.)., ARSC(Lond.)

Dean, JIS University,
81, Nilgunge Road, Kolkata-700109

Former Research Scientist (UGC, Govt. of India)
Department of Pharmceutical Technology,
Jadavpur University, Kolkata.

Former Director,
Clinical Research Centre (CRC),
Jadavpur University, Kolkata.

Former Professor,
Division of Pharmacology,
Department of Pharmaceutical Technology,
Jadavpur University, Kolkata.

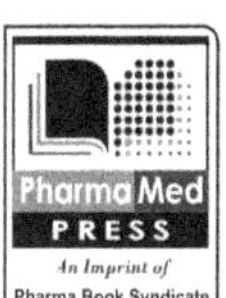
PharmaMed Press
An imprint of Pharma Book Syndicate
A unit of BSP Books Pvt. Ltd.
4-4-309/316, Giriraj Lane,
Sultan Bazar, Hyderabad - 500 095.

Essentials of Herbal Options *by*
Prof (Dr.) Tapan Kumar Chatterjee

Published by

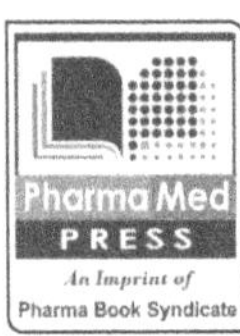

PharmaMed Press

An imprint of Pharma Book Syndicate

A unit of BSP Books Pvt. Ltd.

4-4-309/316, Giriraj Lane, Sultan Bazar, Hyderabad - 500 095.

Phone: 040-23445688/600; Fax: 91+40-23445611

E-mail: info@pharmamedpress.com

www.pharmamedpress.com/pharmamedpress.net

ISBN: 978-93-88305-52-5

Dedicated to:

LATE SARDAR JODH SINGH
(1920-2018)

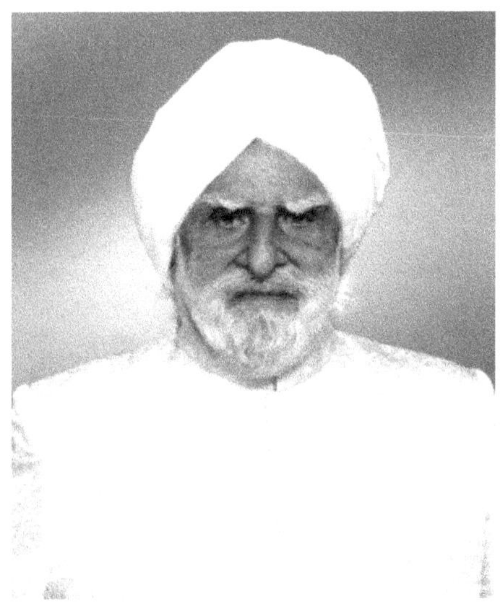

Chairman and Founder - JIS Group

PREFACE

At the beginning, I candidly express my belief that it is needless to emphasize too strongly, the need for quest of indisputable knowledge in the use and utility of medicinal plants, in the field of curative treatment of various diseases and prevention thereof.

Since time immemorial, human beings have leaned on plants/herbs/shrubs etc. for curative treatment of diseases and to secure prevention and care against manifestations of various ailments. The same herbs, plants and shrubs etc. which were being put to use by the people of ancient days and used appreciably by the Egyptians, Grecians, Chinese, Romans as well as Indians have been continuing to be valued to combat diseases. Many of these plants and herbs are being used till today and some are even being introduced in the manufacture of indigenous medicines following extensive researches after clinical studies and trials.

For quite some time in the past, I felt the urge of compilation of a Handbook on medicinal plants, with up-to-date scientific information and educative/discovered, formulae, after being persuaded by the requests from Pharmaceutical Researchers for a comprehensive compilation on this subject. I have therefore been prompted to venture for compilation of the Book-named/styled as *"ESSENTIALS OF HERBAL OPTIONS"*.

The aim of this compilation is to highlight the information on scientific nomenclature, local names, distribution, parts used, pharmacological activities and chemical constituents of the different medicinal plants, meant for use for medicinal purposes. The information collected from different unpublished data, books, scientific journals, available up to the date of publication of this compilation (August, 2018) have been detailed systematically to provide accurate scientific informative data.

This Hand-Book embraces nine chapters. Chapters I to VII enunciate anti-cancer, anti-diabetic, anti-fertility, hepatoprotective, anti-inflammatory, anti-microbial and anti-ulcer medicinal plants respectively. Chapter VIII deals with Herbs-Food interactions and Chapter IX describes about different analysis techniques to identify the phytochemicals of herbs. Each chapter has been reviewed by way of close probing by the scientists. Unquestionable special help and guidance were rendered by **Prof. B. C. Mal**, Vice-Chancellor, JIS University that enabled me to complete the compilation of this Hand-Book within a short spell of time. Prof Mal being highly interested on this subject of human-welfare, laid hand in carrying out corrections of the manuscript with certain modulations. Exhilarating Counsel and encouragement have been exhibited by **Dr. B. Ruhidas, Mr. S. Karan, Miss. J. Pal, Mr. B. Chakra,**

Mr. S. Debnath, Mr. D. Naskar, Mrs. S. Chakraborty, Mr. M. Chakraborty, Dr. A. Sengupta with expert knowledge over the subject matter caused to enrich the value of this Hand-Book enormously. **Mr. Sanjib Jana** has extended his help in linguistic revision. I am also grateful to **Dr. M. U. Sharief,** Jt. Director of Botanical Survey of India (BSI), Howrah for his immense help to take photographs of medicinal plants from the herbal garden (Charak) of BSI. Acknowledgements are also due to my publisher "BSP Books Pvt. Ltd." and their editorial staff for co-operation, encouragement and valuable suggestions.

This book is also a result of enormous encouragements and sacrifices made by my family. Support from my wife **(Lisa)** and daughter **(Anuja)** has been a determining factor in enabling me to write this book. My late father **Sree K. K. Chatterjee** (who wrote more than 80 informative articles in reputed journals) was also one of my role models for me in providing the courage to undertake this challenging endeavor.

The materials and data compiled in this book may be used by a variety of professionals including pharmacists, pharmacologists, medicinal chemists, toxicologists, pharmacognosists, botanists etc. The book is highly recommended for herbal medicine manufacturers for beneficially using the data available in this compilation.

The author and the Publishers cannot be urged to accept any responsibility in the event of any error or omission creeping in or in compilations or printing, keeping in view, the human errors as well as the ever-changing scientific advancement of knowledge all over the world by continuous penetrating researches, according to developments, which are gradually coming up to surface rapidly.

In fact, I shall be deriving high satisfaction, if this handbook could attract readers/users to utilize the materials and explored data, elaborated in this small handy compilation.

Prof. T.K. Chatterjee,
JIS University
Kolkata-700 109

CONTENTS

Introduction

The word 'herb' has an origin from old French or Latin word 'herba' which means 'plant without solid stem'. Medicines prepared by using herbs are called herbal medicines. Since primitive human existence, many natural resources were used as routine material for human well-being by transparent perception or, more appropriately, by trial and error. Owing to this exercise, practically most of the countries including the epochmaking civilizations of China, Egypt and India redefined its own medical system. Thus, the Indian medical system, Ayurveda ('science of life'), came into permanence which is mainly based on herbal medicines. The raw materials for ayurvedic medicines were mostly obtained from plant sources in the form of crude drugs such as dried herbal powders or their extracts or mixture of products.

Chinese drugs have been in operation for over 5,000 years for the medication of diverse types of fever and respiratory ailments. However, the active principal ephedrine was isolated only in 1887 and placed in modern medicine in 1925. Analogously, Opium was first introduced in Asia Minor, the active principle was later identified as morphine in 1804 and then it came into modern medicine in 1818. Cinchona species was used in Peru by the natives from time immemorial; Countess of Cinchon, cured of a fever by it in 1638, gave it her name, but its active principle was divulged as quinine as late as 1820 followed by introduction in modern medicine five years later. Vinca roses is a plant which grows widely in Indian continent. Embedded on the Ayurvedic lead, Lilly Company of U.S.A. initiated work on *Vinca roses* dried leaves, and ultimately discovered two alkaloids named vinblastine and vincristine which are used in therapy of Leukemia. Many other drugs have also come into existence as reputed medicines in recent years as a result of biological screening. Protuberant among them is gossypol, a competent male contraceptive. Ginsing— a preparation of dried roots of *Panax ginsing*—is known for improvement of memory and also as a general tonic.

Old drugs find new use—in early 1990s China introduced new antimalarial drug (artemisinine) derived from the plant *Artemisia annuta*.

The modern age has seen some decrease in the use of medicinal plants or their extracts as curative agent—especially in developed countries. Modern medicines and herbal medicines are complimentarily being used in areas for health care programme in several developing countries including India. Of late, interest in the plant products increased all over the world due to the fact that many herbal medicines are known to be free from side-effects. Moreover, the truth that the unearthing of new synthetic drugs is a time-consuming, expensive affair, and, if we want to implement "Health for all by the year 2020", possibly the rational choice, would lie in exploring plant products as capable medicines to the maximum conceivable usage.

Indian research based on Ayurvedic medicine has not been substantially blessed, even though screening of plants based on ancient reports have been exceedingly persuaded. It is appropriate to notice that between 1960-1980, CDRI Lucknow and CIBA Research, Mumbai, have screened more than 2,500 plants which have claimed to own some kind of activity—the results were pleasing. While screening, many Indian medicinal plants have shown exciting physiological properties resulting in the isolation of clinically useful compounds. During screening, CDRI was skillful to isolate a new hypotensive agent—forskolin—from its plant. Hoechst R & D center at Mumbai has also recorded a few more interesting biologically active compounds from Indian plants. A contemporary example resulted from the Ayurvedic medicine guggulu, the first work done by the scientists of NCL and thereafter by the researchers of Multi-chem Research Center, Vadodora. They discovered that the gum-resin from guggulu was responsible for hypocholesteralemic activity.

Mother nature has provided ample medicinal plants for her children. Plants have granted mankind a large divergence of potent drugs to alleviate suffering from diseases. In spite of amazing advances in synthetic drugs in recent years, some of the drugs of plant source have still retained their momentousness. The utilization of plant-based drugs in the Western world is flourishing and ever-increasing.

India has a wealthy pedigree of science on plant-based drugs—both for use in remedial and preventive medicines. Ancient Indian scholars—**Charak, Sushruta, Bagavatta** and several others gave remarkably detailed description of Indian medicinal plants in the **Atharva Veda.** The preparation of these are still made in exalted distinction in the medical profession. Our ancient Ayurvedic system of medicine is primarily a plant-based meteria medica making use of our native invaluable plants.

It goes beyond saying that today cancer is a leading cause of mortality globally. Various therapeutic attempts to fight cancer have failed mainly owing to the side effects they pose and also due to the high cost associated with them. In this regard it must be mentioned that natural products are safer than their synthetic counterparts and also are less expensive. In fact plant derived molecules like vinblastine, vincristine, paclitaxel etc proved to be effective as chemotherapeutic agent. With a large number of molecules of natural origin already established, yet so many that have passed preliminary screening and there could still be a huge number of them still concealed within nature that could have potential anticancer activities. Hence, screening of natural products for efficacy against cancer becomes imperative.

Type 1 diabetes, the aggravation and prolongation of hepatitis and onset of liver cirrhosis are associated with cell-mediated allergy such as delayed type hypersensitivity. In spite of this, modern science has not advanced adequately to be able to give a complete answer. Many patients complain of general malaise of unidentified etiology. Symptoms include sleepiness, dizziness, depression, becoming tired easily, cold hands and feet, stiff shoulders, muscle pain and headache. These are the conditions where traditional medicines alone may prove advantageous without causing any harm. It is often impossible to scientifically identify diseases of such obscure symptoms. Traditional systems have an answer to a certain extent.

Glycyrrhizin from Glycyrrhiza for chronic hepatitis and Ginseng radix for complaints of general malaise in patients with circulatory disorders has passed through the Medical Act to undergo double blind studies (Phase III trials) in Japan. Thus a proper scientific approach has to be developed for the traditional formulation to be understood by the Western Medicine. Hence it is obvious that through new and improved understanding of Molecular Biology, Immunology, etc. we will have to understand and evaluate the claimed effects of traditional medicines. Many a times questions are raised as to how a single formula-on can produce so many effects. The answer, it seems, may lie in these studies. The traditional systems of medicines are completely different from Western medicine in their philosophy and history of development. It was, therefore, once thought that they contradict each other. Today, however, combination of Chinese and Western medicine is strongly recommended and practiced in China. In Japan, a Society is set up to develop and unite the two branches of medicine. From the above account it will be observed how much importance is given and how much development works have been done in practicing of the traditional medicine in a country with a known traditional system like Chinese in China and Kampo in Japan.

Inflammatory diseases, including rheumatism, are very common throughout the world. This is one of the oldest known diseases of mankind and affects a large population of the world. The need of antirheumatic drugs will constantly increase as our life expectancy goes on increasing. So-called systematic study of anti-inflammatory effect of Indian medicinal plants was done by many workers. About 40 plants were identified as having definite anti-inflammatory activity.

Flavonoids from *Hibiscus, vitifolius, Ochrocarpus longifolius, Arnebia hispidissinia, Rims Undulata, Scutellaria baicalensis, Rhannius infectioria, Dalbergia voluhilis, Hedychiuni spicatuni, Glycyrrhiza glabra* etc. are found to be active.

Coumarins from 5 plants, Xanthines from 4 plants, Lignins and Triterpenoids from about 10 plants, Alkaloids of 5 plants and miscellaneous compounds from 3 plants have shown such activity. An exhaustive review of this is done by Prof. Handa of Chandigarh.

Until recently it had been accepted, almost as dogma, that there was none—and that there cannot be any—pharmacological treatment for liver disease. The only drugs used were corticosteroids or immunosuppressive agents. Although a number of plants were used in Ayurveda for liver diseases— till the work on *Silybom marianum* was published by Western workers—our medical-scientists were not that alive on the subject. Now, more than 25 plants of Indian origin have been investigated and proved to possess these properties of treating the disease.

Prof. Norman Farnsworth and others in 'Medicinal Plants in Therapy' mention: one of the conditions for the success of primary health care is the availability and use of suitable drugs. Plants have always been a common source of medicaments — either in the form of traditional preparations or as pure active principles. It is thus rational for decision-makers to identify locally available plants or plant extracts that could be usefully added to the national list of drugs or that could even replace some pharmaceutical preparations that need to be imported.

We can just look at the market potentiality of these herbal drugs. As per WHO estimates, 80% or about 7,630 million population rely on plant products. This study covers the market dynamics and trends in major countries that are expected to influence the current market scenario and future status of the Global Herbal Medicine Market over the forecast period. Considering all these factors the market for herbal medicine is expected to reach $ 111 billion by the end of 2023, this market is projected to be growing at a CAGR of ~ 7.2 % during 2018-2023.

We can count on a number of plant products which command a current sale of more than a few billion dollars each. Almost all except a few multinational companies are directly or indirectly connected with companies dealing in plant products all over the world. According to WHO estimates, almost 80% population of many Asian and African countries depend on traditional medicine for primary health care. The market drivers for the global herbal medicine market are growing aging population, increasing consumer awareness, little or no side effects, supplier innovations, and the release of Current Good Manufacturing Practices (CGMP) for dietary supplements by the FDA. Another factor is escalating prices, tighter health budgets of modern medicinal system which has driven consumers towards the more economical and safer herbal medicine systems. The market constraints are lack of research and standardization in herbal medicines, poor legal and regulatory frame work which causes patent problems, poor manufactured herbal products etc.

Therefore, this has upsurged the growth of the market. India's share in the global herbal medicinal market is a miniscule 0.5 percent at \$358.60 million; government informed the Lok Sabha recently.

"Estimated global market is around \$70 billion. As per available information, India's export of AYUSH and value-added products of medicinal plants (herbal drugs) during 2015-2016 was \$358.60 million," Minister of State for AYUSH Shripad Yesso Naik said replying to a question in the House.

The ministry attributed India's poor share to several factors including lack of financial support to the herbal industry, he said. Another reason cited was lack of recognition of the ISM system of medicine (herbal) internationally. Currently, it is recognized only in few countries like Sri Lanka, Nepal, Bhutan, Malaysia and Bangladesh.

The ministry also rued the fact that there was a lack of awareness of international opportunities to export herbal products in different countries.

Essentials of the Herbal Options

- Going back to nature is something that has caught on world over in the last decade. This has seen an ascent in Ayurvedic (herbal) products, an area where India's competency dates back millennia, but it is only in the last decade that the country has truly seen the commercialization on the herbal concept. Herbal has now become a full-fledged wave, encompassing both beauty-care and health-care products. The recent upsurge in use of herbal medicines has led to a sudden increase in herbal manufacturing units. In India, there are about 14 well-recognized and 86 medium scale manufactures of herbal drugs. Other than this about 8,000 licensed small manufactures in India are on record. In addition, thousands of Vaidyas also have their own miniature manufacturing facilities. The estimated current annual production of herbal drugs is around Rs. 3500 crores. This section gives an overview of the rapidly growing Indian herbal industry followed by the legal parameters encompassing the manufacturing of herbal drugs. Herbal over the counter (OTC) drugs have gained considerable ground. Currently, according to industry estimate, Indian pharmaceutical market grew 5.5 per cent in the year 2017 in terms of moving annual turnover. In March 2018, the market grew at 9.5 per cent year-on-year with sales of Rs 10,029 crore (US$ 1.56 billion).

The reason for the take-off of herbal products has been gradual and can be ascribed to many reasons. The origins, according to many, can be sourced to the World Health Organization's Canberra conference in 1976, which promoted the concept of "traditional" medicines for the developing countries.

In India, almost a decade later, herbal cure began to be accepted, as alternative therapies with minimal side-effect gained in precedence elsewhere.

The herbal drug market itself is growing at a rate of 20 to 30% annually, with individual companies registering different growth rates.

While the domestic market is opening up to the herbal phenomenon, the export market is also showing promise. Many pharmaceutical companies are targeting export as the prime source in the coming years.

'Health is Wealth' says the Western scholar; 'Attainment of health is the highest attainment' (Lavanant Shreya Arogyam) says the Eastern scholar. Both agree on the point. So, the time has come for a new synthesis—a synthesis of Western and Eastern systems of medicine. The whole world will be benefitted by it.

PHOTOGRAPHS OF MEDICINAL PLANTS (PLATE 1.1 TO 1.40)

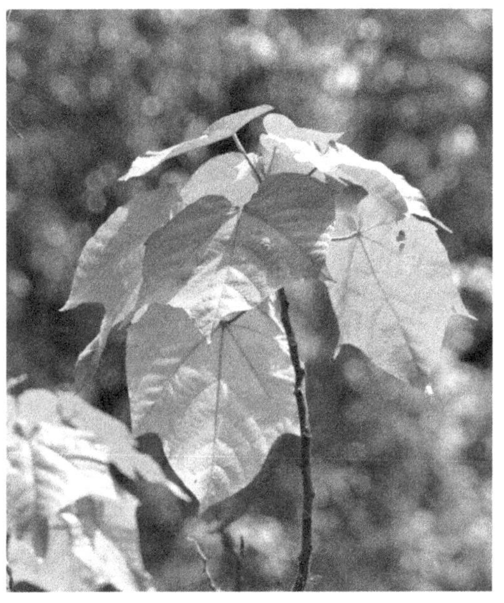

Plate 1.1 *Abroma Augusta*

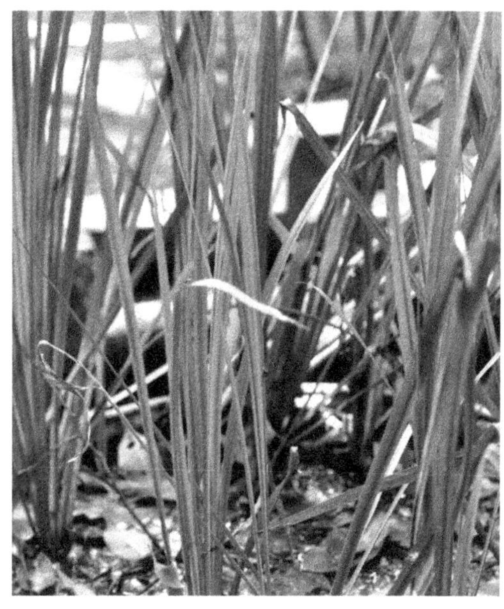

Plate 1.2 *Acorus Calamus*

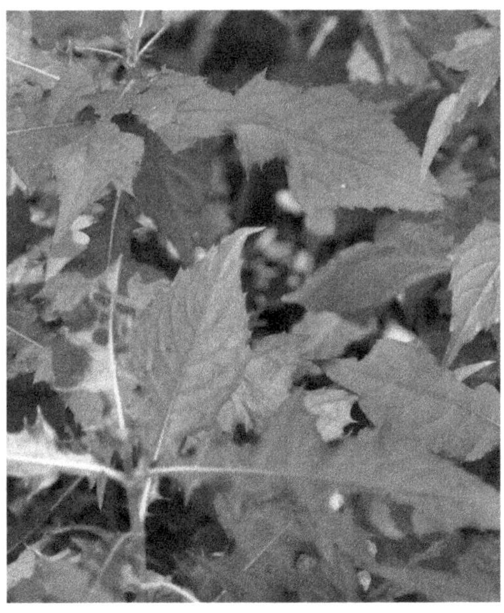

Plate 1.3 *Acunthus Ebractectus*

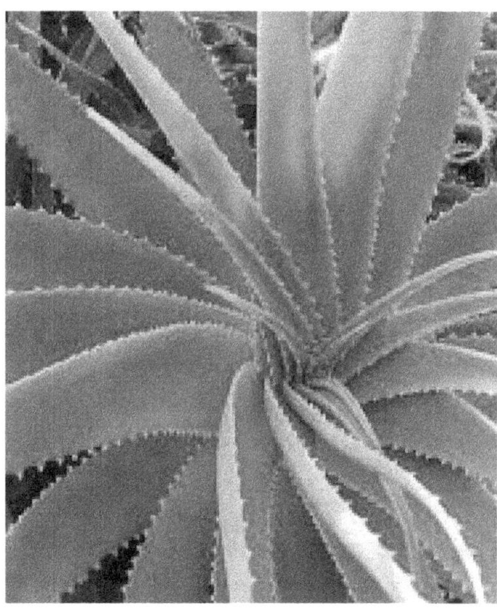

Plate 1.4 *Aloe Vera*

Insert – 1-10

Photographs of Medicinal Plants

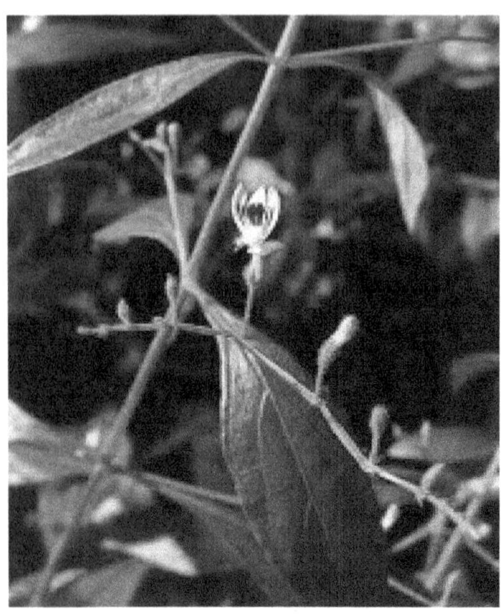

Plate 1.5 *Andrographis Paniculata*

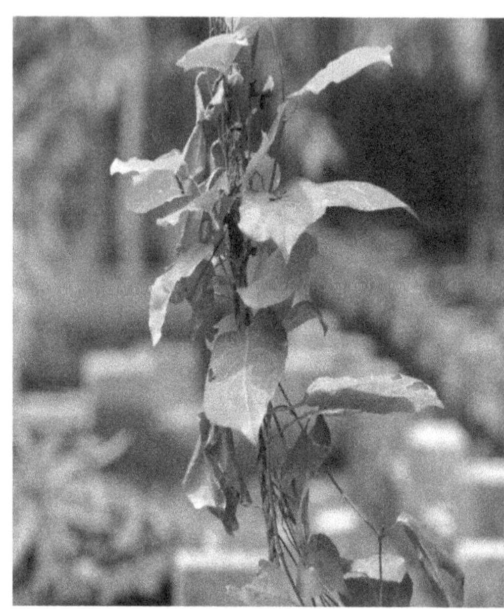

Plate 1.6 *Aristoloca Indica-Iswarmul*

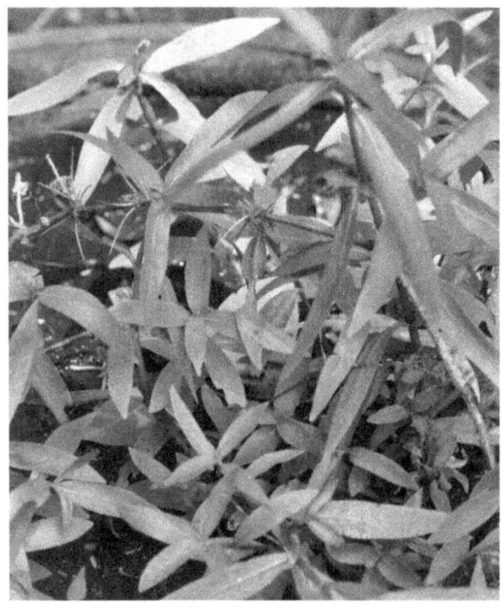

Plate 1.7 *Asteracantha Longifolia*

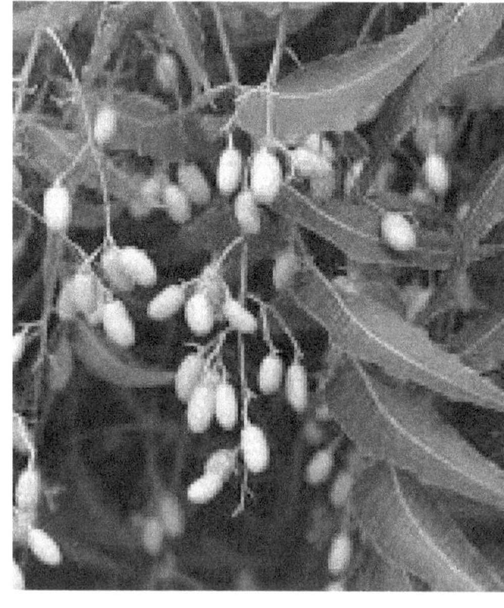

Plate 1.8 *Azadirachta Indica*

Photographs of Medicinal Plants

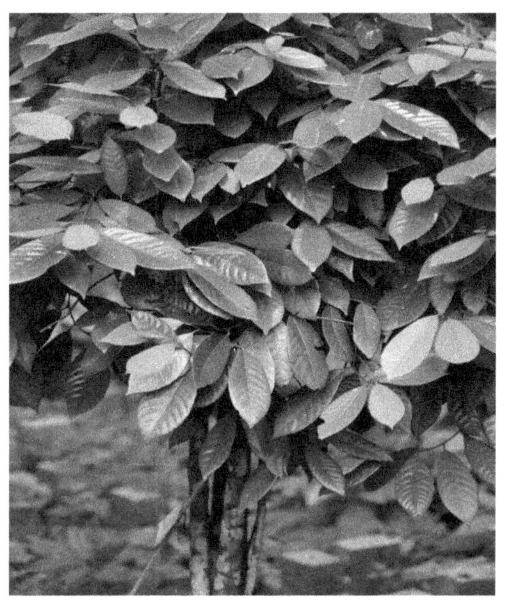

Plate 1.9 *Carissa carandas*

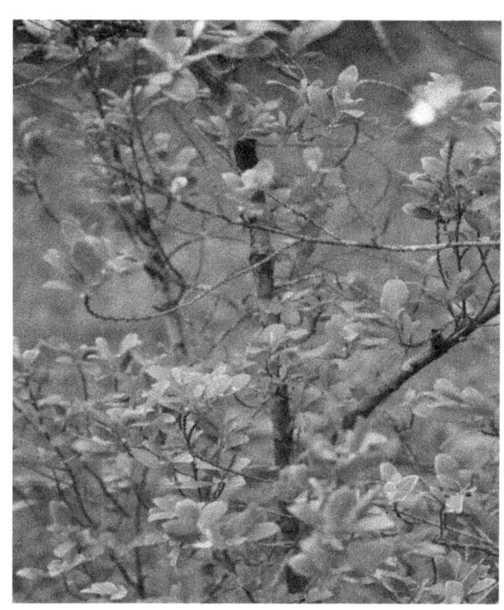

Plate 1.10 *Cinnamomum camphora*

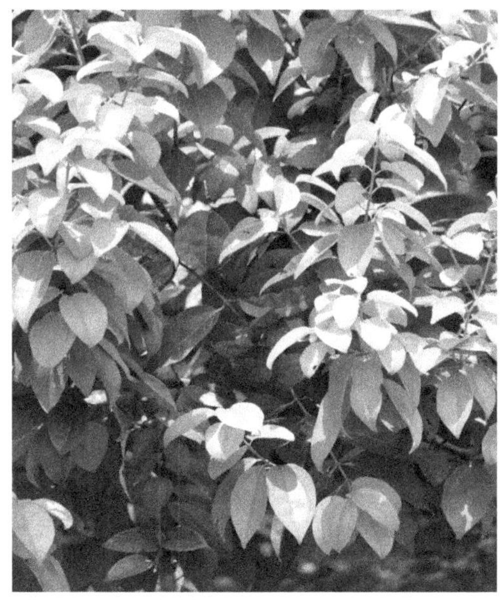

Plate 1.11 *Cinnamomum tamala*

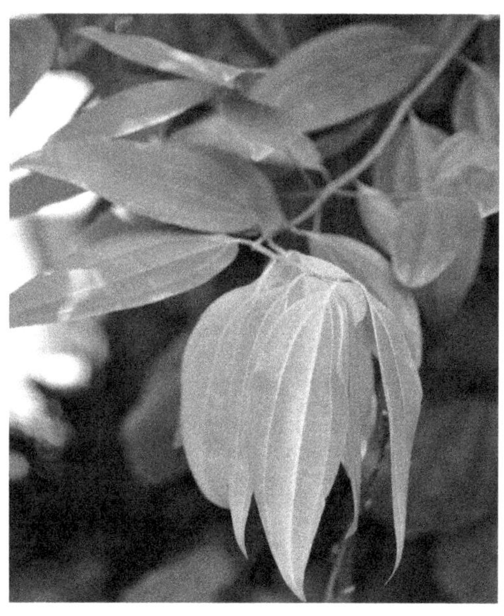

Plate 1.12 *Cinnamomum verum*

Photographs of Medicinal Plants

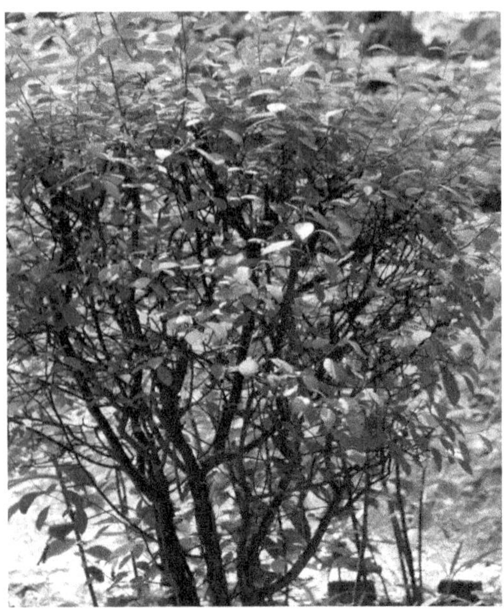

Plate 1.13 *Commiphora wightii*

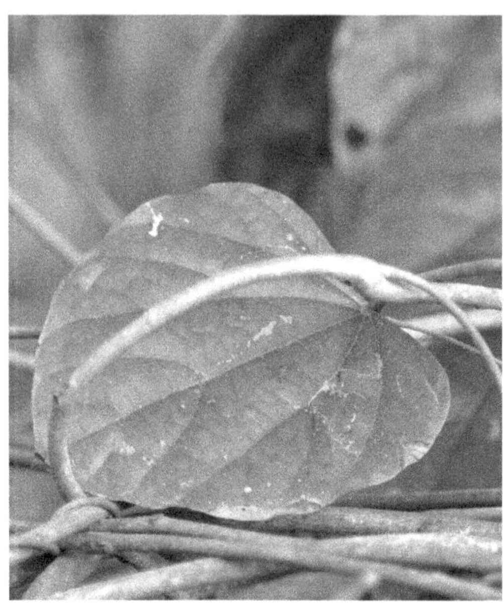

Plate 1.14 *Coscinum fenestratum*

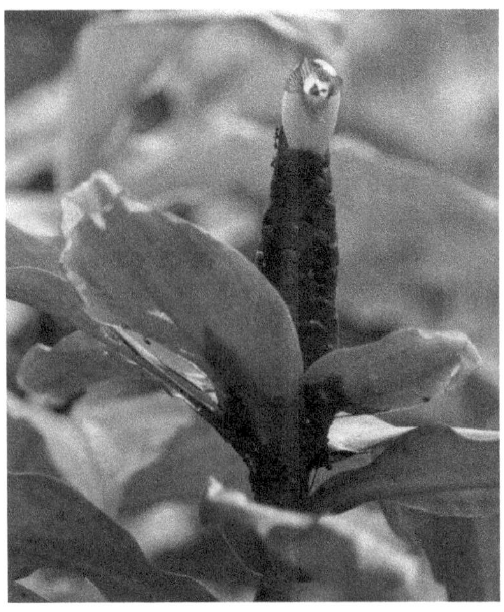

Plate 1.15 *Costus pictus*

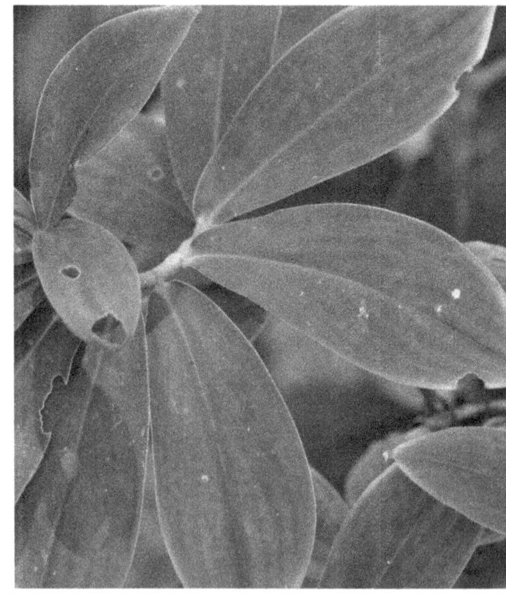

Plate 1.16 *Costus specious*

Photographs of Medicinal Plants

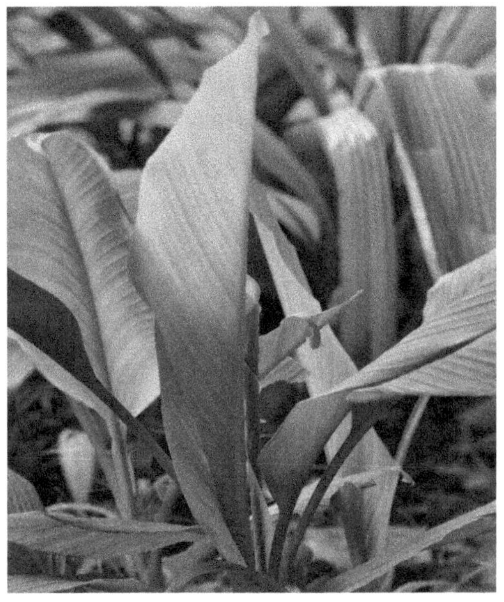

Plate 1.17 *Curcuma longa*

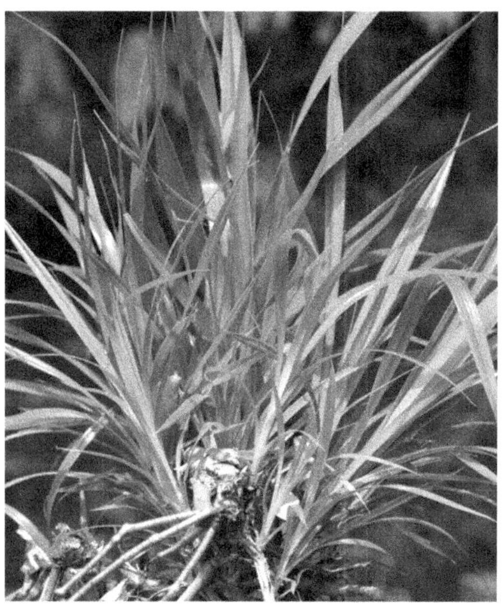

Plate 1.18 *Cymbopogan citrates*

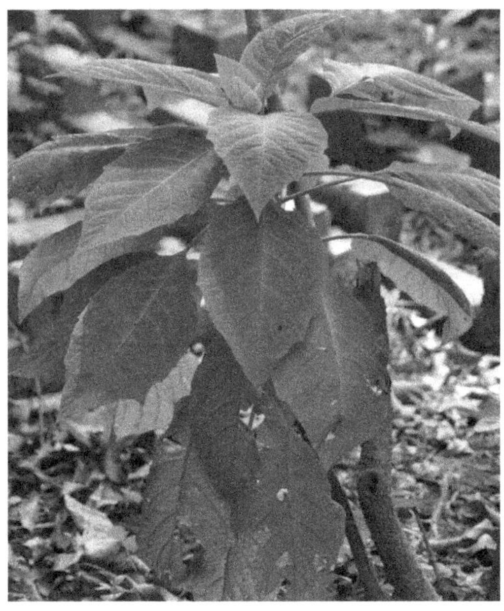

Plate 1.19 *Datura arboria*

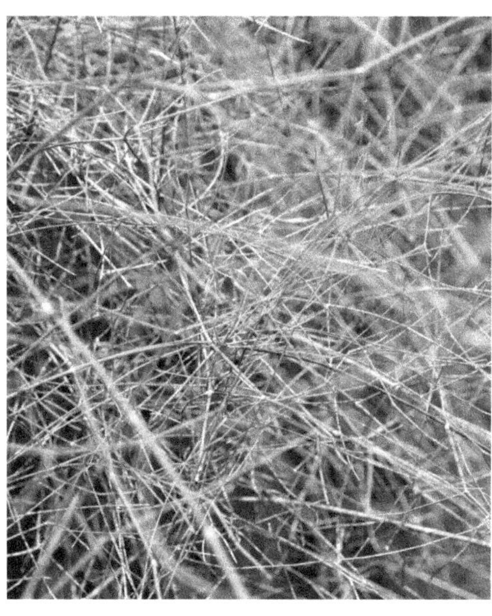

Plate 1.20 *Ephedra sinica*

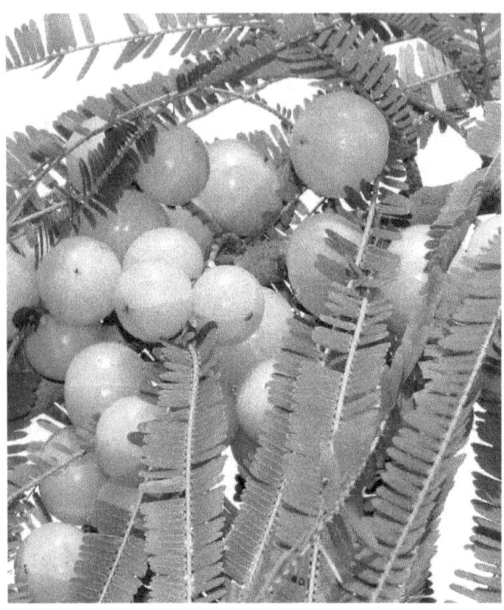

Plate 1.21 *Ephyllanthus emblica*

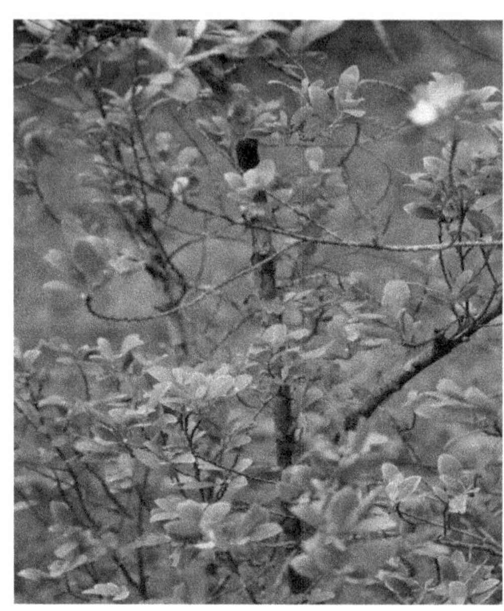

Plate 1.22 *Erythroxylum coca*

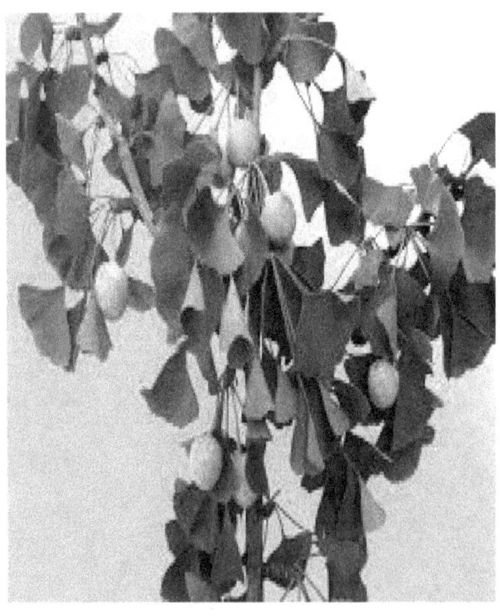

Plate 1.23 *Ginkgo biloba*

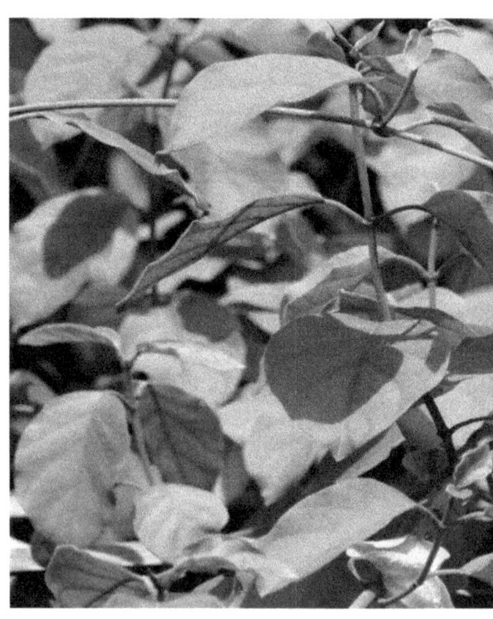

Plate 1.24 *Gymnema sylvestre*

Photographs of Medicinal Plants

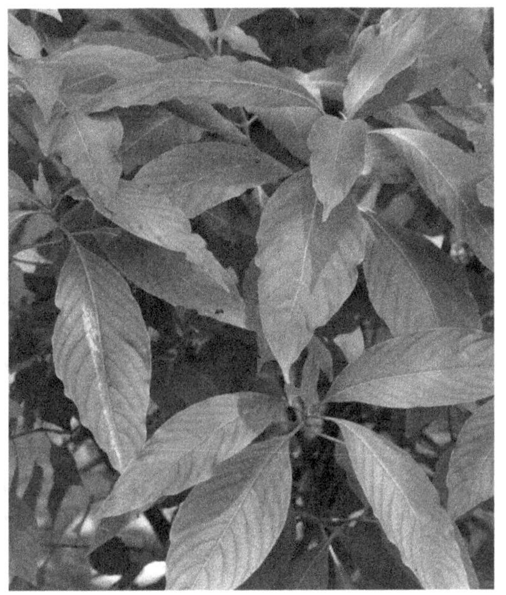

Plate 1.25 *Justicia adhatoda*

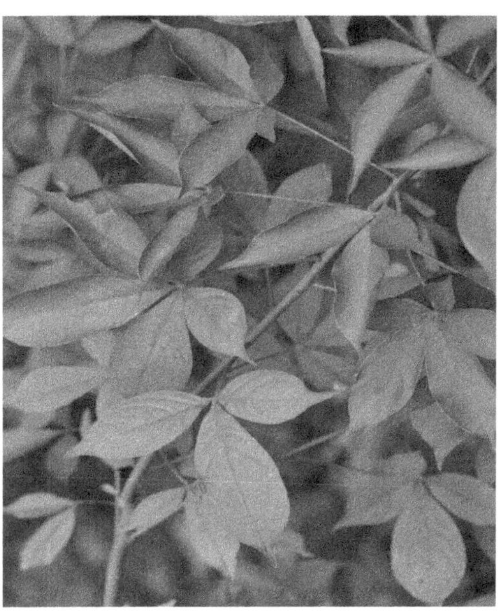

Plate 1.26 *Myristica fragrans*

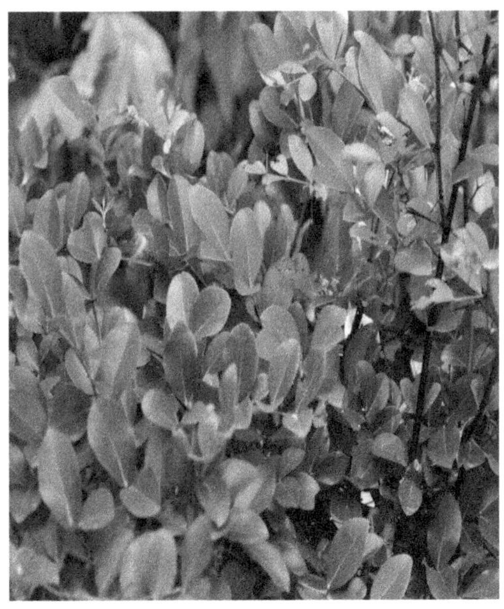

Plate 1.27 *Pandula amralafolus*

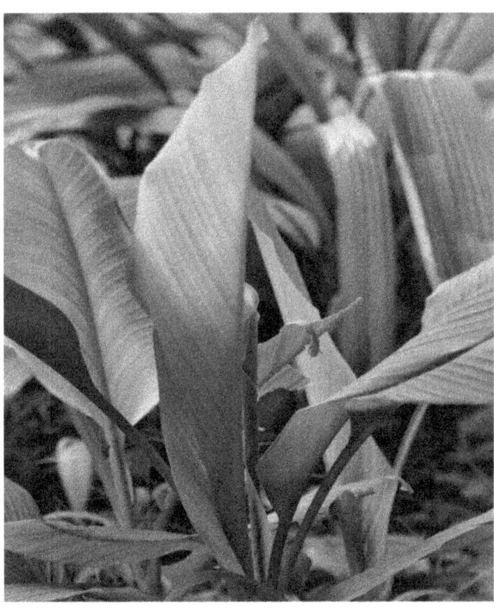

Plate 1.28 *Pimenta diycaia*

Insert – 7-10

Photographs of Medicinal Plants

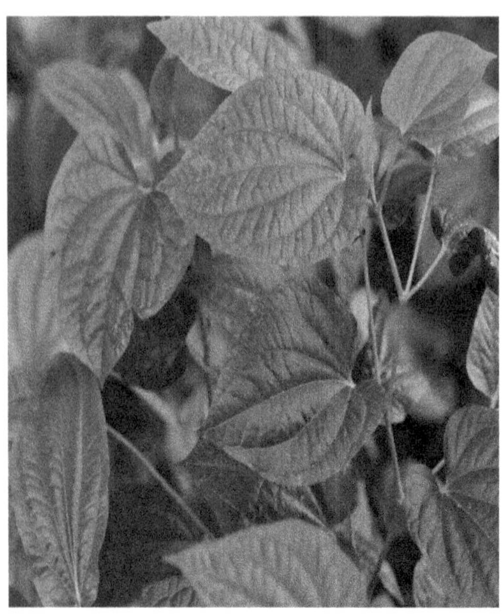

Plate 1.29 *Piper longum*

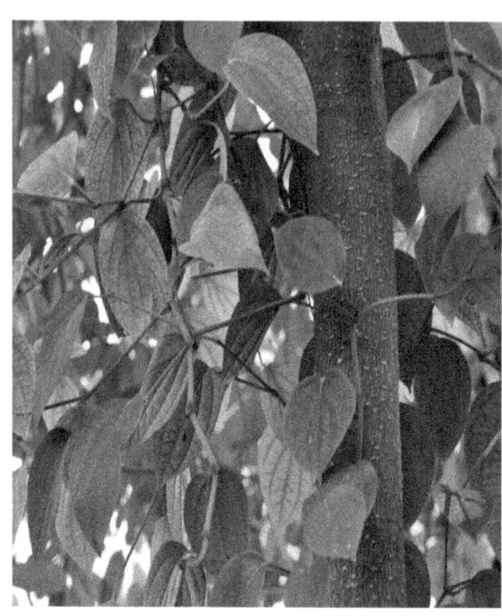

Plate 1.30 *Piper nigrum*

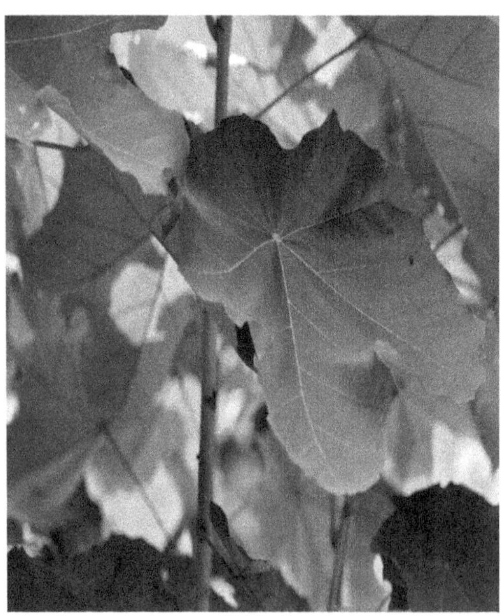

Plate 1.31 *Pterospermum acerifolium*

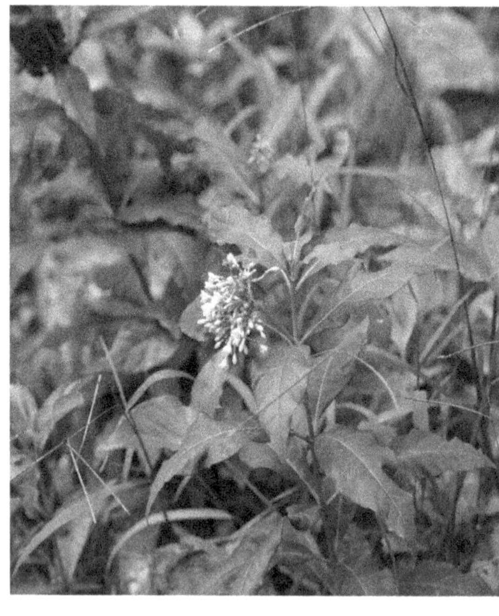

Plate 1.32 *Rauvolfia serpentine*

Photographs of Medicinal Plants

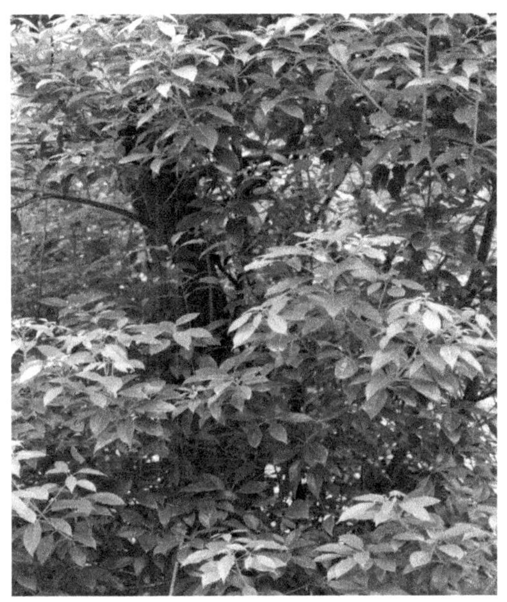

Plate 1.33 *Santalum album*

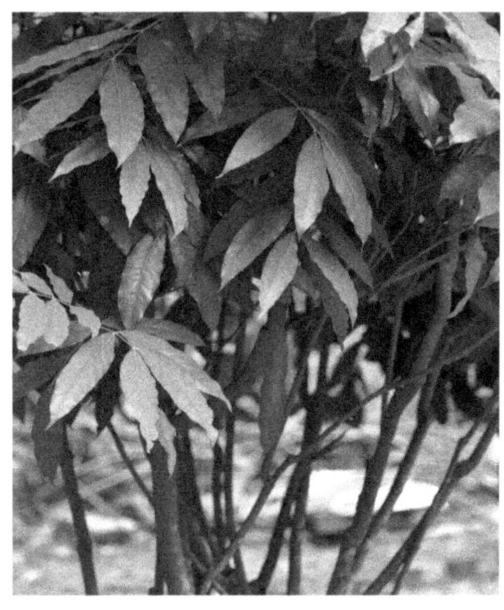

Plate 1.34 *Saraca asoca*

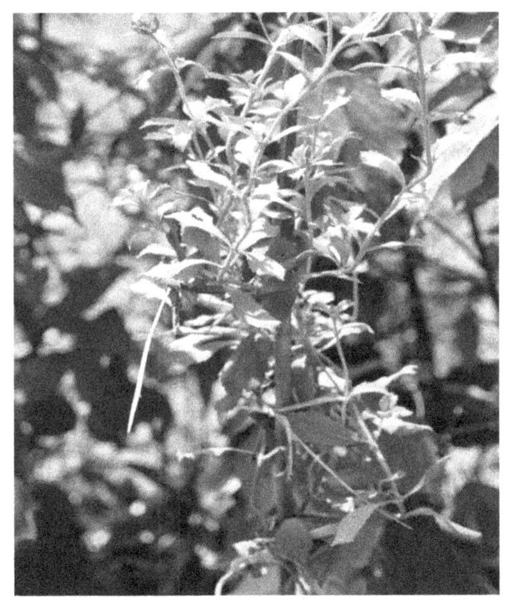

Plate 1.35 *Stevia rebaudiane*

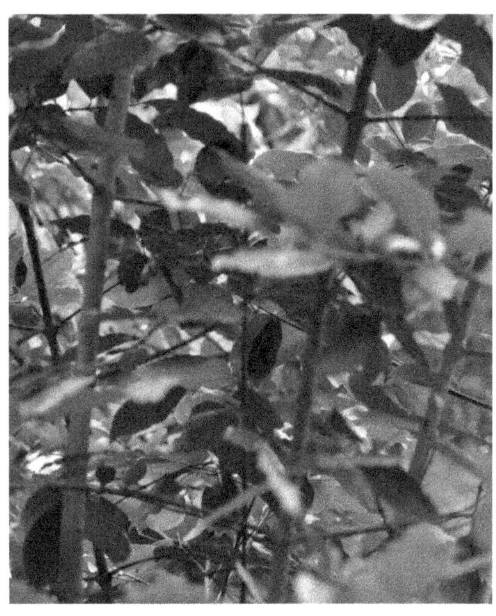

Plate 1.36 *Strychnos nuxvomica*

Photographs of Medicinal Plants

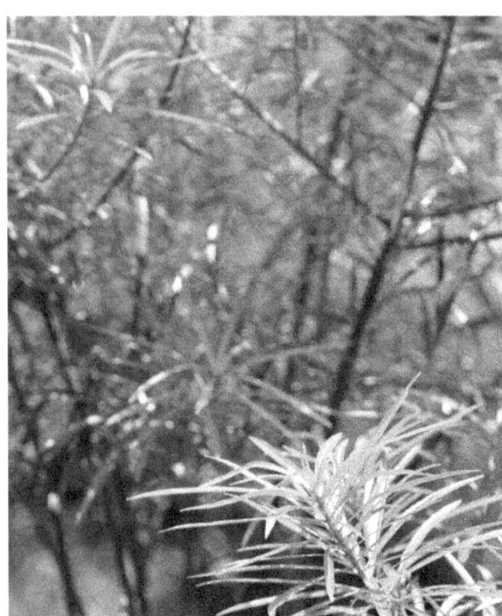

Plate 1.37 *Thevetia perviana*

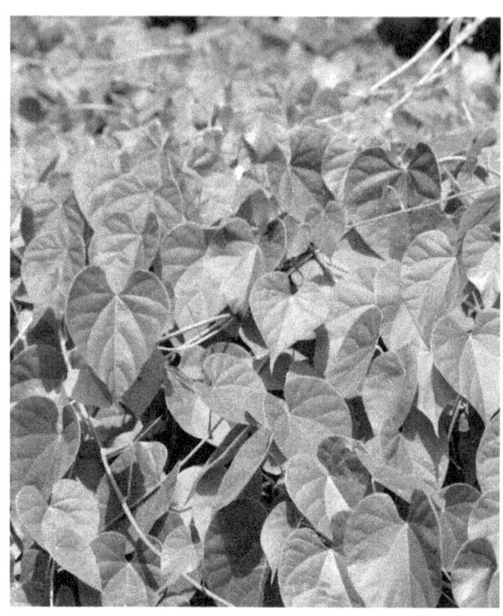

Plate 1.38 *Tinospora cordifolia*

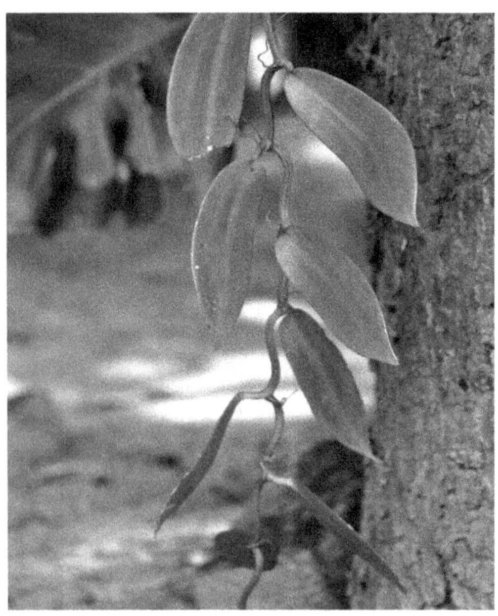

Plate 1.39 *Vanilla cordifolia*

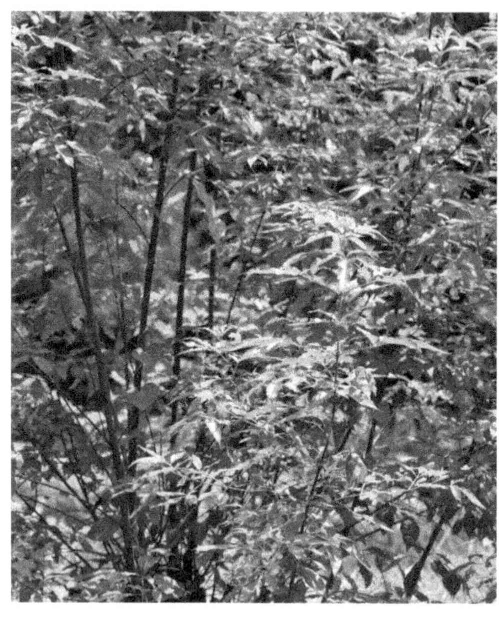

Plate 1.40 *Vitex negundo*

1 *Medicinal Plants with Anticancer Properties*

Introduction to Cancer

Cancer can be defined as a disease in which a group of abnormal cells grow uncontrollably by disregarding the normal rules of cell division. Normal cells are subject to signals that dictate whether the cell should divide, differentiate into another cell or die. Cancer cells develop a degree of autonomy from these signals, resulting in uncontrolled growth and proliferation. If this proliferation is allowed to continue and spread, it can be fatal. In fact almost 90% of cancer related deaths are due to tumor spreading- a process called metastasis.

The foundation of modern cancer cell biology rests on a simple principle- virtually all mammalian cells share similar molecular networks that control cell proliferation, differentiation and cell death. The prevailing theory, which underpins research into the genesis and treatment of cancer, is that normal cells are transformed into abnormal cancer cells as a result of changes in the network of biochemical, molecular and cellular level, and for each cell there is a finite number of ways by which this disruption can occur.

Phenomenal advances in cancer research in the past 50 years have given an insight into how cancer cells develop this autonomy. Now cancer is defined as a disease that involves changes or mutations in the cell genome. These changes (DNA mutations) produce proteins that disrupt the delicate cellular balance between cell division and quiescence, resulting in cells that keep dividing to form cancers.

Insights into Cancer

Initiation and progression of cancer depends on both external factors in the environment (tobacco, chemicals, radiation and infectious organisms), and factors within the cell (inherited mutations, hormones, immune conditions). These factors can act together or in sequence, resulting in abnormal cell behavior and excessive proliferation. As a result, cell masses grow and expand, affecting surrounding normal tissues (such as in the brain), and can also spread to other locations in the body (metastasis). However, it is important to remember that most common cancers take months and years for these DNA mutations to accumulate and result in a detectable cancer.

Cancers occur approximately in one among every 3 individuals. DNA mutations arise normally at a frequency of 1 in every 20 million per gene per cell division. The average number of cells formed in any individual during an average lifetime is 10^{16}(10 million cells being replaced every 16 seconds). It would be therefore logical to assume that human populations anywhere in the world would show similar frequencies of cancer. However, cancer incidence rates vary dramatically across countries. Evidently, some factors seem to intervene to increase cancer incidences in some population. Schematic sketch of cell division is shown in the figure below.

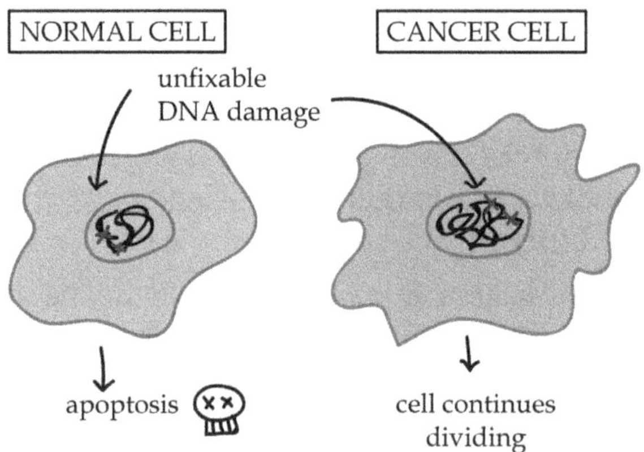

Cancer Cell Division

When it comes to cell division, cancer cells multiply uncontrollably and very rapidly. It can divide without any external signals; cancer cells do not exhibit contact inhibition. M phase starts after completion of S phase, in other words DNA replication must not start until mitosis is complete and mitosis must not begin until the previous round of DNA replication has ended, thus the integrity of genome is maintained. In between S and M phases two gaps, G1 and G2 are there. G1 follows from mitosis and is in a time during the cell cycle when the cell is responsive to both positive and negative growth signals. G2 is the gap after S phase, when the cell prepares for entry into mitosis. Finally, the last stage G0 phase occurs.

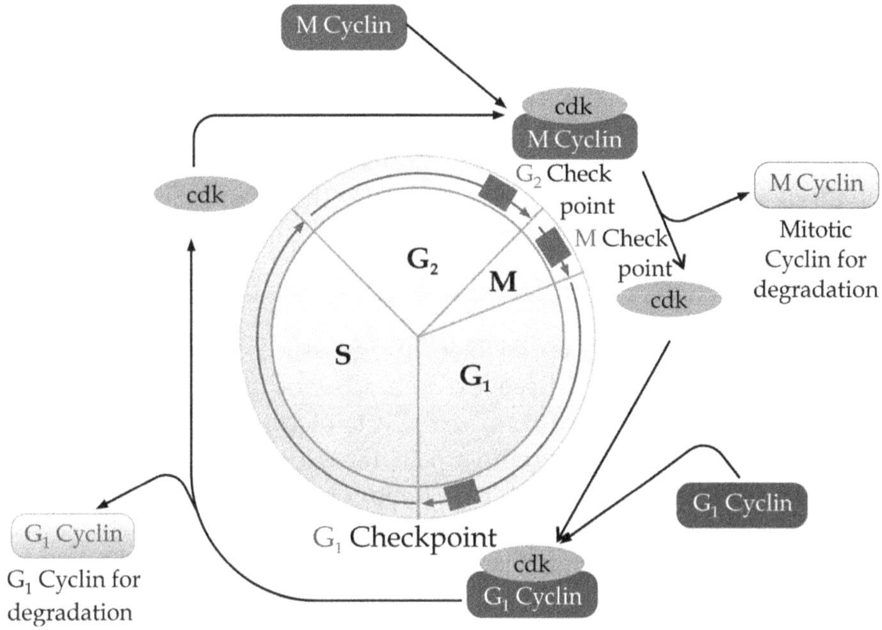

Types of Cancer

There are more than 100 types of cancers. The type of cancer is named according to the organ from where it is originated. The most common of them are sarcoma, adenoma, carcinoma, melanoma, leukemia and lymphoma.

Carcinoma

Carcinomas are the most common types of cancer. They are formed by epithelial cells. There are many types of epithelial cells, which often have a column-like shape when viewed under a microscope. Adenocarcinoma is a cancer that forms in epithelial cells that produce fluids or mucus. Tissues with this type of epithelial cell are sometimes called glandular tissues. Most cancers of the breast, colon and prostate are adenocarcinomas.

Transitional cell carcinoma is a cancer that forms in a type of epithelial tissue called transitional epithelium, or urothelium. This tissue, which is made up of many layers of epithelial cells that can get bigger and smaller, is found in the linings of the bladder, ureters, and part of the kidneys (renal pelvis), and a few other organs. Some cancers of the bladder, ureters and kidneys are transitional cell carcinomas.

Sarcoma

Sarcomas are cancers that form in bone and soft tissues, including muscle, fat, blood vessels, lymph vessels and fibrous tissue (such as tendons and ligaments). Osteosarcoma is the most common cancer of bone.

Leukemia

Cancers that begin in the blood-forming tissue of the bone marrow are called leukemias. These cancers do not form solid tumors. Instead, large numbers of abnormal white blood cells (leukemia cells and leukemic blast cells) build up in the blood and bone marrow, crowding out normal blood cells. The low level of normal blood cells can make it difficult for the body to get oxygen to its tissues, control bleeding, or fight infections.

There are four common types of leukemia, which are grouped based on the rapidity of spread of the disease (acute or chronic) and the type of blood cell on which the cancer starts in (lymphoblastic or myeloid).

Lymphoma

Lymphoma is cancer that begins in lymphocytes (T cells or B cells). These are disease-fighting white blood cells that are part of the immune system. In lymphoma, abnormal lymphocytes build up in lymph nodes and lymph vessels, as well as in other organs of the body.

There are two main types of lymphoma:

Hodgkin lymphoma: People with this disease have abnormal lymphocytes that are called Reed-Sternberg cells. These cells usually form from B cells.

Non-Hodgkin lymphoma: This is a large group of cancers that start in lymphocytes. The cancers can grow quickly or slowly and can form from B cells or T cells.

Melanoma

Melanoma is the cancer that begins in cells that become melanocytes, which are specialized cells that make melanin (the pigment that gives skin its color). Most melanomas form on the skin, but melanomas can also form in other pigmented tissues, such as the eye.

Brain and Spinal Cord Tumors

There are different types of brain and spinal cord tumors. These tumors are named based on the type of cell in which they are formed and where the tumor is first formed in the central nervous system.

Other Types of Tumors

Germ Cell Tumors

Germ cell tumors are a type of tumor that begins in the cells that give rise to sperm or eggs. These tumors can occur almost anywhere in the body and can be either benign or malignant.

Neuroendocrine Tumors

Neuroendocrine tumors form from cells that release hormones into the blood in response to a signal from the nervous system. These tumors, which may make higher-than-normal amounts of hormones, can cause many different symptoms. Neuroendocrine tumors may be benign or malignant.

Carcinoid Tumors

Carcinoid tumors are a type of neuroendocrine tumor. They are slow-growing tumors that are usually found in the gastrointestinal system (most often in the rectum and small intestine). Carcinoid tumors may spread to the liver or other sites in the body, and they may secrete substances such as serotonin or prostaglandin.

Plants having Anti-Cancer Potentials

1. *Betula alba*

   Common name: Birch

   Chemical constituents: The bark of birch contains about 3 percent tannic acid, which is used as a tannic acid. The white epidermis of the bark contains empyreumatic oil, also known as birch tar. The tar is almost identical to Wintergreen oil but contains a high concentration of methyl salicylate. It also contains creosol and guailacol. Besides the tar, the bark also contains salicylate and methyl salicylate. Other constituents include saponins, flavonoids, glycosides, quercitrin, kaempferol etc.

   Pharmacological activities: The betulinic acid has been known to kill cancerous cells and has been especially effective in the treatment of prostate cancer patients[1].

   Distribution: The Birch has sixty species throughout the world, ten of which are native to Canada and the northern part of the United States.

2. *Colchicum autumnale* (Liliaceae)

   Common name: Naked ladies, meadow saffron and colchicum.

   Chemical constituents: Colchicum seeds contain 0.2-1% of amino alkaloids of which colchicine is the main constituent. The seeds contain up to 0.8 per cent of colchicine and in corms, it is up to 0.6%. Colchicum also contains demecolcine. Both the alkaloids contain tropolone or cycloheptatrien-ol-one ring structure.

   Pharmacological activities: Colchicine obtained from Colchicum plant works by interrupting the process of division of cancerous cells[1].

   Distribution: The Autumn Crocus, of the Lily Family (Liliaceae), is a plant with small flowers of varying colors. This plant is indigenous to Europe, Northern Africa and Asian continents. Being a plant with a history of medicinal use, records show that it was used in Ancient Greece, India, and Egypt.

3. *Camptotheca acuminata*

   Common name: Xi Shu, Happy Tree, the Camptotheca

Chemical constituents: The bark and stems of *C. acuminata* contain the alkaloid camptothecin. Several chemical derivatives of camptothecin are under investigation for or used as drugs for cancer treatment, including irinotecan, topotecan, rubitecan. *C. acuminata* also contains the chemical compounds trifolin and hyperoside.

Pharmacological activities: Camptothecin is helpful in brain tumors through the drug Irinotecan. It contains antineoplastic, used to prevent the mutation of cells into cancerous cells with the possibility of preventing or reducing the disease into one that is benign[1].

Distribution: Three living species in the genus Camptotheca are now recognized with the extant natural distribution restricted to remote regions in southern China. However, neither the geographical distribution nor the resource availability in China was investigated prior to the surveys. Consequently, such data are not available in either the government forestry departments or universities, or in the botanical and medical institutions.

4. *Curcuma zedoaria*

   Common name: White turmeric, Zedoary root

   Chemical constituents: (+)- germacrone-4, 1,8-cineole, 5-epoxide, germacrone, furanodienone, curzerenone, zederone, dehydrocurdione, curcumenol, isocurcumenol, curcumenone, curmanolide A, curmanolide B.

   Pharmacological activities: Polysaccharides and protein bound polysaccharides obtained from *C.zedoaria* could inhibit the growth of Sarcoma- 180[2,3]. Essential oil from *C.zedoaria* has an antiproliferative effect on MCF-7, HL-60 and OVCAR-3 cells[4,7].

   Distribution: Zedoary plant is native to India and Indonesia. However, it is widely used as a spice in the West today. It is also found in sub-tropical regions of eastern Nepal.

5. *Cannabis sativa*

   Common name: Marijuana, Bhang, Ganja, and Hashish

   Chemical constituents: Cannabidiol, Tetrahydrocannabinol, Cannabinoids.

   Pharmacological activities: Most of the effects produced by cannabinoids in the nervous system and in non-neural tissues rely on CB1 receptor activation. In contrast, the CB2 receptor was initially described to be present in the immune system, but was more recently shown to be also expressed in cells from other origins. Notably, expression of the CB1 and CB2 receptors has been found in many types of cancer cells, but not necessarily correlating with the expression of those receptors in the tissue of origin[8,9].

Distribution: It is native to Central Asia, and long cultivated in Asia, Europe, and China. Now it is widespread as tropical, temperate and subarctic cultivar and waif. The oldest use of hemp seems to be for fiber, and later the seeds began to be used for culinary purposes. Plants yielding the drug seem to have been discovered in India, cultivated for medicinal purposes as early as 900 BC. In medieval times it was brought to North Africa where it is now cultivated exclusively for hashish or kif.

6. ***Tabebuia Impetiginosa***

   Common Names: Lapacho, Pau D'Arco, Taheebo, and Ipe Roxo

   Chemical constituents: Beta-Lapachone, Lapachol Beta-lapachone

   Pharmacological activities: Beta-lapachone, one quinone compound from the bark of different Tabebuia trees was reported to have anti-cancer activities. Therefore, extensive investigations were carried out with human cell lines for finding new insights into possible molecular mechanisms. So fl-lapachone inhibits the progression and metastasis of hepatoma cell lines by inhibiting the invasive ability of the cells[10]. In human prostate, carcinoma DU 145 cells lapachone induced inhibition of growth and apoptosis in dose-dependent manner as measured by MTT assay, fluorescent microscopy and flow-cytometry analysis.

   Distribution: It is found in the rainforests of South America, especially in Argentina, Paraguay, and Brazil. The Lapacho Tree is an evergreen with blossoms that may be red or purple. It has been proven to be medically useful, even since the time of the Incas.

7. ***Nothapodytes Foetida***

   Common Name: Nothapodytes Tree

Chemical constituents: Acetylcamptothecin, Camptothecin, Scopolectin Camptothecin

Pharmacological activities: Camptothecin itself is not used clinically due to its cytotoxicity, but its derivatives are most effective for the treatment of cancer. Interest in camptothecin congeners was renewed when it was reported that 9-aminocamptothecin exhibits curative activity against human colon adenocarcinoma[11]. Camptothecin and its derivatives inhibit the growth of human breast carcinoma cell *in vitro* and induce complete regression of breast tumors[12].

Distribution: It has its medicinal use whose wood-extract is used in treating cancer. This tree is found in Western Ghats, India. This plant has medicinal properties similar to the camptothecin plant, as they have remarkably similar chemical constituents.

8. *Taxus brevifolia*

   Common Name: Pacific Yew

   Chemical constituents: Taxine, Taxagifine

   Pharmacological activities: Various studies have shown that Paclitaxel is effective anticancer agent against lung, breast, ovarian, leukopenia and liver cancer. Paclitaxel has a role in treating various kinds of cancer by targeting tubulin or inducing cell cycle arrest or enhancing the signaling factors or mutating them[13].

   Distribution: This coniferous tree is native to Southeast Alaska, it also commonly exists in the western part of the United States.

9. *Catharathus roseus*

   Common Names: Madagascar Periwinkle, Periwinkle

   Chemical constituents: Vinblastine, Vincristine, Vindesine, Vinorelbine Vinblastine.

   Pharmacological activities: The leaves and stems are the sources of dimeric alkaloids, vinacristine and vinblastine that are indispensable cancer drugs. The extracts of Vinca have demonstrated significant anticancer activity against numerous cell types[14].

Distribution: The periwinkle plant is located in the southern portion of North America. Its fruit has an ellipsoid structure with pink or purple shaded petals in its flower.

10. *Alpinia galanga*

    Common names: Vacha, Kulanjan

    Chemical constituent: Galangin

    Pharmacological activities: It possesses significant anticancer activity against cancers of breast, lung, stomach, colon, prostate, multiple myeloma and leukaemia. Pinocembrin isolated from *Alpinia galanga* inhibits growth & spread in colon cancer by arresting cell proliferation and inducing apoptosis[1].

    Distribution: It is native to South Asia, Indonesia and cultivated in Malaysia, Laos and Thailand.

11. *Amoora rohituka*

    Common names: Rohituka Tree

    Chemical constituents: Amooranin

    Pharmacological activities: Amooranin (a triterpene acid), isolated from Amoora rohituka inhibits growth & spread of breast and cervical cancers by arresting G2/M phase of the cell cycle and by inducing apoptosis. Amooranin and its derivatives are effective in both chemotherapy-sensitive and chemotherapy resistant cancers. Amooranin has the ability to overcome (reverse) multidrug resistance in breast cancer, colon cancer and leukaemia[1].

    Distribution: It is available throughout India in dense evergreen forests

12. *Bauhinia variegata*

    Common names: Kanchnar

    Chemical constituents: Cyanidin glucoside, malvidin glucoside

    Pharmacological activities: Cyanidin glucoside, malvidin glucoside, peonidin glucoside and kaempferol galactoside isolated from Bauhinia variegata inhibit growth & spread of various cancers such as cancers of breast, lung, liver, oral cavity, larynx and malignant ascites. Bauhinia variegata also possesses significant hepatoprotective activity[1].

    Distribution: It is native to Southeast Asia, China, Burma, Pakistan, Sri Lanka etc.

13. *Berberis vulgaris*

    Common names: Kachnar, Orchid tree

    Chemical constituents: Berberine, berbamine, chelidonic acid, citric acid, columbamine, hydrastine, isotetrandrine, jacaranone, magnoflorine, oxycanthine and palmatine.

    Pharmacological activities: Berberine (an isoquinoline alkaloid), possesses anticancer, immunoenhancing, antioxidant and antiinflammatory properties. Berberine arrests cancer cell cycle in G1-phase and induces apoptosis. It possesses strong anticancer activity against prostate cancer, liver cancer and leukaemia. Berberine interferes with P-glycoprotein in chemotherapy-resistant cancers. Berberine also increases the penetration of some chemotherapy drugs through the blood-brain barrier, thereby enhancing their effect on intracranial tumours. Cannabisin-G protects against breast cancer. Berberis vulgaris also inhibits growth of stomach and oral cavity cancers[1].

    Distribution: It is native to South Asia, Indonesia and cultivated in Malaysia, Laos and Thailand.

14. *Emblica officinalis*

    Common names: Amlaki

    Chemical constituents: Ellagic acid, gallic acid, quercetin, kaempferol, emblicanin, proanthocyanidin.

    Pharmacological activities: It is valued for its unique tannins and flavonoids and possesses powerful antioxidant and anticancer properties. Emblicanin A & B (tannins) possess strong antioxidant and anticancer properties. *Emblica officinalis* inhibits growth & spread of various cancers including that of the breast, uterus, pancreas, stomach, liver and malignant ascites. *Emblica officinalis* protects against cancer, especially, the liver cancer. It also reduces the side effects of chemotherapy & radiotherapy[15].

    Distribution: It is grown in Tamil Nadu, Rajasthan and Madhya Pradesh.

15. *Ginkgo biloba*

    Common names: Maidenhair Tree

    Chemical constituents: Ginkgetin and Ginkgolides (A & B)

Pharmacological activities: Ginkgetin and Ginkgolides (A & B), isolated from Ginkgo biloba inhibits growth and spread of various aggressive cancers such as invasive oestrogen-receptor negative breast cancer, glioblastoma multiforme, hepatocellular carcinoma and cancers of ovary, colon, prostate and liver by inducing apoptosis. *Ginkgo biloba* extract is well known for its antioxidant activity. It also reduces side effects of chemotherapy and radiotherapy[1].

16. *Glycine max*

    Common names: Soya

    Chemical constituents: Genistein, Daidzein, Quercetin

    Pharmacological activities: Isoflavones (such as genistein & daidzein) and saponins isolated from *Glycine max* inhibit growth and spread of various cancers such as cancers of the breast, uterus, cervix, ovary, lung, stomach, colon, pancreas, liver, kidney, urinary bladder, prostate, testis, oral cavity, larynx, and thyroid. Glycine max is also effective in nasopharyngeal carcinoma, skin cancer, malignant lymphoma, rhabdomyo-sarcoma, neuroblastoma, malignant brain tumours and leukaemia. Isoflavones and saponins isolated from *Glycine max* possess wide ranging anticancer properties such as inhibition of cancer cell proliferation, promotion of cell differentiation and induction of apoptosis. Genistein works by blocking angiogenesis (formation of new blood vessel), acting as a tyrosine kinase inhibitor (the mechanism of action of many new cancer drugs) and inducing apoptosis. Genistein is an excellent intracellular antioxidant. It also blocks the supply of oxygen and nutrients to cancer cells, thus killing them by starving. Genistein and quercetin have synergistic anticancer effect against ovarian carcinoma[1].

17. *Gossypium hirsutum*

    Chemical constituents: Gossypol, Gossypolone

    Pharmacological activities: Gossypol isolated from Gossypium hirsutum inhibits growth and spread of various cancers such as cancers of the breast, oesophagus, stomach, colon, liver, pancreas, adrenal gland, prostate, urinary bladder, malignant lymphoma, malignant ascites, brain tumours, sarcomas and leukaemia by inducing apoptosis and arresting cancer cell division in G0/G1 phase. The negative isomer of gossypol, (-) gossypol, inhibits growth and spread of chemotherapy and radiotherapy-resistant cancers of prostate, breast, ovary, lung, pancreas, head and neck and brain by inducing apoptosis. Gossypolone, oxidative metabolite of gossypol, inhibits growth and spread of various cancers including that of the breast, cervix, lung, malignant melanoma and leukaemia[1].

18. *Morinda citrafolia*

Chemical constituents: Damnacanthol

Pharmacological activities: Damnacanthol, NB10 and NB11 isolated from Morinda citrifolia possess strong anticancer activity against various cancers particularly lung cancer and sarcomas. Morinda citrifolia, possesses strong antioxidant, hepatoprotective and immunoenhancing properties[16].

19. *Nigella sativa*

Common names: Kalajeera

Chemical constituents: Thymoquinone and dithymoquinone

Pharmacological activities: Thymoquinone and dithymoquinone isolated from Nigella sativa have strong anticancer activity against various cancers including cancers of the colon, prostate, pancreas, uterus, malignant ascites, malignant lymphoma, malignant melanoma, sarcomas and leukaemia. Thymoquinone is effective in both hormone-sensitive and hormone refractory prostate cancer. Nigella sativa kills cancer cells by binding to the asialofeutin (lectin) on the surface of cancerous cells, causing their aggregation and clumping. Nigella sativa also possesses immunoenhancing and anti-inflammatory properties. It protects against liver cancer. Nigella sativa enhances immune function of the body and reduces side effects of chemotherapy and radiotherapy[1].

20. *Panax ginseng*

Chemical constituents: Ginsenosides

Pharmacological activities: Ginsenosides (panaxadiol and panaxatriol saponins) isolated from Panax ginseng inhibits growth and spread of various cancers such as cancers of breast, ovary, lung, prostate, colon, renal cell carcinoma, malignant melanoma, malignant lymphoma and leukaemia. Ginsenosides possesses strong anticancer activity against lung cancer and also prevents lung metastasis by blocking angiogenesis. Compound K (a metabolite of ginsenosides) inhibits growth and spread of chemo-resistant lung cancer. Ginsenosides Rc, Rd, Rg1 and Re-overcome (reverse) P-glycoprotein mediated multidrug resistance to chemotherapy. Ginsenoside Rf helps in reducing doses of morphine in terminally ill cancer patients[17].

21. *Ocimum sanctum*

    Common names: Tulsi

    Chemical constituents: Eugenol, Linolenic acid, Rosmarinic acid and flavonoids such as orientin, vicenin, apigenin.

    Pharmacological activities: Active constituents such as Eugenol, orientin and vicenin inhibit growth and spread of various cancers such as breast cancer, liver cancer and sarcomas particularly fibrosarcoma by blocking supply of oxygen and nutrients to the cancer cells and killing them by starving. It has antioxidant and radioprotective properties, protects against various cancers particularly the breast cancer and reduces side effects of chemotherapy and radiotherapy[1].

22. *Plumbago zeylanica*

    Common names: Chitrak

    Chemical constituents: Plumbagin

    Pharmacological activities: Plumbagin inhibits growth and spread of breast cancer, liver cancer, fibrosarcoma, malignant ascites and leukaemia by inhibiting cancer cell proliferation[1].

23. *Podophyllum hexandrum*

    Chemical constituents: Podophyllotoxin, Podophyllin

    Pharmacological activities: Podophyllotoxin and podophyllin (lignans) isolated from Podophyllum hexandrum (Himalayan May Apple) inhibit growth and spread of various cancers including that of the breast, ovary, lung, liver, urinary bladder, testis, brain, neuroblastoma, Hodgkin's disease, nonHodgkin's lymphoma and leukaemia. Podophyllotoxin is the most active among all the natural anticancer compounds[1].

24. *Rubia cordifolia*

    Common names: Manjistha

    Chemical constituents: Rubianin, Rubiadin

Pharmacological activities: Rubidianin, rubiadin, RA-7, RA-700 and RC-18 isolated from Rubia cordifolia inhibit growth and spread of cancers of breast, ovary, cervix, colon, lung, malignant ascites, malignant lymphoma, malignant melanoma sarcoma and leukaemia[18].

25. *Saussurea lappa*

Chemical constituents: Cynaropicrin

Pharmacological activities: Sesquiterpenes and costunolide dehydro-costuslactone, isolated from Saussurea lappa inhibit growth and spread of breast cancer. Cynaropicrin, isolated from Saussurea lappa possesses strong anticancer activity against malignant lymphoma and leukaemia. Costunolide, isolated from Saussurea lappa inhibits growth and spread of intestinal cancer. Mokkolactone isolated from Saussurea lappa induces apoptosis in leukaemic cells. Shikokiols isolated from Saussurea lappa exhibits anticancer activity against cancers of the ovary, lung, colon and central nervous system[1].

26. *Solanum nigrum*

Chemical constituents: Solamargine, Solasonine

Pharmacological activities: Solamargine and solasonine, isolated from Solanum nigrum (Lo-ing-kue) inhibit growth and spread of various cancers including that of the breast, liver and lung. Steroidal glycosides (spirostane, furostane, spirosolane and pregnane), isolated from *Solanum nigrum* inhibit growth and spread of colon cancer and pheochromocytoma. Glycoproteins isolated from *Solanum nigrum* have antiproliferative and apoptotic effects on colon and breast cancers[19]. Polysaccharides isolated from *Solanum nigrum* have significant inhibitory effect on growth of cervical cancer.

27. *Tinospora cordifolia*

Common names: Guduchi

Chemical constituents: Tinosporaside

Pharmacological activities: Sesquiterpenes obtained from this plant alleviates spread of various cancers including that of lung, cervix, throat and malignant ascites. Polysaccharide fraction isolated from *Tinospora cordifolia* inhibits lung metastasis[20].

28. *Andrographis paniculata*

Common name: Kalmegh

Chemical constituent: Andrographolide

Pharmacological activities: Andrographolide, active diterpine component, isolated from Andrographis paniculata, has immunoenhancing and strong anticancer activity against cancers of breast, ovary, stomach, colon, prostate, kidney, nasopharynx malignant melanoma and leukacmia. Andrographolide exerts direct anticancer activity on cancer cells by arresting G0/G1 phase of cell-cycle and inducing apoptosis[1].

Distribution: It is found throughout India.

29. *Glycyrrhiza glabra*

Common name: Shankhapushpi

Chemical constituent: Glycyrrhizin

Pharmacological activities: Flavonoids (flavones, flavonals, isoflavones, chalcones, licochalcones and bihydrochalcones), derived from Glycyrrhiza glabra possess strong anticancer, antioxidant, antimutagenic, antiulcer, anti-HIV and hepatoprotective properties[1].

30. *Psoralea corylifolia*

Common name: Bavchi

Chemical constituents: Bavachinin, corylfolinin and psoralen

Pharmacological activities: Bavachinin, corylfolinin and psoralen isolated from Psoralea corylifolia (Bu Gu Zhi), possess strong anticancer activity against lung cancer, liver cancer, osteosarcoma, fibrosarcoma, malignant ascites and leukaemia. Psoralen enhances immunity of the body by stimulating natural killer cell activity. Psoralidin isolated from Psoralea corylifolia inhibits growth and spread of stomach and prostate cancers by inhibiting G2/M phase of cell cycle[1].

Chemical Structures of Anti cancer plants

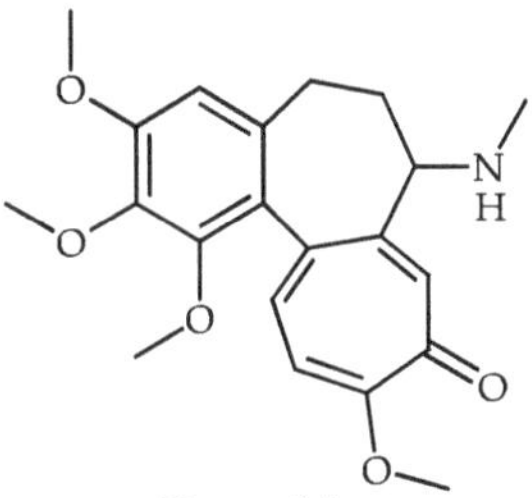

Demecolcine

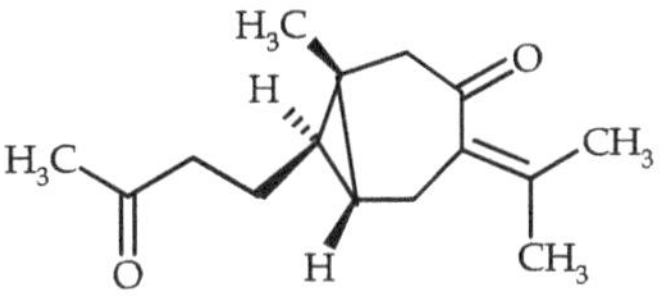

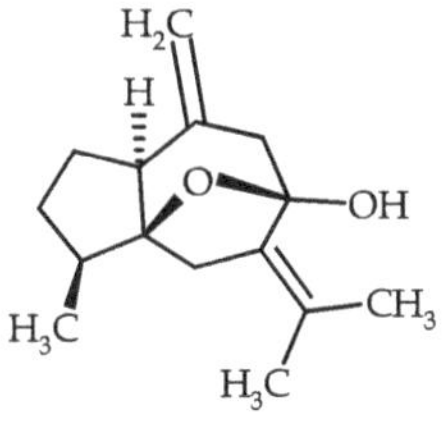

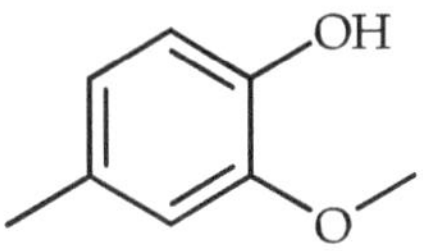

Creasol

Camptothecin

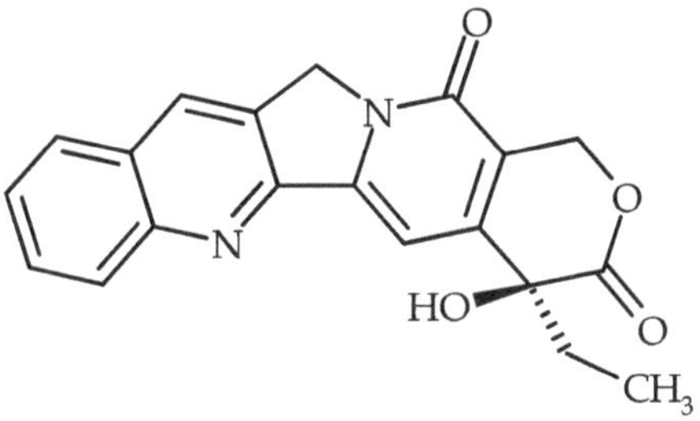

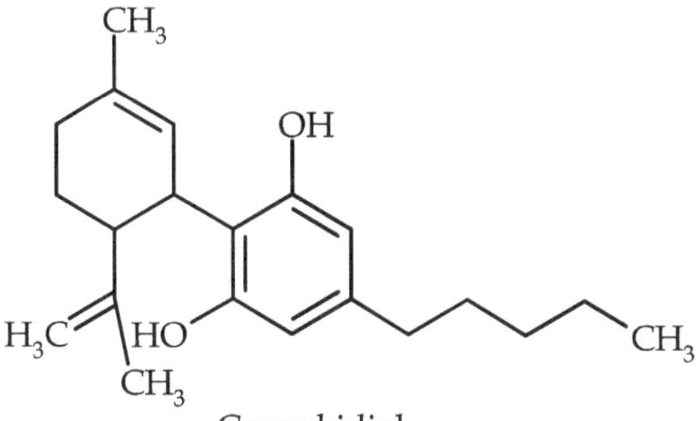

Cannabidiol

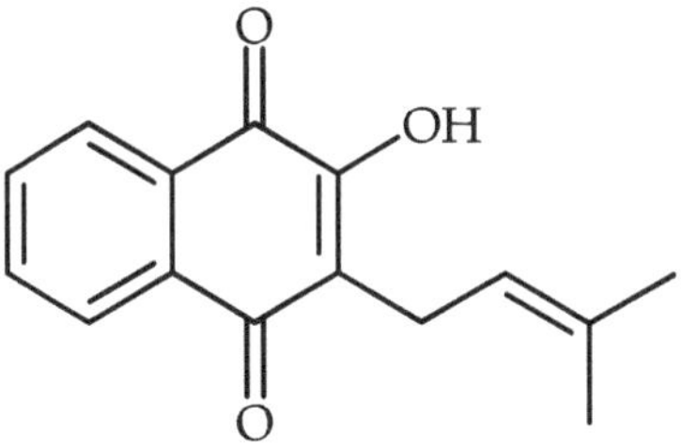

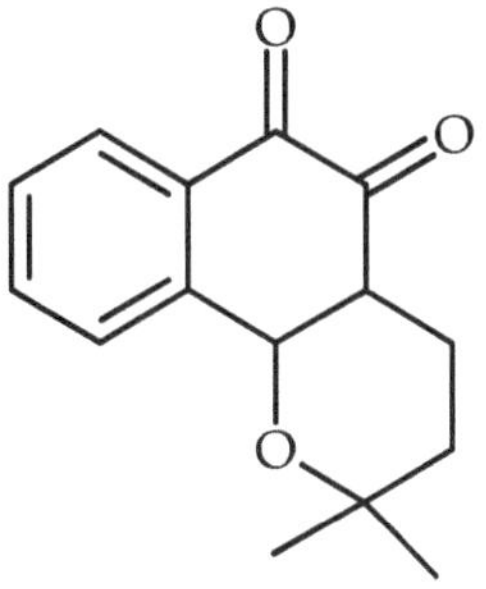

Lapachol

Beta-Lapachone

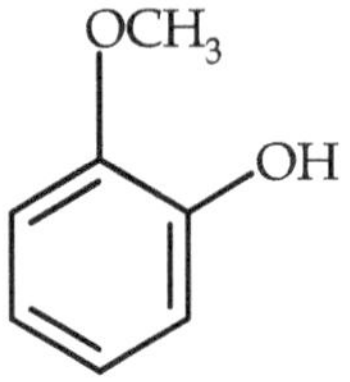

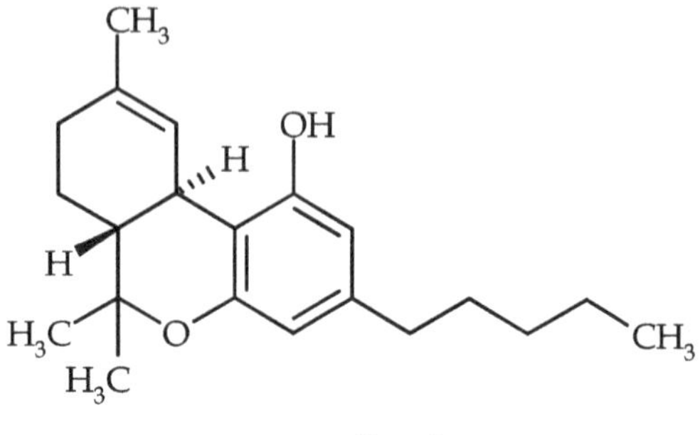

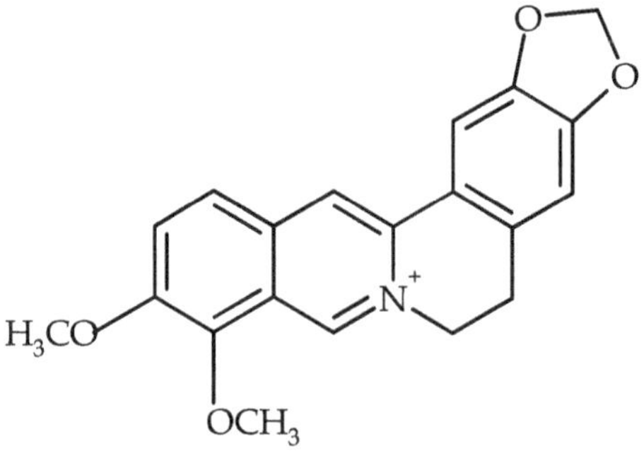

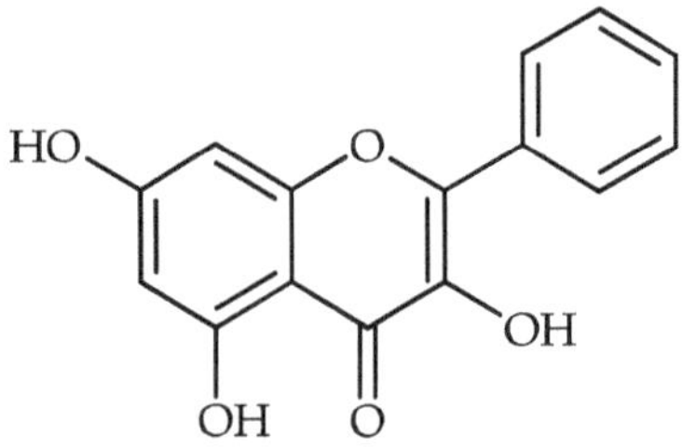

Berberine

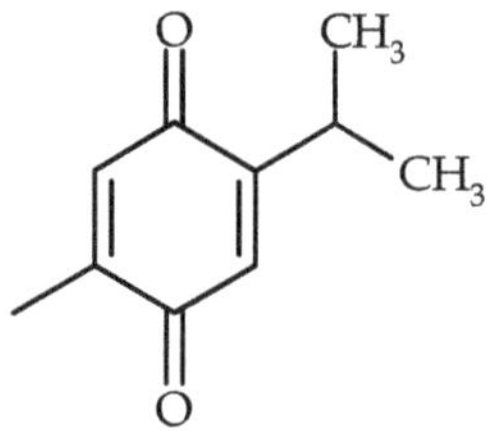

Thymoquinone

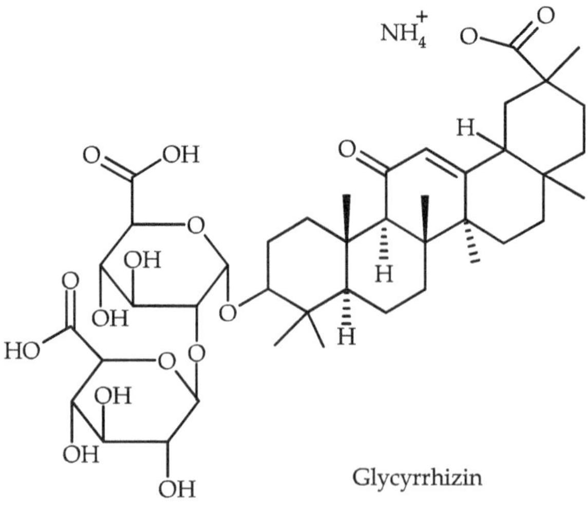

Glycyrrhizin

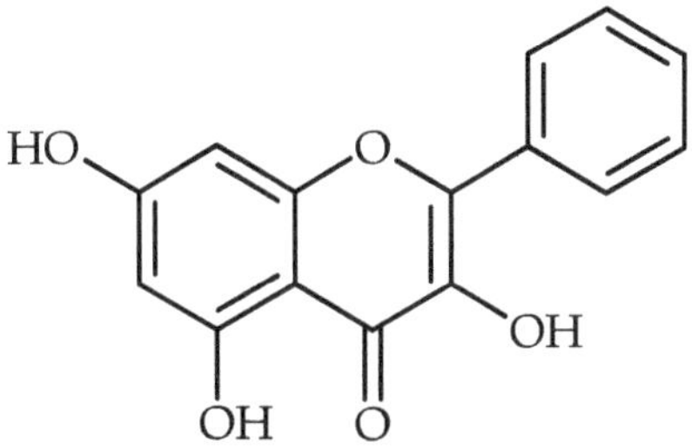

Berberine

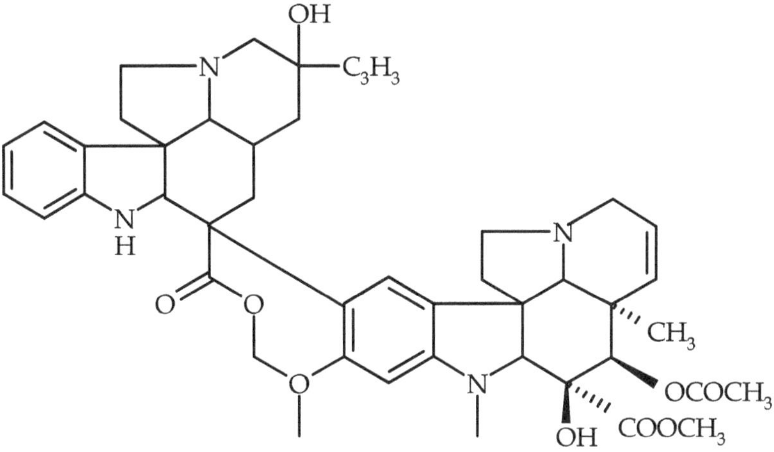

Vinblastine

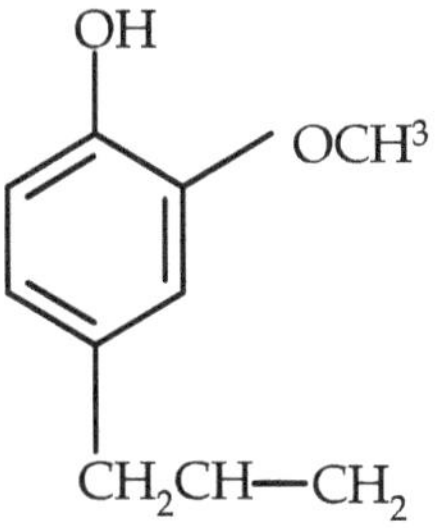

Eugenol

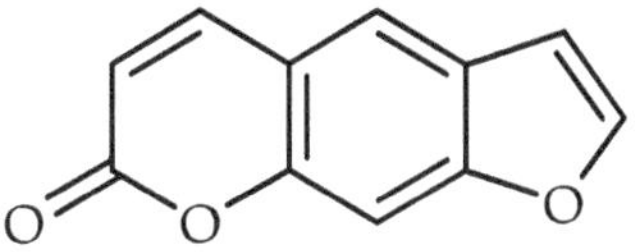

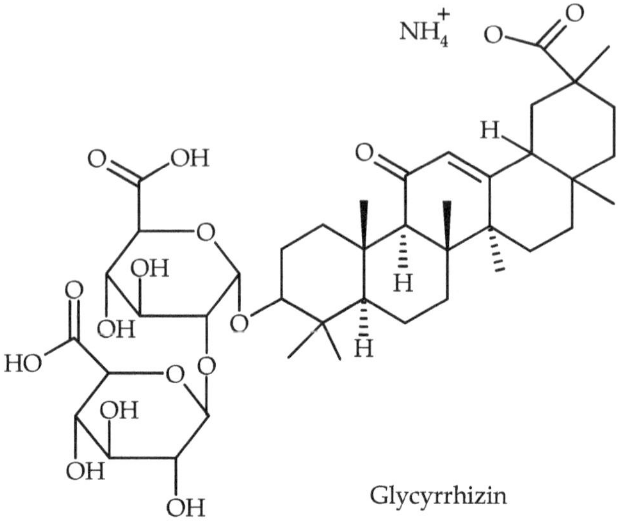

Glycyrrhizin

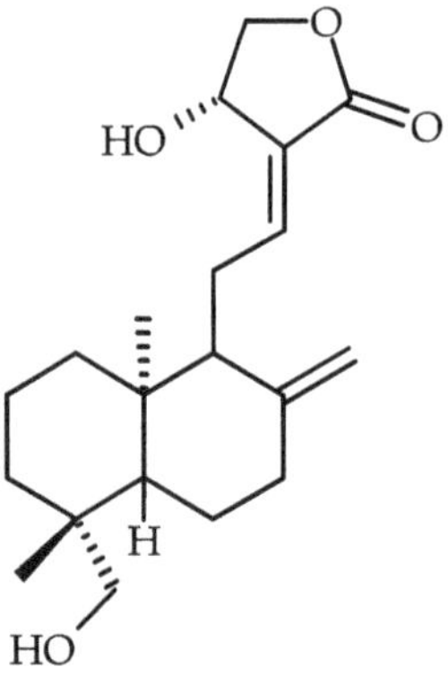

Andrographolide

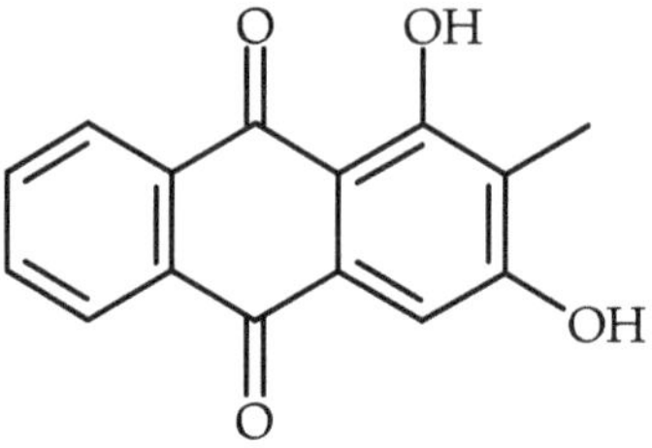

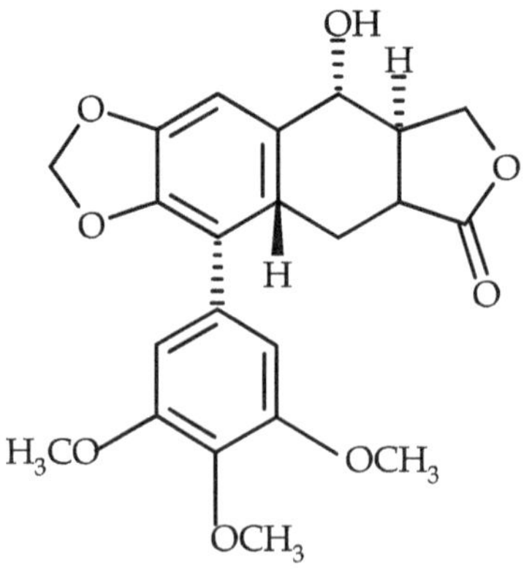

Rubiadin

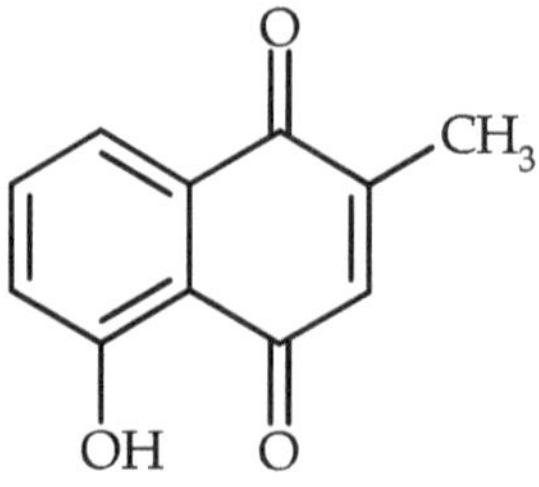

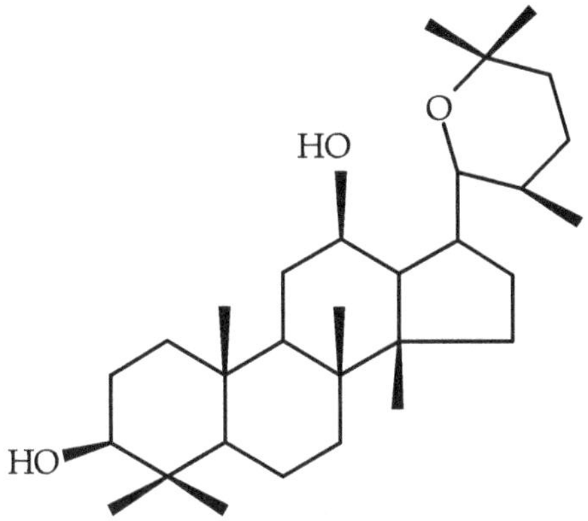

Panaxadiol (aglycone)

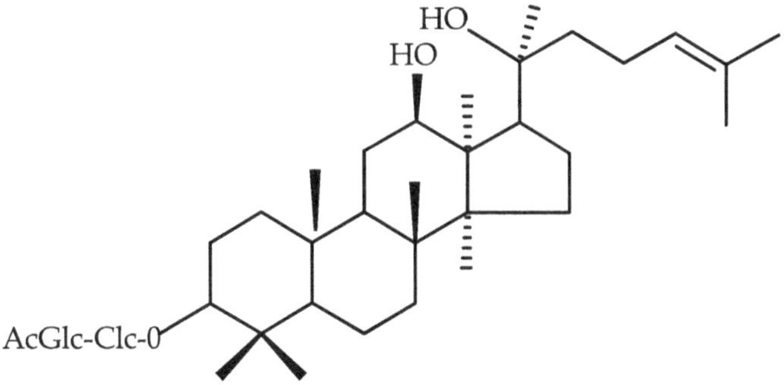

Ginsenoside-R3 (G-re3)

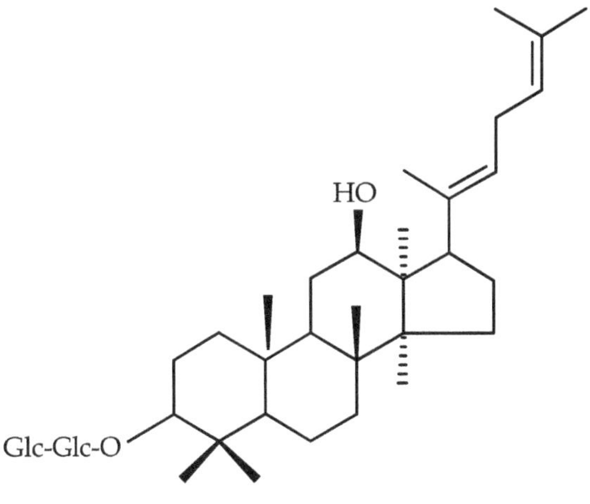

Ginsenoside-Rg5 (G-Rg5)

References

1. Umadevi M, Kumar Sampath K.P, Bhowmik Debjit, Duraivel S. Traditionally used anticancer herbs in India. Journal of Medicinal Plants Studies. (2013), Volume: 1, Issue: 3: 56-74.

2. Moon C.K., Park K.S., Lee S.H., Yoon Y.P. Antitumor activities of several phytopolysaccharides. *Arch. Pham. Res.* (1985); 8: 42-44.

3. Kim K.I., Kim J.W., Hong B.S., Shin D.H., Cho H.Y., Kim H.K., Yang H.C. Antitumor, genotoxicity and anticlastogenic activities of polysaccharide from Curcuma zedoaria. *Mol. Cells.* (2000); 10: 392-398.

4. Syu W.J., Shen C.C., Don M.J., Ou J.C., Lee G.H., Sun C.M. Cytotoxicity of curcuminoids and some novel compounds from Curcuma doaria. *J. Nat. Prod.*(1998); 61: 1531-1534.

5. Lay E.Y., Chyau C.C., Mau J.L., Chen C.C., Lai Y.J., Shih C.F., Lin L.L. Antimicrobial activity and cytotoxicity of the essential oil of Curcuma zedoaria. *Am. J. Chin. Med.* (2004); 32: 281-290.

6. Lu J.J., Dang Y.Y., Huang M., Xu W.S., Chen X.P., Wang Y.T. Anti-cancer properties of terpenoids isolated from Rhizoma Curcumaea review. *J. Ethnopharmacol.* (2012); 143: 406-411.

7. Syed Abdul Rahman S.N., Abdul Wahab N., Abd Malek S.N. *In vitro* Morphological assessment of apoptosis induced by antiproliferative constituents from the rhizomes of Curcuma zedoaria. *Evidence Based Complement Alternat. Med.* (2013); 2013: 257108.

8. Munro S, Thomas KL, Abu-Shaar M. Molecular characterization of a peripheral receptor for cannabinoids. *Nature.* 1993; 365: 61-5.

9. Fernandez-Ruiz J, Romero J, Velasco G, Tolon R, Ramos J, Guzman M. Cannabinoid CB2 receptor: a new target for controlling neural cell survival? *Trends Pharmacol Sci.* 2007; 28: 39-45.

10. Kim SO, Kwon JI, Jeong YK et al. (2007). Induction of Egr-1 is associated with anti- metastatic and anti-invasive ability of fl-lapachone in human hepatocarcinoma cells. Biosc Biotechnol Biochem 71, (9): 2169-76.

11. B.C. Giovanella, M.E. Wall, M.C. Wani, A.W. Nicholas, L.F. Liu, R.Silber, *et al. Science,* 246 (1989), p. 1046

12. P. Pantazis, A.J. Kozielski, D.M. Vardeman, E.R. Petry, B.B. Giovanell Oncol Res, 5 (1993), p. 273.

13. Priyadarshini K, Keerthi Aparajitha U, Paclitaxel against Cancer: A Short Review. *Med Chem* 2012, 2-7.

14. El-Sayed A, Cordell GA. Catharanthamine, a new antitumor bisindole alkaloid from Catharanthus roseus. *J. Nat. Prod,* 1981; 44(3): 289-293.

15. Sairam K, Rao CV, Babu MD, Kumar VK, Agarwal VK and Goel RK. Antiulcerogenic effect of ethanolic extract of Emblica officinalis: An experimental study. *J Ethnopharmacol.* 2002; 82: 1-9.

16. P. Muralidharan and Srikanth J. Antiulcer Activity of Morinda Citrifolia Linn Fruit Extract. *J Sci Res.* 2009; 1(2): 345-352.

17. Yun TK. Experimental and epidemiological evidence of the cancer-preventive effects of Panax ginseng C.A. Meyer. *Nutr Rev,* 1996; 54: S71-81.

18. Son JK, Jung SJ, Jung JH, et al., Anticancer constituents from the roots of Rubia cordifolia L. *Chem Pharm Bull* 2008; 56: 213-216.

19. Sanjay Patel, Neerav Gheewala, Ashok Suthar, Anand Shah. *In-vitro* cytotoxicity activity of Solanum nigrum extracts against Hela Cell-line and Vero cell-line. *International Journal of Pharmacy and pharmaceutical sciences.* 2009; 1(1), 38-46.

20. Rumana Ahmad, Shrivastava AN, Mohsin Ali Khan. Evaluation of *In-vitro* anticancer activity of stem of Tinospora cordifolia against human breast cancer and vero cell lines. *Journal of Medicinal Plant Studies.* 2015; 3(4): 33-37.

2 *Medicinal Plants with Antidiabetic Properties*

The disease of all age-groups virtually in all parts of the world: the DIABETES/DIABETES *MELLITUS* (Madhumeha), has been appropriately known as a wasting disease due to insulin insufficiency in human beings. The pancreas secretes insulin. Carbohydrate metabolism is fundamentally under the control of insulin. Insulin insufficiency occurs in a person due to the functional disturbance of the pancreas.

The Pancreas

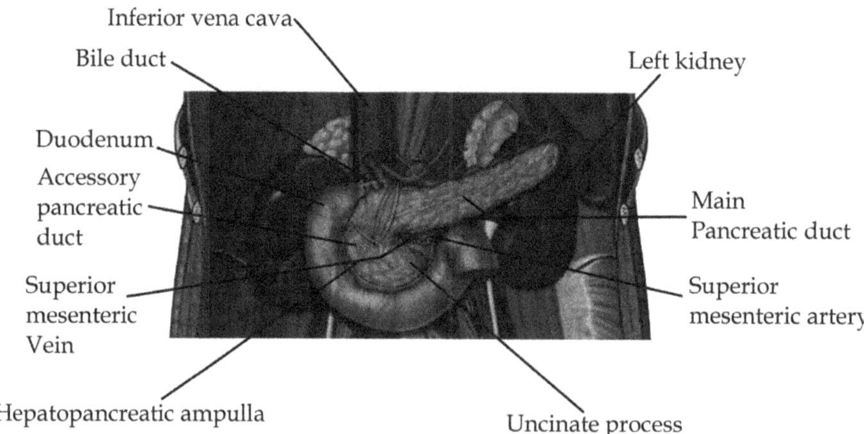

Fig. 2.1 Pancreas.

A mixed gland, the pancreas, a gland of the; digestive system, has both exocrine as well as endocrine functions and is therefore called mixed gland. The endocrine part consists of a group of cells forming the Islets of Langerhans which releases hormones related with carbohydrate metabolism and the exocrine part secretes the digestive juice, known as the pancreatic juice, containing proteolytic, lypolytic and amylolytic enzymes.

The pancreas is devoid of distinct connective tissue capsules and is covered by a thin layer of the loose tissue which passes into the gland as septa and subdivides the gland in many lobules. The main pancreatic duct or the duct of Wirsung extends from the left to the right of the organ to open into the duodenum. Within the duodenal wall at the ampulla of vater, this main pancreatic duct and the common bile duct fuse to form a common duct which opens into the duodenal lumen.

In the pancreas the main pancreatic duct receives many inter-lobular ducts from each lobule.

The Endocrine Part of the Islets of Langerhans

The normal human adult pancreas contains, on an average 5,00,000 islets, scattered with the gland, comprising 1 to 3 per cent of the total tissue. As each group of cells of the endocrine part is encircled by the acini of the exocrine part, they gaze like islands and are hence termed as islet. The distribution of islets is maximum in the tail and minimum in the head of the gland.

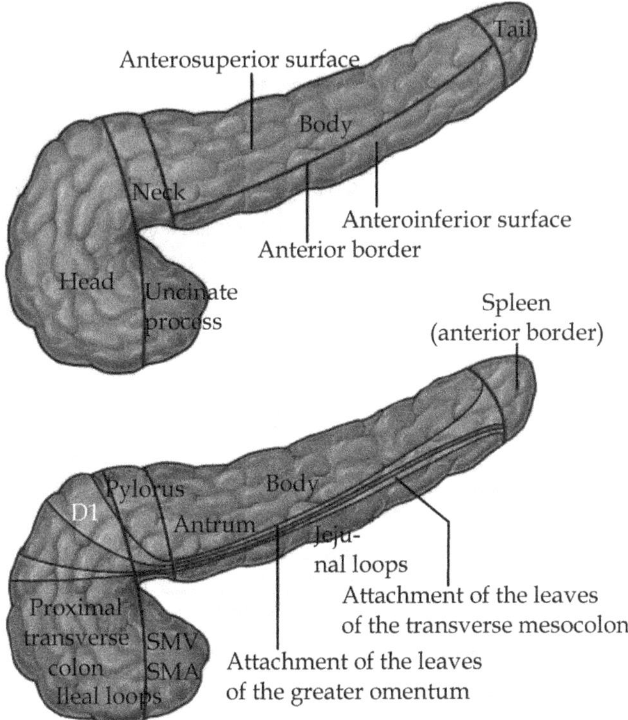

Fig. 2.2 Different parts of Pancreas.

Three types of cells are detected in the islets. These are called the alpha (α), beta (β) and the delta (8) types. The alpha cells are fewer in number (about 20%) and they dwell peripherally in the islet, while the most abundant beta cells (about 75% to 80%) are situated centrally in the appearance of lumps.

The formation of two hormones insulin and glucagon take place in the β cells and the α cells respectively in the Islet of langerhans. Both hormones play significant roles in carbohydrate metabolism. The function of the delta cells (about 5% in number) is not clearly known. It is presumed that they may secrete serotonin but some others believe that gastrin is secreted by these cells.

Biosynthesis, Storage, and Catabolism of Insulin

It is already established that insulin is synthesized by the β cells of Islets of Langerhans but details of the synthesis are unfamiliar. After synthesis, insulin is stored in the β cells of the pancreas and the hormone is released in a controlled and graded mode. The insulin in β cells appears to be allied with granules of the cells. Insulin is released from the β cells into the plasma by the action of glucose and certain other sugars. Growth hormone appears to arouse insulin secretion. Tolbutamide and other sulfonylureas amplify insulin secretion but C7 sugar, mannoheptulose, may discourage its secretion. Several studies suggests that glucose use in the β cells is more or less affiliated to insulin release. Insulin is inactivated in tissues by pair enzymic and nonenzymic reductive cleavage of disulfide bonds and by proteolysis. The glutathione reductase enzyme system may be specially involved in the reductive inactivation.

The Role of Insulin in Carbohydrate Metabolism

By depancreatizing an animal or in diabetes that occurs in human beings, the insulin insufficiency manifests itself in the following fashion:

1. Hyperglycemia and glycosuria.
2. Depletion of glycogen stores in the liver tissues.
3. Lowered respiratory proportion indicating the lack of carbohydrate oxidation.

4. Increase in urinary nitrogen excretion characteristic of the conversion of protein into carbohydrate.

5. The incident of acetone and beta hydroxy butyric acid in the blood and urine payable to faulty fat metabolism.

The injection of insulin will alleviate these symptoms and reinstate to normalcy the deformed metabolic pattern.

The main effect of insulin is to increase the utilization of glucose by most body tissues. In the whole animal the most important overall effect of insulin quantitatively is to increase the rate of glycogen formation and oxidation of carbohydrate in muscles. The primary effect of insulin in increasing glucose utilization is to transport glucose across the cell membrane into the cell. Insulin has been shown to increase the penetration into cells of many monosaccharides. Insulin appeared to promote the entry into cells of such sugars which possess the same chemical configuration at carbon atoms 1, 2 and 3 as does 5-glucose. The insulin effect has been demonstrated in cats, dogs, rats, rabbits and man and on diaphragm, erythrocytes, heart and skeletal muscles, but not in brain. It is of interest that insulin is not necessary in the metabolism of brain tissue.

In relation to the action of insulin in increasing the passage of sugar into the cells the concept of a membrane carrier system as the functional mechanism governing the transport of glucose and other sugars is considered the most valid. According to the theory, the sugar on the outside of the cell membrane is postulated to form a complex with a "Carrier" substance in the membrane. The complex then moves across the membrane. Within the cell the "sugar-carrier" complex dissociates and releases free sugar. The free carrier may either combine with free sugar in the cell and transport it to the extracellular fluid or may move back to the outside membrane to complex with free sugar and transport it into the cell.

Nothing is known about the chemical nature of the carrier. Presumably it may be a lipid character which combines reversibly with sugar molecules, the complex formed possessing membrane solubility.

As primary action of insulin on carbohydrate metabolism appears to reduce blood sugar concentration by greatly enhancing the rate of entrance of sugar to the intracellular compartment and considering the carrier theory of sugar transport to be valid, the action of insulin may be implied to occur upon some component of the carrier system. Insulin particularly facilitates the transport of glucose into the skeletal and cardiac muscles and possibly into the adipose tissues. In the transport of glucose into the tissues such as liver, brain, kidney, intestinal mucosa etc. insulin does not appear to be involved. These tissues offer much less resistance to glucose penetration.

Within the cell, glucose enters the metabolic stream. At the initial stage the metabolism of glucose generally involves phosphorylation by ATP to the glucose-6-phosphate in a reaction catalyzed by the glucokinase enzyme in the hexokinase reaction.

$$\text{Glucose} + \text{ATP} \rightarrow \text{Glucose - 6 - phosphate} + \text{ADP}$$

The activation of glucokinase and glucose phosphorylation is partly affected by insulin and opposes the inhibitory influence of the pituitary growth hormone and adrenal steroids in transformation of glucose to glucose-6-phosphate. Insulin has been found to increase glucagon synthetase activity in muscle.

The Role of Insulin in Fat Metabolism

Insulin is indirectly accountable for the conversion of glucose to fat in the liver and in the adipose tissue. The fundamental steps of biosynthesis of fat from glucose are conversion of glucose to fatty acid and combination of fatty acids with glycerol to form neutral glycerides which are stored largely in the adipose tissue in the liver.

In this course, pyruvic acid formed from glucose reacts with coenzyme A to form acetyl coenzyme A which is reduced to fatty acid at the cost of hydrogen, derived from reduced nicotinamide adenine dinucleotide phosphate or NADPH2. Reduction of NADP to NADPH2 is concluded by hydrogen derived from the glucose-6-phosphate. Hydrogen of NADPH2 receives oxygen from the glucose and water is formed during the biosynthesis of fatty acids from glucose. Fatty acids thus formed combine with glycerol to form neutral fat. Again, glycerol is formed from the glucose-6-phosphate. Thus, the storage of fat is also affected by insulin.

The Role of Insulin in Protein Metabolism

Investigations testify that insulin stimulates protein creation by increasing transport of amino acids into cells and at the same time stimulating nucleic acids - particularly RNA and the messenger RNA, which is especially implicated in protein synthesis. Insulin has been shown to stimulate RNA synthesis in many cases. Thus, it appears that insulin primarily promotes protein synthesis through its effect upon the RNA synthesis. Moreover, the secondary effect of insulin is in increasing carbohydrate metabolism and formation of ATP supply energy for protein synthesis.

In the diabetic patient, glucose cannot be fully utilized for the production of energy and the deficiency of glucose is compensated by the utilization of fat and protein. Breakdown of protein serves as a second source of energy. In the diabetic patient, tissue catabolism and increased excretion of nitrogen produce a negative nitrogen balance.

Thus, it has been instituted that the anabolic and catabolic processes of the three essential food constituents (carbohydrate, fat and protein) are insulin dependent.

The role of insulin, therefore, appears to be as follows:

1. It facilitates the movement of glucose through cell barriers into the cell.
2. It effects the phosphorylation of glucose.
3. It also plays a role in oxidative phosphorylation
4. And it is fundamental to lipid and protein catabolism and anabolism.

Diabetes Mellitus

It was referred to as honey urine and melting away of the flesh in the urine. In 1776, Matthew Dobson discovered a chemical method of evidence that the sweetness of diabetic urine was due to the occupancy of glucose. The disease is characterized by clinical symptoms resulting from genuine or perceptible insufficient pancreatic secretion of insulin or perhaps over-abundance of some insulin inhibiting factors such as hypersecretion of anterior pituitary or adrenal gland. The result is an elevated blood sugar level (normal range is 80 - 120 mg/100 mL of whole blood) which results in pronounced glycosuria tending towards Ketosis. The loss of carbohydrate results in polyphagia and asthenia; water balance is disturbed and polyuria and polydypsia follow.

The deficiency of normal utilization of glucose in the tissues is accompanied by lack of energy production which is gratified by the utilization of fat and protein.

Excessive breakdown of fat causes production of Ketone bodies in excess than can be utilized in the body which results in the accumulation of the Ketone-bodies in the blood. Ketone-bodies like beta hydroxybutyric acid and acetoacetic acid are strong acids and they displace bicarbonate in the blood resulting in a metabolic acidosis and ketosis.

The protein loss in the diabetic results from the breakdown of amino acids to form glucose (gluconeogenesis). It has already been stated that breakdown of protein serves as a second source of energy. Catabolism of tissue protein causes increased excretion of nitrogen, potassium, magnesium phosphate and sulphate. These inorganic anions also displace bicarbonate and a metabolic acidosis develops. The kidney makes every attempt to compensate this metabolic acidosis by excreting an excess of anions in combination with H^+ and NH_4. Loss of electrolytes, acidosis and increased fluid loss due to polyuria seriously affect salt and water balance of the electrolytes excreted. The increased excretion of potassium specially affects the cerebral tissue by reducing its capacity to utilize oxygen. The result of such an extensive alteration of metabolic pattern is hypotension, shock, and finally death.

Diabetes mellitus is classified broadly as Type-I (insulin dependent diabetes mellitus) which typically occurs in younger people who cannot secrete insulin as there are no beta cells in the Islet of Langerhans (Juvenile diabetes) and Type-II (non-insulin dependent diabetes mellitus), which typically occur in older, often corpulent people who retain capacity to secrete insulin but the beta cells of the pancreas are decreased in number, the reduction in number of beta-cells corresponding to the lack of insulin. The onset of the Type-I diabetes is sudden and requires insulin for the treatment.

The disease diabetes mellitus appears to exhibit a hereditary tendency.

Treatment of Diabetes Mellitus

No remedial medicine capable of ensuring radical cure of diabetes has yet been discovered.

A. Insulin in the treatment of Diabetes mellitus:

The principal intention of insulin therapy in diabetes mellitus is the hindrance of diabetic symptoms and complications and accomplishment of sugar free urine. All patients of diabetes don't require insulin. Mild diabetes of older age group may be controlled by dietary regulation. But most diabetic patients require some hypoglycemic agents for leading a symptom free life.

Insulin is the oldest and the best drug in the treatment of diabetes mellitus. Administration of insulin causes disappearance of sugar from the urine and lowers down the above level of sugar to the normal level of blood, within twenty-four to forty-eight hours. Insulin promotes a better utilization of carbohydrate, accordingly raising the respiratory quotient.

In Juvenile diabetes and in patients of younger age group (Type-I) soluble insulin is the drug of choice. In all cases of diabetic coma soluble insulin is the only lifesaving drug and it should be administered as early as possible. About 40 to 60 units of insulin is given intravenously and the same dose is concurrently administered by subcutaneous route.

Soluble insulin (un-modified insulin) is short acting and exerts its effect for a period of six to eight hours and several injections are required per day to maintain blood sugar at normal level.

There are some long acting preparations of insulin also. Names of some long acting preparations of insulin, also known as modified insulin, are Insulin Zinc suspension, B.P., Insulin Zinc suspension (Crystalline), B.R, Insulin Zinc suspension (amorphous), B.P., Injection of protamine Zinc insulin, B.P., I.P., Isophane insulin injection, B.P., Injection of globin Zinc insulin, B.R, I.P., etc.

Hypoglycemic Shock: One of the hazards of insulin administration is the production of hypoglycemic shock. The hypoglycemic symptoms which occur in man are hyperirritability, trembling, incoordination, muscular weakness, disorientation, convulsions, unconsciousness and death.

B. Oral hypoglycemic agents:

Oral hypoglycemic agents are of two kinds

    (i)   sulfonamide derivatives (sulphonyl ureas), and

    (ii) guanidine derivatives (biguanides).

Mode of Action

  (i) Sulphonyl ureas stimulate receptors on the beta-islet cells of the pancreas to release more stored insulin in retort to glucose. They do not increase insulin formation. They are unavailing in totally insulin deficient patients and for successful therapy probably requires about 30% of normal beta-cells' function to be present. They cause hypoglycemia in normal subjects as well as diabetics.

  (ii) The cellular mode of action of biguanides is ambiguous but the most important effect seems to be to degrade the production of glucose in the liver i.e. gluconeogenesis. Other effects comprise enhancement of peripheral insulin effect (they don't act in the absence of insulin) and increase glucose uptake in the peripheral tissues. They do not (used alone) cause lactic acidosis.

Both groups of drugs are effective only in the presence of insulin. Drugs of the two groups may be used together.

A. The drugs of sulphonyl ureas

    1. *Tolbutamide:* Tolbutamide was the first compound available for the treatment of diabetes other than insulin. Upon oral administration it is easily absorbed from the gastrointestinal tract. Administration of 3 gm of tolbutamide to nondiabetic fasting individuals will cause about a 30 per cent fall in blood sugar in about 1 hour. In the diabetic patient the hypoglycemic is of more progressive onset.

        Tolbutamide is prescribed in initial dose of 0.5 gm twice daily to be taken before breakfast and tea.

2. *Toxic effects:* There may be malaise, digestive disorders e.g. anorexia, nausea and vomiting and epigastric discomfort. There may be also be skin rashes.

3. *Chlorpropamide:* Chlorpropamide is an oral hypoglycemic agent intimately related structurally to tolbutamide. It is quickly absorbed from the gastrointestinal tract, and while circulating in the blood it is bound partially by serum protein. Chlorpropamide is a more effective hypoglycemic agent than tolbutamide and needs to be given only once a day.

   It is administrated in a single dose of 250 mg given before breakfast.

4. *Toxic effects:* Chlorpropamide is more toxic than tolbutamide. Its toxic effects comprise gastrointestinal disturbances like those produced by tolbutamide. There may be reversible leucopenia, eosinophilia and lymphocytosis, drug rashes and intolerance to alcohol.

5. *Glibenclamide:* It is appropriate for use in single daily dose; it is short acting than chlorpropamide and its action is concluded by metabolism.

6. *Other sulphonyl ureas include:* Glipizide, Gliquidone, Gliclazide, Glibornuride.

B. **The drugs of biguanides (diaguanides)**

1. *Metabolism:* Lesser adverse gut reactions are common, which comprise diarrhea, and a metallic taste in the mouth, and protracted use may cause vitamin B_{12} deficiency due to malabsorption. It is not metabolized. It is excreted by the kidneys. It should not be used in the attendance of renal dysfunction. It's most common use is in combination with a sulphonyl urea when the latter alone has failed. It is taken with meal.

Dietary Fibre and Diabetes

On summation of un-absorbable gel-forming, hydrocolloidal polysaccharide fibers (such as guar gum from the seeds of 'Cluster bean') to the diet of diabetics reduces carbohydrate absorption and flattens the post prandial blood glucose curve, and requirements of insulin and oral hypoglycemic agents are reduced, which has been reported. But large amount causes displeasure due to flatulence.

Precautions with Oral Hypoglycemic Agents

Hypoglycemia occurs with sulphonyl ureas compounds, but occurrences are much more fewer than with insulin therapy.

A biguanide should not be used in patients with renal disease.

Medicinal Plants with Antidiabetic Properties

1. *Abroma augusta Linn.* (Sterculiaceae)
   - *Common names:* Eng.: Perennial Indian Hemp, Devil'a Cotton, Hindi & Beng.: Ulat Kambal.
   - *Distribution: A shrub, found throughout the hot parts of India & Pakistan. Cultivated mainly in Uttar Pradesh and Assam.*
   - *Parts used:* Leaves.
   - *Pharmacological activities:* Leaves used for uterine disorders, rheumatic pains, sinusitis and diabetes[1].
   - *Chemical constituents:* Taraxxeryl acetate, taraxerol, and p-sitostero! are found in leaves. Choline, betaine and alkaloid, p-sitosterol and stigma sterol are obtained from roots, p-sitosterol an difriedelin octacosane-1,28-diol from heartwood.

2. *Acacia melanoxylon R. Br.* (Fabaceae)
   - *Common names:* Eng: Australian Black Wood.
   - *Distribution:* Introduced around 1840 in the Nilgiris and has become naturalized.
   - *Parts used:* Roots.
   - *Pharmacological activities:* Seeds produced marked hypoglycemia and hypochlolesterolaemic effects in normal as well as in alloxan diabetic albino rats[2].
   - *Chemical constituents:* Quercetin-3-galactoside (hyperin or hyperoside) m.p. 227-30° from flowers was isolated. Stigmast-7-enol and a-spinasterol from heartwood was isolated.

3. *Acacia modesta Wall* **(Fabaceae)**

   - *Common name:* Punjab : Phulai.
   - *Distribution:* It is found in Punjab, sub-Himalayan tract and outer Himalayas, ascending up to 4,000 ft.
   - *Parts used:* Seeds.
   - *Pharmacological activities:* Seed diet exhibited hypoglycemic effect in normal rats[3].
   - *Chemical constituents:* It contains gum.

4. *Acacia nilotica Linn.*

   Syn. *A. arab*/cawilld. (Leguminosae)

   - *Common names:* Eng.: Indian Gum Arabic, Hindi, Punjab & U.P. : Kikar. Beng: Babul.
   - *Distribution:* A moderate sized, spiny evergreen tree common all over India, in dry and sandy localities, plentiful in Western Peninsula, the Deccan and coramandal coast.
   - *Parts used:* Seeds.
   - *Pharmacological activities:* Seed diet reduced blood sugar level in normal rats[3].
   - *Chemical constituents:* Bark contains a large quantity of tannin, pods contain also tannin. Gum contains arable acid combined with calcium, magnesium and potassium and small amount of malic acid. A new arabinobiose-2-O-p-L-arabinofuronosyl-L-arabinose-along with known 3-0-p-L-arabinopyranosyl-L-arabinose from gum was isolated.

5. *Aconitum ferox Wall ex. Ser* **(Ranunculaceae)**

   - *Common names:* Eng: Indian Aconite, Monkshood, Hindi: Mithazahar, Beng: Kathbish or Mithavish.
   - *Distribution:* Distributed at sub-Alpine regions of the Himalayas, rat ward of Kumaon, Nepal, Kashmir and Sikkim.
   - *Parts used:* Roots.
   - *Pharmacological activities:* Root has diaphoretic, diuretic, antiperiodic antipyretic and antidiabetic actions in very small doses[4]. For internal administration of the tincture of the roots must be used with great caution on account of the high

toxicity. It should not be used in the case when heart disease is present.

- *Chemical constituents:* The tuberous root contains crystalline toxic alkaloid called napelline or pseudo - aconitine, similar to aconitine, and small- quantity of aconitine, picro - aconine, benzyl aconine and homo napelline.

6. *Adhatoda vasica Nees* **(Acanthaceae)**

- *Common names:* Hindi: Arrisha, Beng: Basak or Vasaka.
- *Distribution:* It is sub-herbaceous bush, found thought the year in plains and sub-Himalayan tracts in India, ascending up to 1200 metre, flowers during February-March and also at the end of rainy seasons.
- *Parts used:* Leaves.
- *Pharmacological activities:* Leaves are commonly used in bronchial troubles.
- Oral administration of the leaves reduced blood sugar in rabbits for a short period of time[5].
- *Chemical constituents:* The chief principles of leaves are alkaloids vasicine (MW 188, C HNOJ, vasicinone and vasicinol. Beside these p-sitosterol, tritriacontane, vasinine, an essential oil and a resin are also obtained from leaves. Beside these new quinazoline alkaloids such as adhatodine, anisotine, vasicoline and vasicoiinone were isolated.

7. *Adiantum capillus- veneris Linn.* **(Polypodiaceae)**

- *Common names:* Eng: Maidenhair Fern, Hindi & Kan: Hansraj, mubaraka, pursha.
- *Distribution:* Chiefly obtained in the Punjab bazar and in some parts of South India.
- *Parts used:* Whole plant.
- *Pharmacological activities:* The fern is used as an expectorant and tonic. Whole plant produced hypoglycemic activity in normal rabbits[8].
- *Chemical constituents:* The fern contains 3cc,4a-epoxy-filicane, 21-hydroxy-adiantone, and adiantone. It also contains an essential oil.

8. ***Adiantum incisum Forsk.***

   Syn. *A. caudatum* Linn. (Polypodiaceae).

   - *Common names: Hindi:* Morshikha (talmurga); Beng.: Mayurshikha.

   - *Distribution:* A Himalayan form, also cultivated in garden as ornamental plants.

   - *Parts used:* Roots.

   - *Pharmacological activities:* Used in hemicramia and diabetes[7].

   - *Chemical constituents:* It contains adiantone iso-adiantone, fernene, hentriacontane hentriacontanone-16, and (3-sitosterol.

9. ***Aegle marmelos Coor. (Rutaceae)***

   - *Common names:* Eng.: Bael Tree, Hindi, Beng. & Mar.: Bel.

   - *Distribution:* A tree, attaining a height of 12m growing wild and also cultivated through out the country, particularly in the dry regions.

   - *Parts used:* Leaves and Roots.

   - *Pharmacological activities:* Marmelosin of the fruit acts as a laxative and diuretic. Unripe and half ripe fruits are stomachic, digestive and used in diarrhea and dysentery.

   - Leaves and roots exhibited hypoglycemic activity in albino rats[8]. Fruit pulp produced no hypoglycemic activity in normal rabbits[9].

   - *Chemical constituents:* Umbelliferone, skimmianine, marmin, p-sitosterol lepeal and y-sitosterol from immature bark and roots. Leaves contain tannin phlobtannins aegeline, flavon -3- ols, leucoanthocyanins, anthocyanins. Fresh leaves yield on distillation a yellowish -green volatile oil with a peculiar odour. Four alkloids, 0-(3, 3-dimethyl allyl)- half ordinol, N-2-ethoxy-2-(4-methoxy-phenyl) ethyl cinnamamide, N-2-methoxy-2-[4-(3,3-dimethyl-allyloxy)   phenyl]   ethyl cinnamamide   N-2-methoxy-2-(4-methoxyphenyl)   ethyl cinnamamide, isolated from leaves. Infruit pulp in addition with normal substance contains a body named marmelosin, which is considered to be one of the most important active principle of the fruit.

10. *Albizia stipulata Sensu Baker* **(Mimosaceae)**

    Syn. A. chinensis (Osbeck) Merr.

    - *Common names:* Hindi: Siran; Beng.: Chakua.
    - *Distribution:* Distributed in the sub-Himalayan tracts, Assam, Bengal, South India and the Andamans, extensively cultivated for shade in the coffee and tea garden.
    - *Parts used:* Seeds.
    - *Pharmacological activities:* Marked hypoglycemic activity was produced in normal albino rats by the seed died but no hypoglycemic effect was found in alloxan-diabetic albino rats[10].
    - *Chemical constituents:* It yields gum.

11. *Allium cepa Linn.* **(Liliaceae)**

    - *Common names:* Eng.: Onion, Hindi: Piyar; Beng.: Pyanj.
    - *Distribution:* Cultivated all over India. Parts used: Bulbs.
    - *Pharmacological activities:* Onion has diuretic, stimulating and expectorant actions, it is also used as antiflatulence.
    - Allyl propyl disulphide from the bulbs reduced blood sugar level of alloxan-diabetic rabbits[17].
    - Significant hypoglycemic effect was produced in mice by onion oil and synthetic dipropyl disulphide oxide[25].
    - Oral administration of allicin (diallyl disulphide oxide) exhibited significant reduction of the blood sugar levels in alloxan diabetic rabbits[15].
    - Hypoglycemic activity was produced by the ether extract of juice expressed onion bulbs in diabetic rabbits[30].
    - Oral administration of allyl propyl disulphide to the human volunteers caused significant full in blood glucose level[11].
    - Petroleum ether extract of bulbs exhibited fall of blood sugar in rabbits[18].
    - Hypoglycemic activity was produced in rabbits by the light petroleum extract of dried onion[28].
    - Onion tops caused the fall of fasting blood sugar level in alloxan and adrenaline-diabetic rats[13].

- Total extract of dried onion bulb produced hypoglycemic activity in rats and rabbits[12].

- Petroleum ether and chloroform extracts caused a significant full is blood sugar at the time of glucose tolerance lost[21,22]. Ingestion of onion bulb juice caused the lowering of the blood sugar level in diabetes mellitus patients[26].

- Two fractions, fractions A and B from the onion bulb juice produced lowering of blood sugar level in rabbits[16].

- Antidiabetic activity was produced by onion bulbs extracts in rabbits[14].

- On oral application of hypoglycemic fraction from the onion bulbs to alloxan diabetic rabbits increased glucose tolerance. The juiced expressed residue of the bulb showed hypoglycemic activity in diabetic patients[29].

- Significant hypoglycemic activity was produced in test animals by onion bulb[20].

- The non-dialyzable fraction from the lipid free juice of the onion bulb exhibited hypoglycemic activity in rabbits[31].

- Insulin like activity was observed in onion bulbs extracts, in rabbits[27].

- Onion bulbs extract produced lowering of the blood sugar level in human volunteers during the glucose tolerance test, but no hypoglycemic effect was observed on fasting blood sugar level[23,24].

- Hypoglycemic activity was observed in the extracts of green sprouting taps, roots and bulbs of onion in rabbits[19].

- ***Chemical constituents:*** Essential oil of whole plant is 0.05%. Chief constituent of inude oil is allyl-propyl disulphide. A new amino acid cycloallin was isolated. (+) S-propyl-L-cysteine sulphoxide isolated as N-2,4-dinitrophenyl derived from bulb. Propyl sulfanic acid was obtained from bulb.

12. *Allium sativum Linn.* (Liliaceae)

- ***Common names:*** Eng.: Garlic, Hindi & Guj: Lasan, Beng. & Mar: Lasum.

- ***Distribution:*** Cultivated all over India.

- ***Parts used:*** Bulbs.

- *Pharmacological activities:* Garlic juice is applied in skin troubles and used as car drops. This juice is also used in dyspepsia and flatulence. Garlic is considered stimulant, expectorant and diuretic. Ethyl ether extract of dried garlic bulb powder exhibited hypoglycemic activity in glucose feeding normal fasting rabbits[35].

- Hypoglycemic activity was exhibited by the Diallyl disulphide oxide (allicin) from garlic bulb in mild alloxan-diabetic rabbits[34].

- Hypoglycemic activity was produced by the garlic bulb in alloxan- diabetic rabbits[33].

- Hyperglycemic effect of glucose feeding in rabbits was controlled by the garlic juice[32].

- *Chemical constituents:* See Hepatoprotective chapter.

13. *Aloe barbadensis Mill.*

Syn. *A. veraTourn. exlinn. (Liliaceae)

- *Common names:* Eng.: Curacao Aloe, Barbados Aloe, Indian Aloe, Jaffarabad Aloe, Hindi: Ghee-kunvar, Beng: Ghrita-kumari.

- *Distribution:* It is xerophylic, arborescent or herbaceous, the fleshy and strongly cuticularised leaves usually prickly at the margin and arranged in dense rosettes. It naturalized in India. Propagated by sucker. It is planted in many Indian garden and available at all over India.

- *Parts used:* Leaves.

- *Pharmacological activities:* Fresh juice is used as cathartic. It is also very useful in x-ray burn and any other radiation burns.

- Semi-transparent, amorphous solid of the fresh leaves produced hypoglycemic effect in normal albino rabbits when administered intravenously and significant hypoglycemic effect was also found in alloxan-diabetic rabbits[36].

- *Chemical constituents:* Leaf latex contains aloin, isobarbaloin, emodin, aloe-emodin, (3-barbaloin.

14. *Alpinia galanga Willd.* **(Zingiberaceae)**

- *Common names:* Eng: The Greater Galangal, Hindi & Beng: Kulanjan. Distribution: Found in South India and Bengal. Parts used: Rhizomes.

- *Pharmacological activities:* Dried rhizomes used as carminative and stimulant.

- Essential oil from rhizomes used in perfumery. It is also used in dyspepsia, fever and diabetes mellitus[37].

- *Chemical constituents:* Compheride, galangin and alpinin. From the green rhizome a pale yellow volatile oil with a pleasant odour can be obtained by distillation. This volatile oil contains methyl cinnamate, cincole, camphor. Seeds contain caryophyllene oxide, caryophyllenol II, 1'-acetoxychavicol acetate, 1'-acetoxyeeugenol acetate pentadecane and 7-heptadecene.

15. *Anacardium occidentale Linn.* **(Anacardiaceae)**

- *Common names:* Eng.: Cashen Nut Tree, Hindi & Mar.: Kaju; Beng.: Hiyli-badam.

- *Distribution:* An evergreen tree, generally cultivated and naturalized in the hotter parts of India especially near sea. Flowers are yellow with pink stripes.

- *Parts used:* Leaves and barks.

- *Pharmacological activities:* Oral application of the tincture or extract of the bark produced hypoglycemic activity in normal individuals[39]. Leaves exhibited hypoglycemic activity in albino rats[40]. Intravenous administration of bark extract reduced the hyperglycemia of alloxan diabetes in dogs and rats[38].

- *Chemical constituents:* A gum containing bassorin, partially soluble in water exudes from the bark. Leaves contain p-hydroxy benzoic, protocatechuic, gentisic, gallic acids, and glycosides of kaempferol and quercitol.

16. *Arctium lappa Linn.* **(Asteraceae)**

- *Common names:* Eng: Burdock.

- *Distribution:* Found at W.Himalayas from Kashmir Simla.

- *Parts used:* Leaves.

- *Pharmacological activities:* Extracts caused sharp long-lasting hypoglycemic effect with increase in carbohydrate tolerance in rats[41].

- *Chemical constituents:* Eremophilence, fukinone, beta-sotolone, fukinanolide (3-endesmol, taraxasterol its acetate and palmitate and dehydro-fukinone and aretior (8cc-hydroxyendesmol) obtained from leaves.

17. *Areca catechu Linn.* (**Arecaceae**)

   - *Common names:* Eng: Areca Nut, Betel Nut, Hindi & Beng: Supari.

   - *Distribution:* Cultivated throughout tropical India. It flourished in dry plateau of Mysore. Canara, Malabar, Assam etc. Areca nuts are most commonly used as a musticatory.

   - *Pharmacological activities:* Alkaloid fraction exhibited hypoglycemic activity[42].

   - *Chemical constituents:* See Antifertility chapter.

18. *Avena saliva Linn.* (**Cyperaceae**)

   - *Common names:* Eng: Oat, Common Oat, Hindi & Beng: Jai.

   - *Distribution:* Annual or perennial grasses. Cultivated to a limited extent in W. Himalayas, Sikkim and N. West Bengal. Available in Indian bazar and many other countries.

   - *Parts used:* Seeds.

   - *Pharmacological activities:* Seed is used in diabetes[43].

   - *Chemical constituents:* See Anti-fertility chapter.

19. *Azadirachta indica A. Juss.*

   Syn. *Melia azadirachta* Linn (Meliaceae)

   - *Common names:* Eng.: Neem Tree, MargosaTree, Hindi & Beng.: Nim.

   - *Distribution:* A large tree with rough bark. Native to India, grown all over India. Grows wild in the dry forests of the Deccan.

   - *Parts used:* Leaves.

   - *Pharmacological activities:* The loss in body weight of rats caused by prolong administration of anterior pituitary extract was prevented by "Tribang shila" a composite drug containing neem leaves[46].

- The hyperglycemic response of anterior pituitary extract in rats, reduced significantly by Tribang Shila" a composite drug containing neem leaves[44].

- Aqueous extract of leaves produced significant reduction of the blood sugar level in diabetic dogs[45].

- *Chemical constituents:* See Anti-inflammatory chapter.

20. *Bauhinia semla Wunderlin.*

Syn. *B. retusa* Roxb. (Mimosaceae)

- *Common name:* Hindi: Semla.

- *Parts used:* Seeds.

- *Pharmacological activities:* Hypoglycemic as well as hypocholesterolemic activities were produced in normal and alloxan - diabetic albino rats by seeds[47].

- *Chemical constituents:* Bark contains quercetin-3-0-(3-D-glucoside and rutin.

21. *Benincasa hispida*

(Thunb) Cogn. Syn. *B.cerifera* Savi. (Cucurbitaceae).

- *Common names:* Eng.: Ash Gourd, Hindi: Petha; Beng.: Chalkumra.

- *Distribution:* A large climber and annual plant. Cultivated through out India, fruits used as vegetable. Flowers are large yellow.

- *Parts used:* Fruits.

- *Pharmacological activities:* An Ayurvedic medicine. "Kushmanda lehyam" is used for diabetes[48].

- *Chemical constituents:* p-Sitosterol, lupeol, n-triacontanol, manitol, arginine, aspastic acid, protine, hydroxyprotine, isoleucine cystoine, glutamic acid, glucose rhamnose found in fruits.

22. *Bougainvillea spectabilis Willd.* **(Nyctaginaceae)**

- *Common names:* Eng.: Baugainvilla, Beng.: Baganbilas.

- *Distribution:* A shrub, flowers are small, usually enclosed by large, purple, or white or orange coloured bracts, commonly grown in gardens.

- *Parts used:* Leaves.

- *Pharmacological activities:* Hypoglycemic action of the leaf-juice was established in alloxan induced diabetic rabbits on oral administration. Moreover, leaf juice also increased liver and muscle glycogen in alloxan diabetic rats on repeated administration[49].

23. ***Brassica oleracea Linn. Var. capitata Linn.* (Brassicaceae)**

- *Common names:* Eng.: Cabbage, Hindi: Band-gobi, patagobhi, Beng.: Bandhakapi.

- *Distribution:* Cabbage is a commonly used vegetable, like cauliflower and available throughout India.

- *Parts used:* Leaves.

- *Pharmacological activities:* No extract was able to prepare from cabbage containing hypoglycemic activity[51]. No significant hypoglycemic effect was produced in morning blood sugar level on application of cabbage extracts orally and subcutaneously[52]. One of the two fractions of cabbage extract caused an increase in blood sugar, associated with glycosuria and decrease of the liver glycogen content but the other fraction exhibited hypoglycemic effect in normal rabbits and caused apparent replacement of insulin in the depancreatized dog[50].

- *Chemical constituents:* Leaves contains quercetin, iso-rhamnetin, and 3-sophoroside-7-glucosides of kaempferol. Moreover cyanidin-3-p coumaryl sophoroside-5-glucoside, cyanidin-3-ferulylsophoroside 5-glucoside, cyanidin-3-sinapy-sophoroside-5-glucoside, cyanidin-3-(disinapyl)-sophoroside-5-glucoside, cyanidin-3-sophoroside-5-glucoside etc.

24. ***Casearia esculenta Roxb.* (Samydaceae)**

- *Common names:* Mar: Mori, kulkulta, Tarn: Kottargovai.

- *Distribution:* Found at W. Peninsula. Parts used: Roots.

- *Pharmacological activities:* Roots used in diabetes and piles[53]. The active hypoglycemic principles a resin fraction and a crystalline compound (m.p. 182) have been isolated from the roots[55]. The water soluble crystalline fraction and the resin part of the root produced hypoglycemic effect[56]. Significant lowering of blood sugar was observed in rats by the decoction of the roots, and glucose tolerance was favourably influenced on chronic administration[54]. Alcoholic extract of the roots caused hypoglycemic effect in albino rats. Aqueous and alcoholic extracts influenced favourably the glucose tolerance[57].

- *Chemical constituents:* Leucopelargonidin, m.p. 220°C and two ster-ols of m.p. 120°C and 132°C are obtained from roots.

25. *Cassia auriculata Linn.* (Mimosaceae).

- *Common names:* Eng.: Tanner's Cassia, Avaram, Hindi: Tarwar, Guj: Awal, Mar: Tarwad.

- *Distribution:* Found at Madhya Pradesh and W.Peninsula. Cultivated elsewhere.

- *Parts used:* Seeds, Leaves and Flowers.

- *Pharmacological activities:* Hypoglycemic effect was observed on application of water extract of the seeds in normal rabbits and alloxan rabbits and dogs[58].

- *Chemical constituents:* p-Sitosterol and kaempferol were isolated from flowers leaves contain saturated higher fatty ketoalcohols and emodin. 4,5,7 - trihydroxy flavan - 3,4- diol also known as leucoanthocyanin-goratensidine and (-) auriculacacidin were detected.

26. *Cassia fistula Linn.* (Leguminosae)

- *Common names:* Eng.: Indian Laburnum, Beng.: Amaltas, kalkasunda, Hindi: Bandarlathi.

- *Distribution:* A moderate sized diciduous tree, common throughout India, as wild and cultivated. Fruits are collected when ripe.

- *Parts used:* Seeds.

- *Pharmacological activities:* Seed diet produced marked hypoglycemic effect on normal albino rats but caused no hypoglycemic effect on alloxan diabetic albino rats[59].

- *Chemical constituents:* See anti-inflammatory chapter.

27. *Cassia occidentalis Linn.* **(Fabaceae)**

- *Common names:* Eng.: Negro Coffee, Hindi: Kasondi; Beng.: Baro-kalkesunda.

- *Distribution:* A common weed found from the Himalayas to the West Bengal and South India.

- *Parts used:* Roots and leaves.

- *Pharmacological activities:* Leaves and roots possessed antidiabetic activity in animals[60].

- *Chemical constituents:* Roots contains anthraquinones, a plytosterol, a hydroxyanthraquinone, m.p. 128°C 1, 8-dihydroxyanthraquinone, emodin, quercetin, an antraquinone m.p. 179°C and a substance similar to rhein and leaves contain dianthronic heteroside. Chrysaphanol and emodol from young roots and C-flavonosides of apigenin from pericarp were isolated.

28. *Cassia sophera Linn.* **(Fabaceae)**

- *Common names:* Eng.: Senna Esculenta, Hindi: Kasauns, Beng.: Chhoto-Kalkesenda.

- *Distribution:* A shrub 2-3m high annual or perenniar, found throughout the tropical parts of India.

- *Parts used:* Seeds and balk.

- *Pharmacological activities:* Infusion of bark or powdered seeds with honey are given in diabetes[61].

- *Chemical constituents:* Emodin, and chrysophanic acid flowers contain rhamnetin-3-O-p-D-glucoside and chrysophanol.

29. *Catharanthus roseus G.Don.*

Syn. *Lochnera rosea* (Linn) Reichb,

- *Vinca rosea Linn.* (Apocynaceae)

- *Common names:* Hindi: Sadabahar; Beng: Nayantara.

- *Parts used:* Whole plants.

- *Pharmacological activities:* It is used in diabetes[62]. Ether and chloroform soluble alkaloid fraction of the whole plant caused marked anti-diuretic activity in rats[66]. It produced hypoglyconic activity[65].

- Main alkaloides fraction from the plant reduced blood sugar level in rats[63].

- No significant hypoglycemic effect was produced by the water extract of leaves in normal and diabetic rabbits and dogs[64].

- *Chemical constituents:* Four alkaloids possessing antibacterial activities from leaves and two glycosidal principles and urosolic acid, leurosine, isoleurosine, previne, mitraphylline, lochnevin perosine.

30. *Cichorium intybus Linn.* (Asteraceae)

- *Common names:* Eng.: Cuicory, Wild Endive, Hindi: Kasani, Kasni.

- *Distribution:* The chicory is native of Europe, found in India, cultivated at elsewhere.

- *Parts used:* Leaves.

- *Pharmacological activities:* Leaves produced no hypoglycemic activity in alloxan diabetic rats[67]. Water extract of leaves produced hypoglycemic activity in rabbits (unpublished work).

- *Chemical constituents:* Aerial parts contain quercitrin, apigenin, hyperin, luteolin-7-p-D-glucopyranoside, caffeic, dicaffeoyltar acids, apigenin-7-O-L-arabinoside, chlorogen and neochlorogenic and inflorescence contains umbelliferne, 6,7-dihydroxy coumarin, cichoriin and esculin.

31. *Citrus aurantium Linn.* (Rutaceae)

- *Common names:* Eng.: Common Orange, Hindi: Narengi. Beng.: Kamla-neboo.

- *Distribution:* Found in northern India, and different varieties are distributed chiefly in the warmer moist regions of India such as Assam.

- *Parts used:* Fruits.

- *Pharmacological activities:* The laevulose, which found in orange is beneficial in diabetes[68].

- *Chemical constituents:* Rind contains volatile oil, hesperidin, isoheperidin etc. Orange fruit contains laevulose.

32. *Clerodendrum phlomidis Linn. f.* **(Verbenaceae)**

- *Common names:* Hindi, Guj & Mar.: Ami.
- *Distribution:* It is found at the Gangetic valley.
- *Parts used:* Whole plant.
- *Pharmacological activities:* Roots are aromatic and astringent. Decoction and alcoholic extract of the crude drug, "Ami" is useful for diabetic mellitus patients[69]. Alcoholic extract of the whole plant exhibited hypoglycemic effect in normal and diabetic mellitus patients[70].
- *Chemical constituents:* Scutellareim and pectolinarigenin (4',6-dimethyl scutellareim) obtained from leaves. Leaves also contain p and y- sitosterols, a monoglucoside mp. 213° ceryl alcohol, palmitic and cerotic acids, and ansteros mp. 155°. Stem contains p-sitosterol-p-D-glucoside, ceryl alcohol and p-sitosterol.

33. *Coccinia indica Wight & Arn.*

Syn. *Cephalandra indica* Nand. (Cucurbitaceae)

- *Common names:* Eng.: Ivy Gourd, Hindi: Kanduri; Beng.: Telakuncha.
- *Distribution:* Found throughout India, wild and cultivated.
- *Parts used:* Roots.
- *Pharmacological activities:* Water soluble fraction of alcoholic extract of fat free roots exhibited hypoglycemic effect in alloxan - diabetic rabbits[71]. Alcoholic extract of roots produced hypoglycemic activity in alloxanized rats and rabbits[72]. Aqueous and ethanolic extracts of the defatted powdered root significantly reduced blood sugar level in alloxan- diabetic rabbits comparable to tolbutamide[73]. No antidiabetic action was observed neither in blood sugar nor in urine of patients suffering from glycosuria by the fresh juice of leaves, stem and roots.
- No hypoglycemic activity was produced by the amytolytic emzyme, a hormon and an alkaloid isolated from the whole plant in rabbits[74,75].
- Acute hyperglycemic condition produced by the anterior pituitary extract in rats was inhibited by the alcoholic extract of fruit[76].

- Corticotropin-and somatotropin induced hyperglycemia was inhibited by the alcoholic extract of fruit in rats[77].

- Alcoholic extract of the drug exhibited better hypoglycemic effect than its aqueous counterpart in normal and alloxan diabetic rabbits[78].

- Hypoglycemic activity for a short duration and activity on glucose tolerance test, were observed in normal guinea pigs caused by a quaternary base isolated from this herb. A moderate lowering of blood sugar was also produced in alloxan-diabetic rats[79].

- *Chemical constituents:* (3-amyrin, lupeol, and cucurbitacin B are found in fruits. Aerial parts contain cephalandrol, mp. 81° tritriacontane, p-sitosterol, cephalandrine A and cephalandrine B. Stigmost-7-en-3-one mp. 154° isolated from roots.

34. *Cryptostegia grandiflora R.Br.(Asclepiadaceae)*

- *Common names:* Mar: Vilayati vakhandi: Tarn: Palai.

- *Distribution:* Cultivated mostly as a hedge plant in gardens.

- *Parts used:* Aerial parts.

- *Pharmacological activities:* Alcoholic extract of the aerial parts produced significant hypoglycemic effect on normal rabbits but no reduction of blood sugar was occurred in alloxan diabetic rabbits. It was hepato-toxic[80].

35. *Cyamopsis tetragonoloba Linn. Taub. (Fabaceae)*

- *Common names:* Eng: Cluster Bean, Hindi: Gowar; Tam: Kothaveray.

- *Distribution:* It is found from the plains of the Himalayas southward to W. Peninsula. Widely cultivated, pods used as vegetable.

- *Parts used:* Seeds.

- *Pharmacological activities:* Significant reduction of blood sugar levels were observed in diabetic and non-diabetic adults after taking meals containing seed gum[84].

- Blood glucose levels were remained unaltered with gum and the post prandial blood glucose curve was flattened[86].

- Excretion of glucose through urine decreased significant in diabetic patients[82].

- The rise of blood glucose level reduced significantly after taking meal containing seed gum[85].

- No significant difference was found between the mean blood sugar levels of healthy volunteers after ingestion of gelled or non-gelled seed gum[81].

- An insignificant effect on post-prandial glucose level was observed in human beings after ingestion of seed gum (guar gum)[83].

36. *Cynara scolymus Linn.* (Asteraceae)

- *Common names:* Eng: Burr Artichoke, Hindi & Beng: Hathichoke.

- *Distribution:* Cultivated to a limited extend throughout India. Young flower heads are eaten as a vegetable. Leaves are bitter.

- *Parts used:* Whole plant.

- *Pharmacological activities:* Flower head produced no hypoglycemic effect on normal rabbits[86]. Hypoglycemic activity was observed when a dialyzed extract of the artichoke was injected into rabbits[87].

- *Chemical constituents:* Leaves contain cynarin mp. 235°, cynaropicrin, cynarolide mp. 126°, Caffeic acid, 7-|3-rutinoside, 1, -3,-4,-5 caffeoyl, luteolin-7-p-D-glucoside, and cynarotrioside, mp. 274°. Cynarogenin, taraxasterol, stigmasterol and p-sitosterol are obtained from receptacles.

37. *Caucus carota Linn.* (Apiaceae)

- *Common names:* Eng: Carrot, Hindi: Gajar, Beng.: Gajar.

- *Distribution:* The carrot is cultivated throughout the greater part of India. Roots are edible.

- *Parts used:* Roots.

- *Pharmacological activities:* Marked lowering of blood sugar was produced without any toxicity, by an amorphous yellow coloured fraction of petroleum ether extract of the dried tuberous roots, in human beings, rabbits and dogs[88].

- *Chemical constituents:* See Antifertility chapter.

38. *Dolichos biftorous Linn.* **(Leguminosae)**

- *Common names:* Eng: Horse Gram, Hindi: Kulthi; Berg: Kurtikalai.

- *Distribution:* It is found throughout the greater part of India. An important crop-plant in southwards Maharashtra.

- *Parts used:* Seeds.

- *Pharmacological activities:* Hypoglycemic as well as hypocholesterotemic effects were caused when seed diet was fed to normal rats[89].

39. *Dolichos lablab Linn.* **(Fabaceae)**

- *Common names:* Eng: Indian Butter Bean, Lablab Bean, Hindi: Sem, Beng: shim.

- *Distribution:* A climbing herb, cultivated throughout India. Pods are eaten as vegetable. Seeds are also used as food.

- *Parts used:* Pods.

- *Pharmacological activities:* Reduction of fasting blood sugar level in alloxan diabetic rats, as well as antagonism of the adrenaline induced hyperglycemic response were produced by the green pods[90].

- Hyperglycemic effect due to the administration of dextrose with adrenaline, fasting blood sugar level were reduced in experimental animals, by the green pods. Green pods diet also exhibited antiglycosuria, antiacetonuria and antiacetonemia activities in diabetic patients[90].

- *Chemical constituents:* L-Pipecolic acid was obtained from pods.

40. *Embtica officinalis Gaertn.* **(Euphorbiaceae)**

- *Common names:* Eng: Emblic Myrobalan, Hindi: Amla, amlika, Beng: Dhatri, amlaki.

- *Distribution:* A small or medium sized tree, found throughout tropical part of India, ascending up to 1300m, cultivated in gardens and home yards.

- *Parts used:* Seeds.

- *Pharmacological activities:* Infusion of seeds is used in diabetes[91].

- *Chemical constituents:* In addition, with vitamin C fruits contain corilagin, ellagic acid, and Trigalloyl glucose.

41. *Enicostemma tittorale Blume.* **(Gentianaceae)**

- *Common names:* Hindi: Chola-chirayata.

- *Distribution:* It is found throughout India flowers are white in auxillary cluster.

- *Parts used:* Whole plants.

- *Pharmacological activities:* 'Tribang shila"- composite drug, contains E littorale extract, inhibited significantly the hyperglycemic activity of anterior pituitary extract in rats[92]. Fresh juice of whole plant exhibited lowering of fasting blood sugar level in diabetic patients without any toxic effect[93]. Oral application "Tribang shila" prevented the loss in body weight in rats caused by the prolonged application of anterior pituitary extract[94].

- *Chemical constituents:* It contain gentiocrucine, a mixture of three compounds and a monoterpene alkaloid-enicoflavine.

42. *Ensete superbum (Roxb) Cheesman Syn. Musa superba Roxb.* **(Musaceae)**

- *Common names:* Mar: Chowani.

- *Distribution:* Distributed from Bombay to Western Ghats to Travancore hills and ravine slopes and in Assam.

- *Parts used:* Seeds.

- *Pharmacological activities:* Hypoglycemic action was produced in experimental animals without any harmful effect by a fraction of seed extract[95].

- *Chemical constituents:* In the seeds three constituents were detected.

43. *Eriodendron anfractuodum DC.*

Syn. Ceapenfandra(Linn) Goertn. (Bombacaceae)

- *Common names:* Eng: Kapok Tree, White Silk Cotton Tree, Hindi: Safedsimul, Beng: Safet shimul.

- *Distribution:* The tree is found in the hotter parts of India, Srilanka etc.

- *Parts used:* Seeds.

- *Pharmacological activities:* Extract used in diabetes[96].
- *Chemical constituents:* Seeds contain fixed which is triglycerides of palmitic, linoleic, and oleic acids. Gum produce by tree contains gallic and tannic acids.

44. *Erythrina indica Lam.* (Fabaceae)

- *Common names:* Eng: Indian coral tree, Hindi: Dadap, Beng: Palita-mandar, Palidhar.
- *Distribution:* A common tree of Bengal, Southern India and many other parts of India, generally planted for shade and support.
- *Parts used:* Root bark.
- *Pharmacological activities:* A decoction of the root bark with a dose of 'vasanta Kusumaker' Rasa is said to reduce the quality as well as sugar of usine on an application on every morning in diabetes cases[97].
- *Chemical constituents:* Bark contains (i-sitosterol, y-sitosterol, mp.148°, S-sitosterol, m.p. 147°, docosyl alcohol and three other substances having m.p. 135°, 126° and 142°.

45. *Eucalyptus citriodora Hook.* (Myrtaceae)

- *Distribution:* It is an aromatic evergreen tree. Grown at North India, Kerala and Nilgin. Leaves yield essential oil.
- *Parts used:* Leaves.
- *Pharmacological activities:* Leaves extract, on oral administration, caused lowering of blood sugar in normal and alloxan-diabetic rabbits and it also flattened the blood sugar curve in glucose tolerance test, action is considered due to myrtillin in extract[98].
- *Chemical constituents:* Citronellal, citronellol, and p-pinene, p-cymene, citronellyl acetate, eucalytin, geraniol isolulegol, linalool, cineole and many other essential oils were detected in leaves.

46. *Ficus bengalensis Linn.* (Moraceae)

- *Common names:* Eng: Banyan Tree, Hindi: Bar, bargad, Beng: Bot, Bar.

- *Distribution:* The banyan tree is a large branching tree with numerous aerial roots occurring all over the plain part of India. Planted for shade.

- *Pharmacological activities:* Hypoglycemic activity was observed in normal and moderately diabetic rabbits produced by the bengaranoside isolated from the bark[104]. Ethanolic extract of bark exhibited hypoglycemic activity in rabbits[103]. Flavonoids A, B & C from bark produced hypoglycemic effect in normal rabbits[102]. No appreciable difference in blood sugar levels was caused in diabetic rabbits by the decoction of bark[101]. Hypoglycemic action was produced by the ethanolic extract of bark in normal male albino rats[100]. Aqueous extract of the bark caused no significant hypoglycemic action on normal fasting rabbits but produced moderate lowering of fasting blood sugar levels in alloxan diabetic rabbits[105,106]. Shilajit and milky sap from the plant produced initial lowering of blood sugar in anterior pituitary extract treated albino rats[107,108].

- Bark extract delayed glucose absorption significantly in mice but without any toxicity, on oral application[109,110]. Hypoglycemic activity was observed only in few cases of human beings on application of aqueous extract of bark[111]. Hypoglycemic activity was produced in rats by the glycosidal fraction, from the aqueous extract of bark[112]. Aqueous extract of bark exhibited hypoglycemic effect in normal and diabetic patients[113]. Aqueous extract of the bark showed hypoglycemic effect in normal and alloxan rabbits[114].

- *Chemical constituents:* Quercetin-3-galac-to side, rutin, friedelin and (3-sitosterol were isolated from leaves, and taraxasterol tiglate from east wood. Stem bark contains three methyl ethers of leucoanthocyanins-delphinide-3-0-a-L-rhamnoside, pelargonidin-3-0-a-L-rhamnosideand leuco-cyanidin -3-0- (J-D-gallactosyl cellobioside and methyl ether of leucoanthocyanidin.

47. *Ficus racemosa Linn.*

Syn. *F. glomerata* Roxb. (Moraceae).

- ***Common names:*** Eng: Cluster Fig, Country Fig, Hindi: Gular; Beng: Jagyadumur.

- ***Distribution:*** A large deciduous tree distributed throughout India, particularly in evergreen forests, moist localities. It is cultivated in village for shade and edible fruits.

- ***Parts used:*** Bark and stem bark.

- ***Pharmacological activities:*** Stem bark caused hypoglycemic activity in albino rats[116]. Bark exhibited hypoglycemic effect in normal rabbits[115]. Aqueous decoction of the bark produced no effect on blood sugar levels of rabbits[117].

- ***Chemical constituents:*** Leaf contains glycoside and bark contains tannin.

48. *Ficus religiosa Linn.* (Moraceae)

- ***Common names:*** Eng: Pipal Tree, Hindi: Pipli, pipal; Beng: Ashathwa.

- ***Distribution:*** A large perennial tree, mostly planted as roadside tree particularly near temples. It is found all over the plains of India.

- ***Parts used:*** Bark and roots.

- ***Pharmacological activities:*** Bark contains tannin used in skin troubles. Aqueous extract of bark produced hypoglycemic activity in rabbits[118]. Water extract of root bark exhibited hypoglycemic effect in rabbits[119]. Sitosterol glucoside of bark decreased blood sugar level of rabbits[120]. No effect was produced on the blood sugar level of rabbits by the aqueous decoction of bark[121].

- ***Chemical constituents:*** Bark contains tannins, p-sitosterol-D-glucoside was isolated.

49. *Glycyne max Merrill.*

Syn. G. soya Sieb. & Zuce. (Fabaceae)

- ***Common names:*** Eng: Soyabean, Soya, Hindi: Bhat, bhatwar, Beng: Garjkalai.

- *Distribution:* Soya bean is a suberect herbs, cultivated mainly in Punjab, Himachal Pradesh, Kashmir, Bengal, Bihar and Assam, seeds are used as a pulse.

- *Parts used:* Seeds.

- *Pharmacological activities:* Seeds produced hypoglycemic activity in normal albino rats[122].

- *Chemical constituents:* Roots contain flavonoid daidzein and on isoflavone glycoside. Genistin and two galactomannans were isolated from soya bean hulls.

50. *Gymnema sylvestre R.Br.* (Asclepiadaceae)

- *Common names:* Hindi: Gur-mar, merasinge; Beng.: Merasingi.

- *Distribution:* A woody climber, distributed at peninsular India. Flowers are minute greenish-yellow in colour, orange spirally in lateral corymbs. Leaves when chewed paralyses the sense of taste for sweet and bitter substance for few hours.

- *Parts used:* Leaves.

- *Pharmacological activities:* Alcoholic extract of leaves produced hypoglycemic effect in mild diabetic animals[123]. An insignificant reduction of blood sugar was occurred in normal rats but significant and marked hypoglycemic effect was observed in hyperglycemic animals caused by the alcoholic extract of leaves[124,125,126,127]. Leaf extract produced hypoglycemic activity in rabbits, on oral administration and in vitro also[128].

- No effect on blood sugar was observed in rabbits caused by the leaves extract, gymnemic acid and sodium salt of gymnemic acid[129]. Aqueous and alcoholic extract of leaves, on oral administration, produced hypoglycemic activity in normal human, dogs and diabetic dogs[130]. Whole plant exhibited hypoglycemic effect on rabbits[131]. Powder and decoction of leaves prevented loss of sugar through urirv in human beings[132].

- Hypoglycemic effect was caused in normal and diabetic rabbits and albino rats by the aqueous extract of leaves on oral application[133]. Leaves and stems parts showed hypoglycemic activity in diabetic human beings but without any toxicity[134]. Aqueous infusion of leaves caused glucose tolerance in albino rats[135].

- Prevention of the loss in body weight in rats caused by the prolonged administration of anterior pituitary extract as well as an increase the glucose tolerance was caused by the alcoholic extract of leaves[136,137,138]. Leaf powder produced hypoglycemic activity in normal and diabetic subjects of age group of 43 to 68 years[139].

- *Chemical constituents:* Triterpene-gymnestrogenin and gymnemagenin were detected in leaves. Beside these leaves contain anti-saccharin principle, gymnemic acid, characterised as hexahydroxy-olean-12-ene-p-glucuronide m.p. 328° and from the hydrocarbon fraction of the leaf extract triacontane and hentriacontane were isolated.

51. *Helicter esisora Linn.* (Sterculiaceae)

- *Common names:* Eng: East Indian screw tree, Hindi: Marori, Marophali, Beng: Atmora.

- *Distribution:* A shrub, found at the Central Peninsula, Central and Western India to Jammu.

- *Parts used:* Root bark.

- *Pharmacological activities:* Juice of root bark or decoction of root bark is applied in diabetes to reduce sugar[140].

- *Chemical constituents:* An orange-yellow coloured crystalline matter, a hedroxy-carboxylic acid (m.p. 178-79"), saponin, phlobotannins, sugar and phytosterol were detected in bark.

52. *Hordeum vulgare Linn.*

Syn. *H. sativum* Jessen (Gramineae)

- *Common names:* Eng: Barley, Hindi: Jau, jav; Beng: Jab.

- *Distribution:* An erect herb. It is cultivated in North-India, Madhya-Pradesh, West-Bengal and Bihar as a food-crop. Barley grain is easily assimilable.

- *Parts used:* Roots.

- *Pharmacological activities:* Hypoglycemic action was exhibited in rabbits by the water-soluble fraction of fermented rootlets of barley[141].

- *Chemical constituents:* Two flavour glycosides orientin and orientoside and a luteolin glycoside were isolated. An arabinogalacto-(4-0-methylglucurone) xylan was isolated from leaves.

53. *Indigofera arecta Hochst.* (Leguminosae)

- *Common names:* Bengal Indigo.

- *Distribution:* A shrub, yield a dye-indigo, principal indigo producing plant of Ethiopia.

- *Parts used:* Whole plant.

- *Pharmacological activities:* The plant extract reduced plasma glucose levels of normal fasting rats, and also increased plasma insulin levels[142].

- *Chemical constituents:* A flavonol glycoside - kaempferitrin (m.p. 201 -03°) was isolated from leaves. Kaempferitrin on hydrolysis gives rhamnose and kaempferol. Beside this the plant contain indigotin (approx.)

54. *Ipomoea nil (Linn) Roth. / hederacea auct. non Jacq.* (Convolvulaceae)

- *Common names:* Hindi: Kaladana, Beng: Hilkalmi, kaladanah.

- *Distribution:* It is a showy plant and found throughout India.

- *Parts used:* Whole plant.

- *Pharmacological activities:* Extracts reduced blood sugar levels in rats[143].

- *Chemical constituents:* Arachidic, stearic palmitic, oleic, linoienic and linoleic acids are obtained from seed oil. Seeds also contain chanoclavine, lysergol, xylose, arabinose and galactose.

55. *Kickxia ramosissima (Wall) Janchen*

Syn. L/nariaramos/ss/maWall (Scrophulariaceae)

- *Common names:* Guj: Kanodi, bhintgalodi.

- *Distribution:* A perennial herbs, found throughout India, on walls, rocky and stony places. Leaves are membranous, and flowers are yellow.

- *Parts used:* Aerial part.

- *Pharmacological activities:* Used in diabetes[144]. Hot water extract of the whole aerial parts had hypoglycemic activity in rabbits[145].

56. *Lagerstroemia speciosa Pers. L flosreginae Retz. (Lythraceae)*

- *Common names:* Eng: Queen Crape Myrtle, Hindi: Jarul, Beng: Jarul.

- *Distribution:* Found from Assam, south wards to Peninsular India. Planted in gardens for ornament. Wood is used to a limited extent for furniture, casts, wheels and boxes.

- *Parts used:* Leaves and fruits.

- *Pharmacological activities:* Leaves and ripe fruits produced hypoglycemic activity on oral administration[146].

- *Chemical constituents:* Alanine, methionine, a-aminobutyric acid and isoleucine were detected. Leaves contain 3, 3', 4-tri-O-methylellagic acid, lageracetal, 3-0-methylellagic acid, ellagic acid amyl alcohol, (3-sitosterol and tannin-lagertannin characterised as 3, 4-di-0-methl-4'-0- (3-D-glycosylellagic acid.

57. *Lupinus albus Linn.* (Leguminosac)

- *Common names:* Eng: White Lupine, Hindi: Turmas, Beng: Turmur.

- *Distribution:* An erect annual herb with white flower. Grown in gardens. Seeds are used as food also as cattle feed after soaking in water for removing toxic alkaloids.

- *Parts used:* Seeds.

- *Pharmacological activities:* A fraction of seed extract caused lowering of blood sugar level in rabbits[147].

- *Chemical constituents:* Lupanine, spartein and hydroxy-lupanine were detected in various parts of the plant. Seedlings and stems are rich source of asparagine. Seeds yield fatly oil. Tiglic, cinnamic and benzoic acid esters of acyloxylupanines and alkaloid angustifoline were isolated from seeds.

58. *Mangifera indica Linn.* (Anacardiaceae)

- *Common names:* Eng: Mango, Hindi: Am, Amb, Beng: Am.

- *Distribution:* A tree, indigenous to India, cultivated widely in many varieties in the plain parts of India for its edible fruits.

- *Pharmacological activities:* Dried powder of tender leaves is useful in diabetes[148].

- *Chemical constituents:* Mangiferolic acid, m.p. 181°, hydroxymangiferolic acid, isomangiferolic acid, hydroxy mangiferonic acid m.p. 190°, ambolic acid, ambonic acid, amyrin, lupeol, acetates of cyloartanol, homomangiferin, mangiferin, m.p. 278°, protocatechuic acid, friedelin, (3-sitosterol, catechin, ellagic acid, gallic acid, m-digallic acid, m-trigallic acid, galotanin, quercetin, leucocyanidin, desetin and butin were isolated. In leaves galactose, glucose, arabinose rhamnose, xylose, tannin, two phenolic compounds and two flavonoids were detected. From resin triterpenes-oleanolic aldehyde, m.p. 168°, a diol m.p. 154°, and an aldehyde, m.p. 166° were isolated and in unripe fruits, a polysaccharide, glucan was *detected.*

59. *Momordica charantia Linn.* (Cucurbitaceae)

- *Common names:* Eng: Bitter Gourd, Hindi: Karela, Beng: Karela.

- *Distribution:* A climbing herb, found throughout India. Often cultivated for fruits, which are used as vegetable.

- *Parts used:* Fruits.

- *Pharmacological activities:* Fresh juice of fruit produced significant hypoglycemic effect in experimental animals[149,150]. "Plant Insulin", the hypoglycemic principle which exhibited a consistent hypoglycemic activity in diabetes mellitus patients was isolated from fruits[151]. Aqueous extract of fruits suppressed the hyperglycemia in albino rats[152]. Fruits produced hypoglycemic activity in alloxan-diabetic rabbits[153].

- Tablets, prepared from the powder of fruits, or the fresh juice of fruits caused significant lowering of blood sugar levels in patients[154,155]. On oral administration of fruit juice showed hypoglycemic effect in normal as well as diabetic rabbits. But toxicity was observed, in the animals[156]. No glycosuria was observed in a diabetic patient, taken fruits along with chlorpropamide[157].

- Fruit juice and the dried extract fruits caused mild hypoglycemic effect in diabetic rabbits[158,159]. Unripe fruits showed hypoglycemic action in rabbits[160]. A non-nitrogenous substance charantin, produced hypoglycemic activity in fasting rabbits was isolated from unripe fruits[161]. No hypoglycemic effect was produced in rabbits only by the fruit extract alone, rather fruit extract potentiatesed the hypoglycemic effects of tolbutamide and Jasadohasma[162].

- Seeds contain a glyco-alkaloid vicine, characterized as 2,6-diaminopyrimidinol-5-beta-D-glucopyranoside, showed hypoglycemic activity in fasting albino rats[163]. No hypoglycemic activity was produced in diabetic and normal human beings by the alcoholic extract of the drug[164].

- Marked hypoglycemic effects were exhibited both by a crude crystalline substance and an infusion of the crude, drug. The drug showed toxicity in fish, rats and rabbits[165,166].

- *Chemical constituents:* Fruits contain stigmast-5, 25-diene-3p-0-glucoside, p-sitosterol glucoside, and a hypoglycemic substance-charantin mp. 266°. A glycoalkaloid- vicine, was obtained from *seeds.*

60. *Moms alba Linn.* (Moraceae).

- *Common names:* Eng: White Mulberry, Hindi: Tut, Beng: Toot.

- *Distribution:* Cultivated throughout the plain parts of India. Parts used: Leaves.

- *Pharmacological activities:* Leaves produced antidiabetic activity in diabetic animals[167]. Marked hypoglycemic effect in normal and hyperglycemic subjects wac caused by the leaves extract[168].

- *Chemical constituents:* See Antifertility chapter.

61. *Mucuna prurita Hook.*

Syn. M.pruriens Baker.(Leguminosae).

- *Common names:* Eng: Common Cowitch, Hindi: Kiwach, Beng: Alkushi.

- *Distribution:* Found almost throughout India. The fine bristles on the pods caused very intense irritation, which sometimes last for several hours. Flowers are purple in axillary pendulous racemes.

- *Parts used:* Seeds and Fruits.

- *Pharmacological activities:* Seeds produced hypo-glycemic activity in normal albino rats[169]. Fruits also caused hypoglycemic effect in albino rats[170]. Chemical constituents: Indole alkylamines.

62. *Murraya koenigii (Linn.) spreng* (Rutaceae)

- *Common names:* Eng: Curry Leaf Tree, Hindi: Kurry patta, gandhela, mitha neem, Beng: Kariaphulli.

- *Distribution:* It is a small tree, found almost throughout India. It is cultivated also for its aromatic leaves used as flavouring agent of curries and chutneys. Parts used: Leaves.

- *Pharmacological activities:* Aqueous extract of leaves, on oral administration showed hypoglycemic activity in normal and alloxan-diabetic dogs[171].

- *Chemical constituents:* Leaves and fruits contain alkaloids koenimbine, mp. 194°, mahanimbine, mp. 94° and koenigicine, mp 224°. Moreover, leaves contain mahanimbidine, cyclomaha nimbine curryangine and curryanine. Marrayanine, mp. 168° mukoeic acid, mp. 242° and girinimbine, mp. 176° were obtained from bark.

63. *Musa sapientum Linn.*

Syn. *M. paradisiaca* Linn. (Musaceae)

- *Common names:* Eng: Edible Banana, Hindi: Kela, Beng: Kala. Distribution: It is native in India and cultivated for its fruits. Parts used: Flowers.

- *Pharmacological activities:* Flowers produced hypoglycemic activity in rabbits[173]. Maximum degree of hypoglycemic activity was caused in normal rabbits by the chloroform extractive fraction, of flowers[174]. Significant hypoglycemic effect was produced both in normal as well as alloxan diabetic rats by the pectine, isolated from the juice of the inflorescence stalk of plantain[172].

- *Chemical constituents:* See Anti-ulcer chapter.

64. *Nigella saliva Linn.* (Ranunculaceae)

- *Common names:* Eng: Small Fennel, Hindi: Kalajira, Kalaunji, Beng: Kalajira.

- *Distribution:* A small herb of 40-60cm high, cultivated in the Punjab, Bengal, Himachal Pradesh, Bihar and Assam. Seeds used as flavouring, carminative, and stimulant agents.

- *Pharmacological activities:* Volatile oil of seeds produced significant hypoglycemic effects in fasting normal and alloxan diabetic rabbits[175]. Chemical constituents: Seeds contain essential oil, Nifellone was isolated from essential oil. Seed oil contains stigmasterol, cholesterol, a-spinasterol, campesterol and p-stitosterol.

65. *Nymphaea nouchale Burm.f.*

Syn. *N. lotus* Hook. f. & Thorns. (Nymphaeaceae)

- *Common names:* Eng: Indian Red Water-Lily, Hindi: Koka, kanval, Beng: Shaluk.

- *Distribution:* An aquatic herb, common through the hotter parts of India. Flowering stalks used as vegetable, starchy rhizomes eaten raw or boiled.

- *Parts used:* Roots.

- *Pharmacological activities:* Rhizomes are used in dyspepsia, dysentery and diabetes. Roots exerted hypoglycemic activity in rabbits[173].

- *Chemical constituents:* Roots contains tannic, gallic acid, gum and starch.

66. *Ocimum sanctum Linn.* (Lamiaceae)

- *Common names:* Holy Basil, Hindi: Tulsi, kala tulsi, Beng: Tulsi.

- *Distribution:* A strongly scented shrub. It is cultivated throughout India, and also considered a sacred plant to the

Hindu. This plant is of two types, one is purple type, called krishna tulsi, and another is green type called Sri tulsi.

- *Parts used:* Leaves.

- *Pharmacological activities:* Leaves are used as stimulant, expectorant and used in bronchitis. The essential oil of leaves has antibacterial property. Hypoglycemic activity was produced by the aqueous decoction of whole plant[176].

- *Chemical constituents:* See Hepatoprotective chapters.

67. *Olea europaea Linn.* **(Oleaceae)**

- *Common name:* Eng: Common Olive.

- *Distribution:* An evergreen tree, grown in Northern India and elsewhere. Both green and ripe fruits are edible. Mature fruits yield the fixed oil, know Olive oil. The plant is native of Mediterranean region.

- *Parts used:* Seeds and Leaves.

- *Pharmacological activities:* Hypoglycemic effect was produced in normal human beings by Olive oil[177]. Hydro-alcoholic extract of leaves lowered blood sugar level in rabbits[178].

- *Chemical constituents:* Root bark contains, oleuropeic acid, theaglycone of 6-0-leuropeoyl sucrose, characterised as [4-(1-hydroxyisopropyl)-1-cyclohexene-1-carboxylic acid]. A triterpenic acid, m.p. 240° was isolated from olive cakes. Fruits, when just ripe contain oil.

68. *Orchis mascula Linn.* **(Orchidaceae)**

- *Common names:* Eng: Salep Orchio, Hindi: Salap, Beng: Salabmisri.

- *Distribution:* Tuberous roots, found at Western Himalayas. It is indigenous to Afghanistan and was imported to many places in India. Tuberous roots are used in medicine and it yields a large quality of mucilage with water and form a jelly.

- *Pharmacological activities:* It is given in chronic diarrhoea, dysentery and diabetes[179].

- *Chemical constituents:* Tuber contain starch, mucilage, glucoside, trace volatile oil, sugar, a bitter substance and albumen.

69. *Orthosiphon spiralis Merill.*

Syn. *0. stamineus* Benth. (Lamiaceae)

- *Common names:* Eng: Kidney Tea Plant.
- *Distribution:* An herb, found at southern India, Madhya Pradesh, and Assam.
- *Parts used:* Leaves.
- *Pharmacological activities:* Leaf extract reduced the blood sugar levels in diabetic patients but not consistently[180,181].
- *Chemical constituents:* Leaves contain tannin, essential oil and potassium salts. 4',5,6,7-tetramethoxyflavone, 5-hydroxy-6,7,3',4'-tetramethoxyflavone and isosinensetin were isolated.

70. *Pinus roxburghii Sarg.*

Syn. *P. longifolia* Roxb. (Pinaceae)

- *Common names:* Eng: Chir Pine, Hindi: Chir. Sans.: Sarala.
- *Distribution:* An evergreen resinous tree, found at outer Himalayan ranges. Oleoresin, obtained from stem, yields turpentine oil.
- *Parts used:* Barks and roots.
- *Pharmacological activities:* Bark and roots produced hypoglycemic activity in rabbits[173].
- *Chemical constituents:* Longicyclene, dl-longifolene, Swedish turpentine olingipinene and isopimaric acid were isolated. p-Sitosterol, friedelin and ceryl alcohol were isolated from bark.

71. *Portulaca oleracea Linn.* **(Portulacaceae).**

- *Common names:* Eng: Common Purslane, Hindi: Launinonia, Beng: Baraloniya.
- *Distribution:* An herb, usually succulent, flowers are terminal, surrounded by a whorl of leaves. It is found throughout India and used as a vegetable.
- *Parts used:* Whole plant.

- *Pharmacological activities:* Oral administration showed lowering of blood sugar in alloxan-diabetic rabbits[182].

- *Chemical constituents:* 4-(2-amino ethyl) pyrocatechol, catechol, noradrenaline, and 3-(3,4-dihydroxyphenyl) alanine were detected.

72. *Prunus persica Batsch.* (Rosaceae)

- *Common names:* Eng: Peach, Hindi: Shaftalu, Aru.

- *Distribution:* It is cultivated mainly in Northern India. Fruits are edible.

- *Parts used:* Leaves.

- *Pharmacological activities:* Leaves produced hypoglycemic activity in rabbits and dogs[183].

- *Chemical constituents:* Aromadendrin, naringenin, 5,3'-dyhydroxy− 7,4'-dimethoxyflavanone, m.p. 163 degrees, were isolated from bark. Leaves and flowers contain kaempferol and kaempferol-3-galactoside respectively 3, 4', 5-trihydroxyflavanone-7-p-D-glucopyranoside, taxifolin-7-glucoside, 6-0-(p-glucuronopyranosyl)-D-galactose, 2-0-(p-glucuronopyranosyl)-D-mannose, galactose, xylose, and rhamnose were detected in gum.

73. *Pterocarpus marsupium Roxb.* (Leguminose)

- *Common names:* Eng: Indian Kind Tree, Hindi: Bija, Beng: Piyasala, Pitshal.

- *Distribution:* A tree of moderate to large size, up to 25 to 30 metre high. It is found mostly at Madhya Pradesh, Orissa, Bihar, and Gujrat. The tree yields a gum-resin known a kino.

- *Parts used:* Bark and wood.

- *Pharmacological activities:* (-) Epicatechin, an active principle of the water extract of bark increased insulin release in rats[184]. Lowering of blood sugar was caused dogs by the pterostilbene, a constituent of wood[185]. Hypoglycemic effects were produced in rabbits by the alcoholic as well as aqueous extract of the heart wood[186].

- Aqueous extract of wood resisted glucose absorption in mice[187]. Aqueous extract of the drug produced hypogly-cemic effect in rabbits[188]. No affect was exerted on the blood sugar of alloxan-rabbits and rats by the extract of wood[189]. Significant hypoglycemic effect with increase glucose tolerance were caused in rabbits by the alcoholic extract of the drug[190].

- Lowering in the blood sugar levels in diabetic human beings as well as increase glucose tolerence, without any side effect, were occurred by the decoction of the bark[191]. An aqueous infusion of wood increased glucose tolerence in rats[192]. Bark powder lowered the blood sugar levels in diabetes mellitus[193].

- Hypoglycemic activity was produced in alloxan-diabetic rats by the decoction of the bark[194]. Induced hyperglycemia was prevented in rats by aqueous infusion of wood[195]. Reduction in urine sugar but without any effect on blood sugar levels of diabetic patients were caused by the aqueous extract of heart wood[196].

- *Chemical constituents:* The main constituents are alkaloid and resin.

74. *Punica granatum Linn.* (Punicaceae)

- *Common names:* Eng: Pomegranate, Hindi: Anar, Beng: Dalim.

- *Distribution:* Small tree, generally cultivated throughout India. Fleshy test is edible. Bark and fruit shells are used for tanning.

- *Parts used:* Fruit rind.

- *Pharmacological activities:* Rind extract exhibited hypoglycemic effect in mild diabetic albino rats[197].

- *Chemical constituents:* See Anti-ferlity chapter.

75. *Quercus infectoria Olivier.* (Fagaceae)

- *Common names:* Eng: Gall Oak, Hindi: Muphal, majuphal, Beng: Majuphal.

- *Parts used:* Galls.

- *Pharmacological activities:* Hypoglycemic action was produced in rabbits by a fraction of gall extract[198].

- *Chemical constituents:* Ellagic acid, gallic acid, stitosterol, methyl oleanolate, methyl betulate and syringic acid were isolated from galls.

76. *Quercus lancaefolia Roxb.* **(Fagaceae)**

- *Common names:* Assam: Bucklai, Nepal: Patlekatus.
- *Distribution:* It is found at Manipur, Khasi Hills, Sikkim, Bhutan and at the Himalayas at an altitude of 300-600 metre.
- *Parts used:* Stem bark.
- *Pharmacological activities:* A significant hypoglycemic activity was exhibited in albino rats by the stem bark extract[199].
- *Chemical constituents:* Bark, leaves and wood contain tannin, Ferulic acid, Canophyllal, canophyllol, friedelin maslinic acid, lignoceryl ferulate and lignoceryl alcohol were isolated.

77. *Rauvolfia serpentina Benth. ex. Kurz.* **(Apocynaceae)**

- *Common names:* Eng: Serpentina root, Hindi: Chola-chand; Beng: Sarpa-gandha chandra.
- *Distribution:* A small shrub found from the Himalayas southwards to Peninsular India.
- *Parts used:* Roots.
- *Pharmacological activities:* Reserpine stimulated the hypoglycemic effect of insulin as well as the hyperglycemic effect of adrenalin also in normal subjects. Both the total extracts and reserpine suppressed the physiological hyperglycemic activities in diabetic patients[200].
- Both the blood glucose and urine glucose were reduced in diabetic patients by the extracts[201]. Moreover, the extracts also caused a sufficient reduction blood sugar levels of cats[202,203].
- *Chemical constituents:* See Anti-fertility chapter.

78. *Ricinus communis Linn.* **(Euphorbiaceae)**

- *Common names:* Eng: Castor seed, Hindi: Erandi; Beng: Bheranda.
- *Distribution:* A small tree cultivated chiefly in Andhra Pradesh, Maharastra, Karnataka and Orissa. It is also found as wild.
- *Parts used:* Roots.
- *Pharmacological activities:* Root extracts produced significant hypoglycemic activity in albino rats[199].

- *Chemical constituents:* Stearic, palmitic, ricinoleic, arachidic, linoienic linoleic, and oleic acid in castor oil as well as lupeol and 30-norlupan -3p-OI-20-one in castor bean were detected.

79. *Rivea cuneata Wight.* (Convolvulaceae)

Syn. *Argyreia cuneata* Ker-Gawl (Convolvulaceae)

- *Parts used:* Leaves.

- *Pharmacological activities:* Leaves are used in diabetes, Pulverized leaves produced a gradual fall is fasting blood. Sugar in rabbits, but oral administration showed little effect on fasting blood sugar in human beings[205]. Significant hypoglycemic activity was caused by the alcoholic extracts of leaves in diabetic rats[206]. Leaves did not produce any significant hypoglycemic activity in diabetic rabbits and rats[207].

- *Chemical constituents:* Leaves *contain glycoside.*

80. *Rourea santaloides W. & A.* (Conoraceae)

Syn. R. Minor (Gaerin.) Alston (Connaraceae)

- *Common names:* Man: Wakeri, Bom: Vardara, Beng.: Vidhadaki.

- *Parts used:* Roots.

- *Pharmacological activities:* Root is used as a bitter tonic in pulmonary complaints, scurvy rheumatism and diabetes[208].

81. *Salacia macrosperma Wight* (Hippocrateaceae)

- *Common names:* Mar: Lendphal, Mai: Anakoranti.

- *Distribution:* Small tree, flowers are small, Fruits are edible and sweet, found at Konkan and Southwards in Western Ghats.

- *Parts used:* Leaves and roots.

- *Pharmacological activities:* Leaves and roots produced significant hypoglycemic effect in rabbits[209].

- *Chemical constituents:* Salacia quinonemethide, tingenone, hydroxytingenone, pristimerin and three quinones-saptarangi quinones A, B & C were isolated from root bark. A triterpene - salaspermic acid was also isolated.

82. *Saussurea lappa C.B. Clarke* (Compositae)

- *Common names:* Eng: Kuth, Hindi: Kur, kutha, Beng: Kur.
- *Distribution:* A tall, perennial herb, found in Kashmir, and North-West Himalayas at an attitude about 2000 to 3000 metre. Flowers are purple.
- *Parts used:* Roots.
- *Pharmacological activities:* Alcoholic extract of roots showed a significant hypoglycemic response without any increase in plasma insulin in albino rats for a treatment of 7 days[210].
- *Chemical constituents:* Leaves contain taraxasterol, m.p. 222° and taraxasteryl acetate, m.p. 246°, plant contain alkaloids, resins essential oil, 22,23-dihydrostigmasterol and costol. Roots contain an essential oil, a glycoside and an alkaloid saussurine.

83. *Scoparia dulcis Linn.* (Scrophulariaceae)

- *Common names:* Eng: Sweet Broomweed, Santal: Jastimadhu.
- *Distribution:* An herb, common in India on waste lende. Flowers are small and white, branches are twiggy.
- *Parts used:* Stems and Leaves.
- *Pharmacological activities:* "Amellin", the active principle of leaves and stems decreased the high blood glucose levels, urine glucose and urine volume of diabetic patients to normal[211,212,213].
- On application of fresh leaves with little cold water twice daily for four months to a patient, produced sugarless urine[214]. Partial reduction of urine glucose and urine volume were caused in rats, by the methanol and hexane extracts of leaves and stems[215].
- *Chemical constituents:* Dulcitol, amellin from aerial parts, and mannitol and a triterpene, m.p. 288° from roots were isolated.

84. *Securigera securidaca (Linn) Dall a Torre & Sarntheim* (Fabaceae)

- *Distribution:* Native of some parts of Europe and Mediterranean region. In India, its cultivation at Bihar and West Bengal has been reported.

- *Parts used:* Seeds.

- *Pharmacological activities:* Hyperglycemia occurred significantly in mice after administration of seeds[216]. Aqueous extract of seeds exhibited hypoglycemic activity in anesthetized cats[217].

- *Chemical constituents:* Cardenolides securidaside, m.p. 177°, securigenin, m.p. 234° and securiside, m.p. 192° were isolated from seeds.

85. *Spathodea campanulata Beauv.* **(Bignoniaceae)**

- *Common names:* Eng: African Tulip tree, Hindi: Rugtoora, Tel: Patode.

- *Distribution:* It is an evergreen tree, generally grown for its shade in many places, flowers are large, bell-shaped and of orange scarlet colour.

- *Parts used:* Stem bark.

- *Pharmacological activities:* Decoction of stem bark produced hypoglycemic activity in streptozotocin diabetic mice[218].

- *Chemical constituents:* Quercetin and caffeic acid were isolated from leaves.

86. *Strychnos potatorum Linn.* **(Loganiaceae)**

- *Common names:* Eng: clearing-Nut tree, Hindi: Neimal, Beng: Nirmali. Distribution: This tree is found at Bengal, content and Southern India. Seeds, used for clearing muddy water, contain brucine but no strychnine, are non-poisonous.

- *Parts used:* Seeds.

- *Pharmacological activities:* Seeds are used in gonorrhoea, diarrhoea and diabetes[219].

- *Chemical constituents:* Leaves contain triterpene-isomotiol (fern-8-en-3p-ol), leaves and bark contain mixtures campesterol, stigmasterol and sitosterol, Alkaloid-diabotine, stigmasterol, oleanolic acid, p-acetate, p-sitosterol and saponin containing oleanolic acid, galactose, mannose were isolated from seeds. Beside these 2-hydroxy-4-methoxybenzoic, sinapic, vanillic, chlorogenic and syringic acids, free sugars such as galactose, mannose and quercetin were isolated.

87. *Swertia chirayita* (Roxb. ex. Flem) Karst

Syn. *S. chirata* Buch. Ham ex c.B. Clarke (Gentianaceae)

- *Common names:* Eng: Chirayita, Hindi & Beng: Chirayita.
- *Distribution:* Annual herb, found from temperate Himalayas to the Khasi Hills. Leaves are usually opposite, flower are bluish to whitish. It is used as stomachic and laxative.
- *Pharmacological activities:* Hexane extract showed a significant lowering of blood sugar in albino rats[220].
- *Chemical constituents:* Roots and aerial parts contain 1-hydroxy-3, 7,8-trimethoxyxanthone decussatin, 1-hydroxy-3, 5,8-trimethoxyxanthone, 1,8-dihydroxy-3,'5-demethoxy-xanthone, 1,8-dihydroxy-3, 7-dimethoxyxanthone, 1,5,8-trihydroxy-3-methoxy-xanthone, 1,3,8-trihydroxy-5-methoxyxanthone, 1,3,7,8-tetrahydroxyxantjpme. 1,3,6,7-tetrahydroxyxanthone-C2-p-D-glucose (mangiterin) and 1,3,5,8-tetrahydroxyxanthone. Beside these swerchirin, swerchirin, swertianin, swertinin, (3-sitosterol friedelin and isobellidifolin were isolated.

88. *Syzygium Cuminii Linn.* (Skeels)

Syn. Eugenia jambolana Lam. (Myrtaceae)

- *Common names:* Eng.: Black plum, Jambolan, Hindi: Jam, jambu, Beng.: Kalajam, Jam.
- *Distribution:* A tree, found throughout India mostly cultivated for its edible fruits, seed coat, within which two cotyledons are distinct, loosely adheres with pericarp.
- *Parts used:* Seeds.
- *Pharmacological activities:* Hypoglycemia was caused in the diabetic rats to normal levels by an active principle from powdered seeds[221]. Seed extracts produced hypoglycemic response in albino rats[222]. Fall in fasting blood sugar in experimental animals was caused by the aqueous extract of seeds[58].
- No remarkable difference in blood sugar levels were observed in rabbits produced by seeds[223]. The seeds exhibited its utility in diabetic patients[224]. Active principle from seeds exerted strong hypoglycemia activity in mice[225]. Ethanolic extract of bark showed hypoglycemic effect in hyperglycemic rabbits[167]. Fruits and seeds showed

hypoglycemic response in rabbits[226]. Powder of fresh seeds lowered the blood sugar levels in diabetic animals on oral administration[227].

- Different doses of alcohol and acetone extracts of seeds produced significant hypoglycemic activity in alloxan-diabetes albino rats on long term feeding[228]. Seed extract caused hypoglycemic response in male rabbits[229]. Lowering of the blood sugar in alloxan diabetic rats was produced by ethanolic extract of seeds[230].

- *Chemical constituents:* Ellagic acids, isoquercitrin, quercetin, acetyl oleanolic acid, myricetin, kaempferol and two other triterpenoids were detected in flowers. Seeds contain ellagic, gallic acids, corilagin related ellagitannins, 3-gailoylglucose, 1-galloylglucose, quercetin, 3,6-hexahydroxydiphenoyl glucose and its isomer4,60-hexadroxydiphenoyl glucose, beside these ferulic, gallic, caffeic, ellagic, 3,3',4'-tri-0-methylellagic, and 3,4'-di-0-methylellagic acids were detected in seeds. Friedelin, friedelinol, sitosterol, and its glucose and sucrose were isolated from bark. Hentriacontane, heptacosane, octacosanol, triacontane, crotegolic and betulinoc acid from leaves and deiphinidin-3-gentiobioside and malvidin-3-laminaribioside two anthocyanine from fruits were isolated.

89. *Tecoma stans Linn.* **H.B. & K.**

Syn. B/gnon/asfansLinn. (Bignoniaceae)

- *Common names:* Tel: Pachagolla, Tarn.: Sona-patti.

- *Distribution:* An erect shrub, commonly found in gardens, bear, showy flowers in terminal racemes.

- *Parts used:* Stem.

- *Pharmacological activities:* Aqueous and alcoholic extracts of stem reduced fasting blood sugar in rabbits and rats on oral administration[231]. Significant lowering of the blood sugar was caused in rats by the fresh aqueous extract of stem[232]. Glucose tolerance in rats was suitably influenced by the aqueous decoction and alcoholic extracts of stem. These extracts also caused increase glucose tolerance[233].

- *Chemical constituents:* Leaves contain tecostanine, m.p. 85° and tecomanine (tecomine), beside these 4-noractinidine, Nnormethyl-skytanthine, boschniakine and few other alkaloids were isolated.

90. *Tinospora crispa Linn.* **ex.Hook.f.& Thorns**

Syn. T. rumphii Boerl. (Menispermaceae)

- *Common names:* Hindi: Gulancha, Beng: Goloncha.
- *Distribution:* A climbing shrubs, found throughout the tropical parts of India, known by the same regional names as Tinospora cordifolia and used medicinally.
- *Pharmacological activities:* Aqueous extract of stem showed hypoglycemic activity in diabetic rats[234].
- *Chemical constituents:* Two unidentified alkaloids one is hydroxy compound m.p. 95°, y-sitosterol, another sterol, volatile oil, sodium, potassium, calcium, iron, copper and zinc were isolated from leaves.

91. *Trifolium alexandrinum Linn.* **(Febaceae)**

- *Common names:* Eng: Berseen, Egyptian clover.
- *Distribution:* A herb, found as wild in temperate regions, sometimes cultivated for green manure.
- *Parts used:* Seeds.
- *Pharmacological activities:* Hypoglycemic activities were produced in different types of diabetic subjects comparable to tolbutamide by the powdered seeds. Hypoglycemic response also exerted in both normal and alloxan diabetic rabbits by infusion of seeds[235].
- *Chemical constituents:* Seeds contain fatty acids like stearic, palmitic, linoleic, linolenic acids etc. and xanthosine.

92. *Trigonella foenum-graecum Linn.* **(Leguminosae).**

- *Common names:* Eng: Fenugreek, Hindi: Muthi, methi, Beng.: Methi, methuka.
- *Distribution:* A herb, cultivated in Northern India and some other places in India. Leaves are used as fodder and vegetable, seeds are used as spice and condiment. Flowers are whitish. It is native of Southern Europe.
- *Parts used:* Seeds.

- *Pharmacological activities:* Alkaloid trigoneliine hydrochloride with feed extract produced a mild, transient hypoglycemia in alloxan -diabetic rats. Remarkable hypoglycemic activities were caused by nicotinic acid and nicotinamide[236]. Hypoglycemic activity was exhibited in rabbits by the seed extract[237].

- *Chemical constituents:* See Antifertility chapter.

93. *Urtica dioica Linn.* **(Urticaceae)**

- *Common names:* Eng: Stinging-Nettle, Hindi: Bichhu booti, Bichu.

- *Distribution:* Annual herbs with stinging hairs found at several parts of Himalayas.

- *Pharmacological activities:* Extracts, after purified with picric acid, on oral and parenteral application, did not reduce the blood sugar in rabbits[238].

- *Chemicals constituents:* Leaves contain a neutral and an acidic carbohydrate protein polymer which contain serine-0-galactoside glycol peptide bond.

94. *Xanthium strumarium Linn.* **(Compositae)**

- *Common names:* Eng.: Burweed, Hindi: Gokhru, Chhota-gokhuru, banokra, Beng.: Chota-dhatura.

- *Distribution:* Annual herbs, found throughout the warmer parts of India, as generally as weeds.

- *Parts used:* Seeds.

- *Pharmacological activities:* A white crystalline glycoside, patented in USA, obtained from seeds, showed hypoglycemic effect in rabbits[239,240]. A crystalline substance from seeds produced hypoglycemic response in rats[241].

- *Chemical constituents:* Xanthumin, m.p. 100° in aerial parts, strumaroside, m.p. 290° and stigmasterol in fruits, beside these p-sitosterol glucoside, xanthatin, m.p. 109°, xanthanol xanthinin, m.p. 110° isoxanthanol and flavonoid A m.p. 209° were isolated.

95. *Zea mays Linn.* **(Gramineae)**

- *Common names:* Eng.: Corn, Maize, Hindi: Makka, makai, bhutta, Beng.: Bhutta.

- *Distribution:* A tall, stout, annual, monoecious grasses, widely cultivated throughout in India for Maize grain or corn, extensively used as food.

- *Parts used:* Styles.

- *Pharmacological activities:* Hypoglycemic effect of well comparable with that of crystalline insulin was produced in fasting rabbits by the decoction of macerated styles[242]. Hypoglycemic activity was also caused in rabbits by a fermented preparation of styles[237].

- *Chemical constituents:* Three substituted cinnamoyl hydroxy citric acid, characterised 2-0-trans-p-coumaroyl-(2S, 3S)-hydroxy citric acid, 2-0-transferuloyl-(2S,3S)-hydroxycitric acid, and 2-0-trans-caffeoyl-(2S,3S)-hydroxycitric acid were detected. Besides these di-O-(indole-S-acetyl)-myo-inositol and tri-0-(indole-3-acetyl)-myo-inositol from kernal and p-sitosterol from oil were isolated. 2-(2-hydroxy-7-methoxy-1,4-benzoxazin-3-one) -(3-D-glucoside m.p. 228° from root and 3-galactosides-cyanidol coumarate in corn pigment in Peruvian variety were detected. Along with a highly odorous compound - geosmin and a major constituents 2-heptanol sixty-one volatile compound were identified.

96. *Zingiber officinale Rose.* **(Zingiberaceae)**
    - *Common names:* Eng.: Ginger, Hindi: Adrak, Beng.: Ada.

    - *Distribution:* A perennial herb, cultivated in West Bengal, Andhra Pradesh, Uttar Pradesh, Kerala and many other places in India for the rhizomes, used as spice and in medicines as carminative.

    - *Parts used:* Rhizome.

    - *Pharmacological activities:* Fresh juice of rhizomes exerted significant hypoglycemic activity in diabetic rabbits and rats. This juice also caused lowering of blood glucose level in normal animals[243].

    - *Chemical constituents:* See Antiulcer chapter.

97. *Zizyphus Jujuba Mill.*\ **(Rhamnaceae)**
    - *Common names:* Eng.: Indian junube, Hindi: Baer, Beng.: Kool, boroi.

- *Distribution:* A tree, found throughout India, in dry deciduous forests. It is also cultivated for the edible fruits.

- *Parts used:* Leaves.

- *Pharmacological activities:* Significant fall in blood sugar level, same as tolbutarnide was produced by the alkaloid of leaves[244].

- *Chemical constituents:* Leaves contain alkaloid and rutin, and, leucocyanidin, in bark, and ceamothic acid, betulinic acid and leucopelar gonidin in wood were detected. Fruits contain N-nornueiferine, asimilobine and stepharine.

References

1. *The useful plants of India,* Publications & Information Directorate, CSIR., Hillside Road, New Delhi-110012, (1986), p-2.

2. Sing, K.N. & Chandra, V., *J. Indian Med. Ass.,* (1977), 68(10), 201.

3. Sing, K.N., Chandra, V. & Barthwal, K.C., *Indian J. Physiol. Pharmacol.* (1975), 19(3), 167.

4. Nadkarni's, Dr. K.M., *Indian Materia Medica,* Bombay Popular Prakashani, (1976), Vol.1, 23.

5. Modak, AT. & Rajarama Rao, M.R., *Indian J. Pharm.,* (1966), 28(4), 105.

6. Jain, S.R. & Sharma, S.N., *Planta Med.,* (1967), 15(4), 439.

7. *The useful plants of India,* Publications & Information Directorate, CSIR, Hillside Road, New Delhi-110012, (1986), p-15.

8. Deshmukh, V.K., Shrotri, D.S. & Aiman, R., *Indian J. Physiol. Pharmacol.,* (1960), 4(3), 182.

9. Gupta, S.S., Verma, S.C.L., Garg, V.P. & Raj, M., *Indian J. Med. Res.,* (1967), 55(7).

10. Sing, K.N. & Bharadwaj, U.R., Indian J. Pharmacol., (1975), 7(1,2), 47.

11. Augusti, K.T. & Benaim, M.E., Clin. Cltim. Acta, (1975), 60(1), 121.

12. Galal, E.E. & Gawad, M.A., J. Egypt. Med. Ass. Spec. No., (1965), 14.

13. Sharaf, A.A., Hussain, A.M. & Mansour, M.Y., Planta Med., (1963), 11, 159.

14. Jain, R.C. & Vyas, C.R., Brit. Med. J., (1974), 2(5921), 730.

15. Augusti, K.T., Experientia, (1975), 31(11), 1263.

16. Mathew, P.T. & Augusti, K.T, Indian J. Exp. Bid., (1973), 11(6), 573.

17. Augusti, K.T., Naturwissenschaften, (1974), 61(4), 172.

18. Brahmachari, H.D. & Augusti, K.T, J. Pharm. Lond. (1962), 14(9), 617.

19. Ambike, S.H. & Rajarama Rao, M.R., Indian J. Pharm., (1967), 29(3), 91.

20. Jain, S.R. & Sharma, S.N., Planta Med., (1967), 15(4), 439.

21. Gupta, R.K. & Gupta, S., IRGS Med. Sci., Libr. Compend., (1976), 4(9), 410.

22. Gupta, R.K., Gupta, S. & Samuel, K.C., Indian J. Exp. Bid., (1977), 15(4), 313.

23. Sharma, K.K., Gupta, R.K., Gupta, S. & Samuel, K.C., Indian J. Med. Res., (1977), 65(3), 422.

24. Sharma, K.K., Gupta, S. & Gupta, R.K, Indian J. Pharmacol., (1975), 7(1,2), 107,Abstract No.110.

25. Augusti, K.T., Indian J. Exp. Bid., (1976), 14(2), 110.

26. Jain, R.C. & Sachdev, K.N, Curr. Med. Pract. (1971), 15, 901.

27. Janot, M.M. & Laurin, J, Compt. Rend., (1930), 191, 1098.

28. Brahmachari, H.D. & Augusti. K.T, J. Pharm. Lond., (1961), 13(2), 128.

29. Mathew, P.T. & Augusti, K.T, Indian J. Physiol. Pharmacol., (1975), 19(4), 213.

30. Augusti, K.T, Indian J. Med. Res., (1973), 61(7), 1066.

31. Laurin, J, Compt. Rend., (1931), 192, 1289.

32. Jain, R.C., Vyas, C.R. & Mahatma, O.P, Lancet, (1973), 2(7844), 1491.

33. Jain, R.C. & Vyas, C.R, Amer. J. Clin. Nutr., (1975), 28(7), 684.

34. Mathew, P.T. & Augusti, K.T, Indian J. Biochem. Biophys., (1973), 10(3), 209.

35. Mukherjee, S.K., De, U.N. & Mukherjee, B, Indian Med. Gaz., (1963-64), 3(1), 97.

36. Pradhan, T.N. & Saxena, S.P., Curr. Med. Pract., (1977), 21(3), 105.

37. Nadkarni's Dr. K.M, Indian Materia Medica, Bombay Popular Prakashani, (1992), Vol.1, 77.

38. Teodosio, N, et al, An. Fac. Med. Univ. Recife., (1960), 20(1), 6380.

39. Arduino, Francisco & Scares, Maria de Lourdes, N.G., Brasil-Med., (1951), 65(31-32), 305.

40. Dhar, Ml, Dhar, M.M, Dhawan, B.N, Mehrotra, B.N. & Ray, C, Indian J. Exp. Biol., (1968), 6(4), 232.

41. Lapinina, L.D. & Sisoeva, T.F., Farmatsevet. Zh. (Kiev)., (1964), 19(4), 52.

42. Chempakam, B, Indian J. Exp. Biol., (1993), 31(5), 474.

43. Biswas, K, & Ghosh, A., Varatiya Banoushadhi, Part-V, Calcutta University, Calcutta, (2nd Ed.), (1973), p-1337.

44. Gupta, S.S., Seth, C.B. & Variyar, M.C, Indian J. Med. Res., (1962), 50(1), 73.

45. Murty, K.S., Rao, D.N., Rao, O.K. & Murty, L.B.G., Indian J. Pharmacol., (1978), 10(3), 247.

46. Gupta, S.S., J. Indian Med. Ass., (1962), 39(1), 10.

47. Singh, K.N. & Chandra, V, J. Indian Med. Ass., (1977), 68(10), 201.

48. The useful plants of India, Publications & Information Directorate, CSIR, Hillside Road, New Delhi-110012, (1986), p-71.

49. Deshmukh, A.A., Vadlamudi, V.P., Wagh, K.R. & Qureshi, M.T., Indian J. Indig. Med.,(1992), 8(2), 65.

50. Macdonald, A.D. & Wislicki, L, J. Physio/., (1938), 24(2), 249.

51. Lewis, J.J., Brit. J. Phartnacol., (1950), 5, 21.

52. Lewis, J.J., Brit. J. Phamacol., (1950), 5, 455.

53. The useful plants of India, Publications & Information Directorate, CSIR., HillsideRoad, New Delhi-110012, (1986), p-108.

54. Gupta, S.S., Verma, S.C.L., Garg, V.P. & Khandelwal, P., Indian J. Physiol. Pharmacol., (1965), 9, 9.

55. Basu, N.K. & Choudhury, K.D., Curr. Sci., (1960), 29(4), 136.

56. Choudhury, K.D. & Basu, N.K., J.Pham. Sci., (1967), 56, 1405.

57. Gupta, S.S., Verma, S.C.L., Garg, V.P. & Khandelwal, P., Indian J. Med. Res., (1967), 55(7), 753.

58. Shrotri, D.S., Kelkar, M, Deshmukh, V.K. & Aiman, R., Indian J. Med. Res., (1963), 51(3), 464.

59. Singh, K.N. & Bharadwaj, U.R., Wan J. Pharmacol., (1975), 7(1,2), 47.

60. Biswas, K. & Ghosh, A., Varatiya Banoushadhi, Part-V, Published by, Sibendra nathKanjilal, Calcutta University, Calcutta.

61. Nadkarni's, Dr. K.M., Indian Materia Medica, Bombay Popular Prakashani (1976) Vol.1, 290.

62. The useful plants of India, Publications & Information Directorate, CSIR, Hillside Road, New Delhi-110012, (1986), p-111.

63. Trivedi, C.P., Indian J.Physiol. Pharmacol., (1963), 7(3), 11.

64. Shrotri, D.S., Kelkar, M., Deshmukh, V.K. & Aiman, R., Indian J. Med. Res., (1963), 51(3), 464.

65. Pillay, P.P., Nair, C.P.N. & Santa Kumari, IN., Bull. Res. Inst. Univ., Kerala, Ser. A, (1959), 6, No.1, 54.

66. Neogi, N.C. & Bhatt, M.C., Indian J. Pharm., (1958), 18(1), 73.

67. Sharaf, A.A., Hussain, A.M. Mansour, M.Y., Planta Med., (1963), 11, 159.

68. Nadkarni's Dr. K.M., Indian Materia Medica, Bombay Popular Prakashani (1976), Vol.1, 339.

69. Laurin, J., Compt. Rend., (1931), 192, 1289.

70. Bhattacharya, S.K. & Bajpai, H.S., J. Res. Indian Med., (1975), 10(4), 1.

71. De, U.N. & Mukherji, B., Indian J. Med. Sci., (1953), 7(12), 665.

72. Mukherjee, S.K., De, U.N. & Mukherjee, Wan Med. Gaz., (1963-64), 3(1), 97.

73. Brahmachari, H.D. & Augusti, K.T., J. Pharm., Lond., (1963), 15(6), 411.

74. Chopra, R.N. & Bose, J.P., Indian J. Med. Res., (1925), 13(1), 11.

75. Chopra, R.N. & Bose, J.P., Wan Med. Gaz., (1925), 60, 201.

76. Gupta, S.S., Indian J. Med. Res., (1963), 51,716.

77. Gupta, S.S. & Variyar, M.C., Indian J.Med. Res., (1964), 52(2), 200.

78. Trivedi, C.P., Indian J.Physiol. Pharmacol., (1963), 7(3), 11.

79. Mukherjee, K., Patra, B., Sikdar, S. & Dasgupta, S.R., Indian J. Pharmacol., (1972), 4(2), 114.

80. Sharma, A.L., Sapru, H.N. & Chowdhury, N.K., Indian J. Med. Res., (1967), 55(12), 1277.

81. Wolever, T.M.S., Taylor, R. & Goff, D.V., Lancet, (1978), 2(8104), 1381.

82. Jenkins, D.A., Wolever, T.M.S., Hockaday, T.D.R., Leeds, A.R., Howrath, R., Bacon, S., Apluig, E.C. & Dilawari, J, Lancet, (1977), 2, 779.

83. Williams, D.R.R. & James, W.P.T., Lancer, (1979), 1(8110), 271.

84. Goulder, T.J., Lancet, (1979), 1(8116), 612.

85. Wolever, T.M.S., Taylor, R. & Goff, D.V., Lancet, (1979), 1(8113), 435.

86. Jain, S.R.. & Sharma, S.N., Planta Med., (1967), 15(4), 439.

87. Risi, A., Arch, intern. Pharmacodymamie, (1939), 61, 428.

88. Franke, M., Malczynshi, S., Giedosz, B. & Onysymow, Compt. Rend. Soc. Bio., /(1934), 115, 1373.

89. Pant, M.C. Uddin, I., Bharadwaj, U.R. & Tewari, R.D., Indian J. Med. Res., (1968), 56(12), 1808.

90. Sharaf, A.A., Hussain, A.M. & Mansour, M.Y., P/an(a Med., (1963), 11, 159.

91. Nadkarni's, Dr. K.M., Indian Materia Medica, Bombay Popular Prakashani, (1976), Vol.1, 480.

92. Gupta, S.S., Seth, C.B. & Variyar, M.C., Indian J. Med. Res., (1962), 50(1), 73.

93. Barot, K.C., Deshpande, I. & Mehedale, W.B., J. Res. IndianMed., (1975), 10(4), 141.

94. Gupta, S.S., J. Indian Med. Ass., (1962), 39(1), 10.

95. Roy, R.N., Bhagwager, S. & Dutta, N.K., Indian J. Pharm., (1968), 30(12), 285.

96. Nadkarni's, Dr. KM, Indian Materia Madica, Bombay Popular Prakashani, (1976), Vol. 1, 505.

97. Nadkarni's, Dr. K.M., Indian Materia Medica, Bombay Popular Prakashani, (1992), Vol. 1, 508.

98. Revoredo, N.L., Monit, Farm. y. terap. (Madrid), (1958), 64, 37.

99. Deshmukh, V.K., Shrotri, D.S. & Aiman, R., Indian J. Physiol. Pharmacol., (1960), 4(3), 182.

100. Brahmachari, H.D. & Augusti, K.T., J. Pharm., Lond., (1961), 13(6), 3'81.

101. Gujral, Ml., Choudhury, N.K. & Srivastava, R.S., Indian Med. Gaz., (1954), 89,141.

102. Brahmachari, H.D. & Augusti, K.T., Indian J. Physiol. Pharmacol, (1964), 8(1), 60.

103. Brahmachari, H.D. & Augusti, K.T., J. Pharm. Lond, (1962), 14(9), 617.

104. Augusti, K.T., Indian J. Physiol. Pharmacol., (1975), 19(4), 218.

105. Vohora, S.B. & Parasar, G.C., Indian J. Pharm., (1970), 32(3), 68.

106. Vohora, S.B. & Parasar, G.C., Indian J. Physiol. Pharmacol., (1970), 14(2), 62.

107. Gupta, S.S., Indian J. Physiol. Pharmacol., (1963), 7(3), 10.

108. Gupta, S.S., Indian J. Med. Res., (1966), 54(4), 352.

109. Joglekar, G.V., Choudhury, N.Y. & Aiman, R., Indian J. Physiol. Pharmacol., (1959), 3(1), 76; Abstract No. 34.

110. Joglekar, G.V., Shrotri, D.S., Aiman, R. & Balwani, J.H., Indian J. Med. Res., (1962), 50(5), 737.

111. Vad, B.G., Joglekar, G.V., Mutalik, G.S. & Barwani, J.H., Indian Med. J., (1965), 59(4), 94.

112. Kulkarni, R.D. & Aiman, R., Indian J. Physiol. Pharmacol., (1960), 4(2), 120, Abstract No. 12.

113. Joglekar, G.V., Shrotri, D.S., Aiman, R. & balwani, J.H., J. Indian Med. Ass., (1963), 40(1), 11.

114. Shrotri, D.S. & Aiman, R., Indian J. Med. Res., (1960), 48(2), 162.

115. Jain, S.R. & Sharma, S.N., Planta Med., (1967), 15(4), 439.

116. Dhar, Ml., Dhar, M.M., Dhawan, B.N., Mehrotra, B.N. & Ray, C., Indian J. Exp. Bio!., (1968), 6(4), 232.

117. Gujral, Ml., Choudhury, N.K. & Srivastava, R.S., Indian Med. Gaz., (1954), 89, 141.

118. Brahmachari, H.D. & Augusti, K.T., J. Pharm., Lond., (1962), 14(4), 254.

119. Brahmachari, H.D. & Augusti, K.T., J. Pharm., Lond., (1962), 14(9), 617.

120. Ambike, S.H. & Rajarama Rao, M.R., Indian J. Pharm., (1967), 29(3), 91.

121. Gujral, Ml., Choudhury, N.K. & Srivastava, R.S., Indian Med. Gaz., (1954), 89, 141.

122. Pant, M.C., Uddin, I., Bharadwaj, U.R. & Tewari, R.D., Indian J. Med. Res., (1968), 56(12), 1808.

123. Gupta, S.S. & Variyar, M.C., Indian J. Physiol. Pharmacol., (1959), 3(1), 74; Abstract No. 31.

124. Gupta, S.S. & Seth, C.B., Indian J. Med. Res., (1962), 50(5), 708.

125. Gupta, S.S., Seth, C.B. & Mathur, V.S., Indian J. Physiol. Pharmacol., (1961), 5(2), 23.

126. Gupta, S.S., Seth, C.B. & Variyar, M.C., Indian J. Med. Res,, (1962), 50(1), 73.

127. Gupta, S.S. & Variyar, M.C., Indian J. Med. Sci., (1961), 15(8), 656.

128. Java, A.M., Sheikh, M.A. & Muzzaffar, N.A., Pakist. J. Sci. Res., (1978), 30, 65.

129. Chopra, R.N., Bose, J.P. & Chatterjee, N.R., Indian J. Med. Res., (1928), 16(1), 115.

130. Guruswami, M. N., Lalitha, K. & Gopal, S., Curr, Med. Prac., (1959), 3(5), 227; Biol.Abstr., (1959), 34, 14336.

131. Jain, S.R. & Sharma, S.N., Planta Med., (1967), 15(4), 439.

132. Gharpurey, K. G., Indian Med. Gaz., (1926), 61,155.

133. Williams, D.R.R. & James, W.P.T., Lancet, (1979), 1(8110), 271.

134. Mitra, P.P., Chakraborty, T. & Ganguly, N., Bull. Calcutta Sch. Trop. Med., (1975), 23(1-4), 6.

135. Gupta, S.S., Indian J. Med. Sci., (1963), 17(6), 501.

136. Gupta, S.S., Indian J. Med. Sci., (1961), 15(11), 883.

137. Gupta, S.S, J. Indian Med. Ass., (1962), 39(1), 10.

138. Gupta, S.S, Indian J. Med. Res., (1963), 51, 716.

139. Balasubramaniam, K.B, Arasaratnam, V, Nageswaran, A, Anushiyanthan, S., & Mugunthan, N, J. Nationl. Sc. Com. Sri Lanka., (1992), 20(1), 81.

140. Nadkarni's, Dr. K.M, Indian Materia Medica, Bombay Popular Prakashani, (1992), Vol.1, 615.

141. Donard, E. & Labbe, H, Compt. Rend., (1953), p-196.

142. Nyarko, A.K., Sittie, A.A. & Addy, M.E, Phytotherapy Research, (1993), 7(1), 1.

143. Lapinina, l.D. & Sisoeva, IF., Farmatsevet. Zh. (Kiev), (1964), 19(4), 52.]

144. The useful plants of India, Publications & Information Directorate, CSIR., Hillside Road, New Delhi-110012, (1986), p-308.

145. Deshmukh, V.K., Shrotri, D.S. & Aiman, R., Indian J. Physiol. Pharmacol., (1961),5(2), 19; Abstract No.25.

146. Garcia, F, Acta Med. Philippina, (1941), 3, 99.

147. Orestano, G., Arch. Farmacol Sper., (1940), 70,113.

148. Nadkarni's, Dr. K.M., Indian Materia Medica, Bombay Popular Prakashani, (1992), Vol.1, 764.

149. Gupta, S.S. & Seth, C.B., J. Indian Med. Ass., (1962), 30(11), 581.

150. Krishnamurthy, T.R., Antiseptic, (1962), 59(2), 131.

151. Baldwa, V.S., Goyal, R.K., Bhandari, C.M. & Pangafiya, A., Rajasthan Med. J., (1976), 15(1), 54.

152. Chatterjee, K.P., Indian J. Physiol. Pharmacol., (1963), 7(4), 240.

153. Vad, B.G., Maharashtra Med. J., (1959), 5(10), 569.

154. Vad, B.G., Maharashtra Med. J., (1960), 6(12), 733.

155. Sharma, V.N., Sogani, R.K. & Arora, R.B., Indian J. Med. Res., (1960), 48(4), 471.

156. Aslam, M. & Stockley, I.H., Lancet, (1979), 1(8116), 607.

157. Pabrai, PR. & Sehra, K.B., Indian J. Pharm., (1962), 24(2), 48.

158. Pabrai, P.R. & Sehra, K.B., Indian J. Pharm., (1962), 24(9), 209.

159. Jain, S.R. & Sharma, S.N., Planta Med., (1967), 15(4), 439.

160. Lotlikar, M.M., & Rajarama Rao, M.R., Indian J. Pharm. (1966), 28(5), 129.

161. Kulkarni, R.D., Gaitonde, B.B., Indian J. Med. Res., (1962), 50(5), 715.

162. Handa, G., Singh, J., Sharma, M.L., Kaul, A., Neeya & Zafar, R., Indian J. NaturalProds., (1990), 6(1), 16.

163. Rons, J.A. & Stevenson, D.S., Puerto Rico J. Pub. Health Imp. Med., (1943), 19.

164. Rivera, G., Amer. J. Pharm., (1941), 113, 281.

165. Rivera, G, Amer. J. Pharm., (1942), 114(3), 72.

166. Ratsimamanaga, A.R., Loiseau, A., Ratsimamanga-Urverg, S. & Dibal-Prot, P., C.R.Acad. Sci., Ser. D., (1973), 277(20), 2219.

167. Bart, C, Compt. Rend. Soc. Biol., (1932), 109, 897, 992.

168. Pant, M.C., Uddin, I., Bharadwaj. U.R.& Tewari, R.D., Indian J. Med, Res., (1968), 56(12), 1808.

169. Dhar, Ml., Dhar, M.M., Dhawan, B.N., Mehrotra, B.N. & Roy, C., Indian J. Exp. Biol., (1968), 6(4), 232.

170. Narayana, K. & Sastry, K.N.V., Mysore J, Agric. Sci., (1975), 9(1), 132.

171. Gomathy, R., vijayalakshmi, N.R. & Kurpur, P.A., J. Biosci., (1990), 297.

172. Jain, S.R., & Sharma. S.N., Planta Med., (1967), 15(4), 439.

173. Jain, S.R., Planta Med., (1968), 16(1), 43.

174. AI-Hader, A., Aqel, M., & Hasan, Z., Int. J. Pharmacog., (1993), 31(2), 96.

175. Luthy, N. & Martinez-fortun, 0., Ohio J. Sci., (1964), 64, 223.

176. Shimono, Hiroyoshi, Kyoto Furitsu Ika Daigaku Zasshi, (1961), 69, 1534.

177. Manceau, P., Netien, G. & Jardon, P., Compt. Rend. Soc. Biol., (1942), 136, 810.

178. Nadkarni's. Dr. K.M., Indian Materia Medica, Bombay Popular Prakashani, (1992), Vol.1, 873.

179. The useful plants of India, Publications & Information Directorate, CSIR., Hillside Road, New Delhi-110012, (1986), p-414.

180. Seidel, W., Med. Monatsschr., (1954), 8, 535.

181. Sinha, B.P. & Varma, S.D., Hoppe-Seyler's Zeits Physiol, Chem., (1962), 327(2,6), 274.

182. Zaidi, A.H., Afaq, S.H. & Toriq, M., Indian J. Pharmacol., (1975), 7(1,2), 110.

183. Ahmad, F., Khan, M.M., Rustogi, A.K., Chaubey, M. & Kidwai, J.R., Indian J. Exp.Biol., (1991), 29(6), 516.

184. Harnarh, S., Ranganatharao, K., Anjaneyulu, C.R. & Ramanathan, J.D., Indian J.Med. Sci., (1958), 12(1), 85.

185. Shah, D.S., Indian J. Med. Res., (1967), 55(2), 166.

186. Joglekar, G.V., Chaudhary, N.Y. & Aiman, R., Indian J. Physiol. Pharmacol., (1959), 3(1), 76; Abstract No. 34.

187. Trivedi, C.R, Indian J. Physiol. Pharmacol., (1963), 7(3), 11.

188. Mukherjee, S.K., De, U, N. & Mukherjee, B., Indian Med. Gaz., (1963-64), 3(1), 97.

189. Saifi, A.Q., Shinde, S., Kavishwae, W.K. & Gupta, S.R., J. Res. Indian Med., (1971), 6(2), 205.

190. Pandey, M.C. & Sharma, P.V., Med. Surg., (1975), 15(11), 21.

191. Gupta, S.S., Indian J. Med. Sci,, (1963), 17(6), 501.

192. Ohiyha, J.K., Bajpai, H.S. & Sharma, P.V., J. Res. Indian Med. Yoga Homoeop., (1978), 13(4), 12.

193. Pandey, M.C. & Sharma, P.V., Med. Surg., (1976), 16(7), 9.

194. Gupta, S.S., Indian J. Med. Res., (1963), 51, 716.

195. Rajasekharan, S. & Tuli, S.N., J. Res. Indian Med. Yoga Homoeop., (1976), 11(2), 9.

196. Zafar, R., & Singh, J., Sci & Gull, (1990), 56(7), 303.

197. Dar, M.S., Ikram, M. & Fakouhi, T., J. Pharm. Sci., (1976), 65(12), 1791.

198. Dhar, Ml., Dhar, M.M., Dhawan, B.N., Mehrotra, B.N. & Ray, C., Indian J. Exp. Biol.,(1968), 6(4), 232.

199. Ricci, G.C. & Ricordato, M., Arch. E. Maragliano Patol. 0. Clin., (1955), 11, 359.

200. Cazzaroli, L, & Dall. Oglio, D., Progr. Med., (1958), 14, 52.

201. Chatterjee, Ml., Indian J. Physiol. Pharmacol., (1958), 2, 414; Abstract No. 22.

202. Chatterjee, Ml., De, M.S., & Seth, D., Bull. Calcutta Sch. Trop. Med., (1957), 5(4), 172.

203. Chatterjee, Ml., De, M.S. & Seth, D, Bull. Calcutta Sch. Trop. Med., (1960), 8(4), 152.

204. The useful plants of India, Publications & Information Directorate, CSIR., Hillside Road, New Delhi-110012, (1986), p-51.

205. Rajarama Rao, M.R. & De, N.N., Curr, Sci., (1952), 21(3), 105.

206. Mukherjee, S.K., De, U.N., & Mukherjee, B., Indian Med. Gaz., (1963-64), 3(1), 97.

207. Nadkarni's Dr. K.M., Indian Meteria Medica, Bombay Popular Prakashani, (1992), 1075.

208. Arora, R.B., Mishra, K.C. & Seth, S.D.S., J. Res. Indian Med., (1973), 8(4), 17.

209. Chaturvedi, P., Tripathi, P., Pandey, S., Singh, U. & Tripathi, Y.B., Phytotherapy Research, (1993), 7(2), 205.

210. Nath, M.C., Sci & Cult., (1942-43), 8(10), 427.

211. Nath, M.C., Indian J. Pharm., (1943), 5(3), 113.

212. Nath, M.C., Indian, June 9, (1948), 407, 36.

213. Sen, S.K., Man J. Pharm., (1943), 5(1), 37.

214. Diamond, M.J., Dissertation, Standford Iniv., (1953); Biol. Abstr., (1954), 28, 10808.

215. AI-Hachim, G.M., Al-Samarrai, H.T. & Ali, S.A.F., Bull. Biol. Res. Cent., (Baghdad),(1969), 4, 69-75.

216. Chatterjee, Ml., De, M.S. & Roy, A.R., Bull. Calcutta Sch. Trop. Med., (1965), 13(1), 12.

217. Niyonzima, G., Scharpe, S., Van Beeck, L., Vlielinck, A.J., Lackeman, G.M. & Mets,I, Phytotherapy Research, (1993), 64.

218. The useful plants of India, Publications & Information Directorate, CSIR., Hillside Road, New Delhi-110012, (1986), p-606.

219. Chandrasekar, B., Bajpai, M. B. & Mukherjee, S.K., Indian J. Exp. Biol., (1990), 28(7), 616.

220. Sigogneau-Jagodzinski, M., Bibal-Prot., P., Chanez, M. Boiteau, P. & Ratsimamanya,A.R., C.R. Acad. Sci., Paris, Ser. D., (1967), 264(8), 1119.

221. Brahmachari, H.D. & Augusti, K.T., J. Pharm. Lond., (1961), 13(6), 381.

222. Gujral, Ml., Choudhury, N.K. & Srivastava, R.S., Indian Med. Gaz., (1954), 89, 141.

223. Sepaha, G.C. & Bose, S.N., J. Indian Med. Ass., (1956), 27, 388.

224. Chatterjee, Ml., De, M.S. & Roy, A.R., Bull. Calcutta Sch. Trop. Med., (1965), 13(1), 12.

225. Jain, S.R. & Sharma, S.N., Planta Med., (1967), 15(4), 439.

226. Vaish, S.K. & Kehar, N.D, Proc. 41st Indian Sci. Congr., (1954), 41, Pt.lll, 230.

227. Singh, N., Tyagi, S.D., Garg, V., Joneya, S., Agarwal, S.C. & Asthana, A., Agri. & Biol.Res., (1990), 6(2), 80.

228. Vimla Devi, M., Nageswara Rao, L. & Krishna Rao, R.V. Abstr. 24th Annual meeting of International Congress for Research on Medicinal Plants, Section A, 1976.

229. Mukherjee, S.K.,De, U.N. & Mukherjee, B., Indian Med. Gaz., (1963-64), 3(1), 97.

230. Gupta, S.S., Verma, S.C.L, Garg, V.P. & Raj, M., Indian J. Med. Res., (1967), 55(7), 733.

231. Gupta, S.S., Verma, S.C.L., Garg, V.P.& Khandelwal, P., Indian J. Physiol. Pharmacol., (1965), 9, 9.

232. Gupta, S.S., Indian J. Physiol. Pharmacol., (1964), 8(4), 37.

233. Noor, N. & Ashcroft, S.J.H., J. Ethnopharmacol., (1989), 27(1-2), 149.

234. Helmi, R., EI-Mahdy, S.A., Ali, H. & Khayyal, M.A.H., J.Egypt, Med. Ass., (1969), 52(7), 538-51.

235. Shani, J., Goldschnmied, A., Joseph, E., Ahronson.Z. & Sulmar, f.G.,Arch. Int. Pharma Codgn, Therp., (1974), 210(1), 27.

236. Menczel, E., Bull. Res. Coun. Israel Sect. E., (1963), 102, 235.

237. Haznagy, Andras, Bet Unger Pharm. Gas., (1943), 19, 247.

238. Subramanian, P.P., Indian Sci. Abstr., (1967), 3(6), 4196.

239. Turner, C.E. & Craig, J.C. (Jr.), US 3, 922, 263, 18 Nov. 1975 app. 533. 347, 16 Dec.19744pp.

240. Kupiecki, P.P., Ogzewalla, C.D. & Schell, P.M., J. Pharm. Sci., (1974), 63(7), 1166.

241. Menczel, E, & Sulman, F.G., Proc. Soc. Exp. Biol. & Med, (1962), 1110(1), 178.

242. Sharma, M. & Shukla, S., J. Res. Indian Med. Yoga Homeop., (1977), 12(2), 127.

243. Mohapatra, S.N.; Das, B.N. & Sahu, N.C., Indian J. Pharm., (1976), 38(6), 165; Abstract No. C-34.

3 *Medicinal Plants with Antifertility Properties*

Fertility Control

History

The extraordinary growth of the world population stands as one of the significant events of the modern era. The current world population of about 5 billion is expected to be 6 billion by the year 2000; it is worth the effort to mention that most of the growth will be in underdeveloped countries. The Old Testament dictum "Be fruitful, and multiply" (Genesis 9:1) has been religiously followed by readers and non-readers of the Bible alike. In 1798, Thomas Robert Malthus started a great controversy by opposing the accepted view of unlimited progress for man by making two postulates and a conclusion. He postulated that "food is necessary to the existence of man," and that sexual attraction between woman and man is essential and likely to remain, since "towards the extinction of the passion between the sexes, no progress whatever has hitherto been made," barring ".... individual exceptions." Malthus concluded that "the power of population is infinitely greater than the power in the earth to produce subsistence for man," a "natural inequality" that would someday loom "insurmountable in the way to the perfectibility of society." Malthus essay sparked great controversy and investigation into the principle governing the growth of population. In seeking to discover the causes of population increases, T.R. Edmonds in 1832 suggested that "a deterioration in the condition of the English labors...., the destruction of the feeling of self-respect" was such a great distress that "among the great body of the people...., sexual intercourse is the only gratification.... When they are better fed they will have other enjoyments at command than sexual intercourse, and their numbers.... will not increase in the same proportion as at present." Today we understand that our sheer numbers have increased so much that they are straining Earth's capacity to supply food, energy, and raw materials. We also know, perhaps better than T.R. Edmonds, where some of the blames for this growth lie. Advances in medicine and public health have led to a significant decrease in mortality and an increased life expectancy. Thus, medical science has begun to assume a portion of rate of the responsibility for population explosion.

Modern Methods to Control Fertility

A number of methods are available to control fertility. These can be grouped into five categories.

A. Barrier methods

The most widely used barrier mechanism is condom. Technological developments have evolved in extra thin membrane sheaths, marketed in a variety of colors with and without extra lubricants. When used properly condoms have a satisfactory effectiveness, no medication is involved in either male or female. An extra advantage in the use of condom is the lack of overt transference of venereal disease.

Diaphragm: Usable in the female these are sacks to cover the passage of the sperm to the cervix. It has a fairly high failure rate probably because the sizes vary, and optimal fitness is not achieved. Its use is on the wave.

Along with the diaphragm, the use of foams, jellies and creams containing spermicides is invariably recommended to increase the overall effectiveness.

B. Intra-Uterine Devices (IUD)

The antifertility action of a foreign body in the uterus was known since ancient times in Egypt and India. A small stone was inserted in the uterus of caravan camel to thwart pregnancy during long journey, IUD were introduced in the family planning program about 25 years back. A variety of IUD's differing in shape have been pointed at. Most of them are made of silastic polymers with or without additional metallic constituents. Examples are Lippe's coop, the Dalken shield, Soonawala Device etc.

The first-generation IUD had limited acceptors, inspite of advantage of one time penetration for a long period of protection. The bleeding affection and pain are known to occur.

These side effects have been reduced in the 2nd generation of IUD currently offered, which are Cu-IUD and the copper-silver IUDs. The protective efficacy is also superior in comparison to the earlier ones.

Mechanism: It essentially prevents the implantation of the blastocyst. The tool induces an inflammatory reaction in the endometrium. The Cu-IUD also have an additional action where they slow the release of Cu, influencing metabolic reaction of endometrial cells. Silver in turn may give risc to galvanic currents.

C.   Contraceptive Steroids (Oral contraceptives)

Presence of a feedback control between the steroid hormones produced by ovaries and the pituitary gonadotrophins which stimulate their synthesis. This characteristic was the basis of utilizing progesterone and estrogen to inhibit the secretion of gonadotrophins and thereby block the ovulation. Natural hormones, progesterone and estradiol were not employed since they have a short biological half-life. Instead of these, synthetic steroids with progestogenic and estrogenic activity were put to use. Earlier these drugs were administered by the oral route, the oral pills consisting of a combination of a progestogens with small quantities of estrogen, taken daily for 21 days. However, the rate of occurrence of side effects are high. A variety of major and minor side effects have been attributed to the use of oral contraceptives of most worry are cardiovascular side effects and induction or furtherance of tumors. The risk of cardiovascular disorders increases several folds in women who are smokers.

In recent times indictable contraceptive steroids have evolved. These are depot pharmaceuticals dispersed in an oily base.

The steroids generally used are:

1.   Medroxy progesterone acetate or depo-provera
2.   Norethindrone acetate

These two have 2 to 3 months span.

D.   Termination of pregnancy

The premature expulsion of the products of conception from the uterus is known as Abortion. It can be embryo or a non-viable fetus. In simple words, the coding or labeling of the medical report named as spontaneous abortion may be somewhat problematic. The CPT codes properly use the medical term abortion.

For abortion, another term "interrupted pregnancy" is often used. It refers to a pregnancy that did not proceed to full term. A full-term pregnancy is normally between 38 and 42 weeks of gestation. There are numerous ways to classify an interrupted pregnancy. It can be an abortion, or it can be a miscarriage. Abortion or miscarriage both are considered as natural death of an embryo or fetus. A miscarriage is one of the most common complications of early pregnancy.

E. Sterilization, Male/female

New developments and improvements of the presently available methods:

1. The subdermal implants norplant

    The population council has developed this implant, which consists of a pack of six silastic capsules filled with the progestogen levonorgestrel. These are introduced underneath the skin under local anaesthesia. The release of the steroid is at a constant rate and ensures effective contraception for five years. These are useful for young women who have completed their family and who require contraception for a longer term but want to retain the option for another pregnancy. A simpler form of the same consists of two rods instead of six capsules may be available in near future.

2. Progestin releasing IUD

    An Intra-Uterine Device (IUD) is a small, flexible, plastic device placed inside a woman's uterus. Mirena is the brand-name for a type of IUD that releases synthetic progesterone hormone into a woman's body. The IUD makes it harder for sperm and eggs to move, or for a fertilized egg to lodge in the uterus.

New Methods in Trial Stage

1. *Analogues & Antagonist of Luteinizing Hormone Release Hormone (LHRH):*
    Several synthetic analogues of LHRH have extended biological half-life. Repeated intake of these super agonists

have the contradictory action of desensitization of the target tissue receptors resulting in negation of the hormone effect. Daily administration of the agonists by systemic injections or nasal spray results in blockade of ovulation in the females, accompanied by diminuation of ovarian progesterone secretion and ammenorrhoea. Since estrogen secretion however remains. These preparations may be contraindicated if it is spread out for a long term. So, the therapy may be limited to one or two years, a spacing or gap procedure.

2. *Gossypol:*

   This compound extracted from cotton seeds was used by accident in China by several thousand males, thereby causing azospermia. The compound binds with sperm proteins. Its toxicity is high in rodents.

   However, in humans (as reported in China) only hypokalemia was detected. Due to low efficacy versus toxicity ratio in conventional experimental animals, it is unlikely to be authorized for human usage.

3. *Prostaglandins & Antiprogesterone compounds for Menstrual Regulation & termination of pregnancy:*

   These contraceptive vaccines are in the developmental stage. This may emanate as the most advanced birth control vaccine, having activity on HCG.

Herbal Options to Control Fertility

One of the critical problems of the third world particularly countries like India, is its geometrical increase in human population. According to evaluation of WHO estimated that the population in India will reach near about 135.8 crores at the end of 2018. This population explosion will have negative impression on our economic policies and would simultaneously disbalance our socio-economic infrastructures. These would be manifested by unemployment dearth of food and shelter and also problem of soil, water and air pollution would take its own course in the long run. To confront the problem, initiations have been made by Government and non-Government institutions, but progress of the object is far reaching than from its target. In this regard search for safe and inexpensive oral agents for fertility control in human beings to reduce the population size is appreciable. In this context it will be relevant to locate the large number of indigenous plants that are used as oral contraceptives specially by tribal and other sections. Such plants are even recommended in folk medicines and ayurvedic medicines from very ancient times. Already several scientific papers have been published related to fertility control, but still more plants are left. In the present context, a venture has been made to gather information on the geographical distribution of such plants related to fertility control, their parts used, nature of chemical compounds of these plants and their pharmacological effects. Such knowledge will cater industries in laying out projects on commercial basis. This would also help in searching plants in particular localities and know the chemical compounds with their definite identity in relation respect to fertility control.

Medicinal Plants with Antifertility Properties

1. *Abroma augusta Jac.*

   Syn. *Ambroma augusta* Linn. f. (Sterculiaceae)

   - *Common names:* Eng.: Cotton Abroma, Hindi & Beng.: Olat Kambal.

   - *Distribution:* A large shrub or small tree, grown in gardens and widely distributed throughout hotter parts of India.

   - *Parts used:* Roots.

   - *Pharmacological activities:* Estrogenic activity in female albino rats[1], abortification and anti-implantation activity in mice[2]. Uterotonic activity on isolated rat uterus, on humans and dog uterus in situ[3].

   - *Chemical constituents:* See Antidiabetic chapter.

2. *Abrus precatorius Linn.* (Papilionaceae)

   - *Common names:* Eng.: Indian liquorice, Hindi: Chirmiti, glumchi, Beng.: Chunhati.

   - *Distribution:* Occurring throughout the country.

   - *Parts used:* Seeds.

   - *Pharmacological activities:* Seeds have antifertility activity in albino rats and Swiss mice[4], oxytocic activity *in vitro* in guinea pigs[5], petroleum ether extract has 60% activity on late pregnancy in rats[6], antifertility effects on mice and rats[7] indigenous preparations of seeds-adversely influences pregnancy, vaginal haemorrhage[8]. Seeds oil showed post-coital antifertility activity in rats oral contraceptives in mice and rats[9].

- *Chemical constituents:* The roots and leaves contain glycyrrhizin (1.25%). Seeds contains an alkaloid abrine, $C_{12}H_{14}O_2N_2$, a glycoside abralin, $C_{13}H_{14}O_4$ and a small quantity of fatty oil (Saponification value 192, iodine value 95). Abrine, hypaphorine, choline, trigonelline, precatorine and methyl ester of N, N-dimethyltryptophan metho cation isolated from seeds; alcoholic extract of seeds showed presence of carbohydrates and amino acids whereas ammonium oxalate extract showed presence of sugars; 5(3-cholanic acid isolated from seeds; two toxic antitumor proteins-abrin A and B isolated from seeds; three new isoflavan quinones I, II and III isolated from roots and characterised.

3. *Achyranthes aspera Linn.* **(Amranthaceae)**

- *Common names:* Hindi: Puthkunda, chirchitta, Beng.: Apang, Sans: Apamarga.

- *Distribution:* Occurring throughout India up to 3000ft as a weed. It is also available in Beluchistan.

- *Parts used:* Whole plant, stem bark.

- *Pharmacological activities:* Stembark- abortification activity in mice[3].

- Whole plant Benzene extract of whole plant showed 100% abortifacient activity in rabbits[10].

- *Chemical constituents:* Betaine (m.p. 292°) was isolated from the plant. Ecdysterone (polypodine A) from roots; two oleanolic acid based saponins from fruits and ecdysone from roots.

4. *Actiniopteris radiata (Swartz) Link.* **(Actinopteridaceae)**

- *Common name:* Eng.: Wild fern.

- *Distribution:* Confined to tropical Africa.

- *Parts used:* Whole plant.

- *Pharmacological activities:* Antifertility property in women (90%) given along with Ocimum americanum seeds[11].

- *Chemical constituents:* Hentriacontane, hentriacontanol, p-sitosterol, its palmitate and its glucoside, an unidentified glucoside, glucose and fructose from aerial parts.

5. *Adhatoda vasica Nees.*

   Syn. A. zeylanica Medik (Acanthaceae)

   - *Common names:* Eng.: Malabur nut, Hindi- Basak, Beng.: Basak.

   - *Distribution:* Commonly found throughout India, especally in plains of West Bengal.

   - *Parts used:* Leaves.

   - *Pharmacological activities:* Treatment with alkaloid vascine showed abortification activity in guinea pig[12], Uterotonic activity on human myometrium strip, abortifacient activity in gunea pig[13]. Leaves have no antifertility activity in mice and rats[14].

   - *Chemical constituents:* See Antidiabetic chapter.

6. *Aeschynomene indica Linn.* **(Papilionaceae)**
   - *Common names:* Hindi: Laugauni, Beng.: Kath shola.

   - *Distribution:* A shrub occurring in canal banks, distributed in Kashmir,Bengal, Assam, and throughout plains of India, ascending to 1500m in hills.

   - *Parts used:* Whole plant.

   - *Pharmacological activities:* Spermicidal activity in human and rat semen[15], Saponin from whole plant shows spermicidal activity in human semen[16].

   - *Chemical constituents:* Vicenin-2, reynoutrin, rutin, myricitrin and robinin were isolated from plant.

7. *Albizia lebbeck (L.) Benth.* **(Mimosaceae)**
   - *Common names:* Eng.: Kokko, Lebbeck tree, Hindi: Siris, Beng.: Sirish.

- *Distribution:* A common road side tree common in West Bengal, Assam, Tamilnadu, M.P, Punjab and U.P.

- *Parts used:* Seeds, Roots, Pods.

- *Pharmacological activities:* Seed extracts shows anti-ovulatory activity of saponins when employed in rabbits[17]. Roots without any antifertility activity[18]. Pods and root extracts showed spermicidal activity in human and rats semen[19] also saponin from pods and roots responded spermicidal activity in human semen[20].

- *Chemical constituents:* Echinocystic acid and p-sitosterol identified in bark and seeds. A new saponin-lebbekanin C on acid hydrolysis yielded echinocystic acid, glucose and rhamnose. Different saponins (lebbekanin-A, m.p. 205°, lebbekanin-D and lebbekanin E m.p. 125°), were isolated.

8. *Allium cepa Linn.* **(Liliaceae)**

   - *Common names:* Eng.: Onion, Hindi & Beng.: Piyaj.

   - *Distribution:* A biennial herb commonly cultivated all over the country. Important onion growing states are Maharashtra, Tamilnadu, A.P., Karnataka and M.P.

   - Parts used: Bulb.

   - *Pharmacological activities:* Bulb extracts showed ecobolic effect in mice and rats[21].

   - *Chemical constituents:* See Antidiabetic chapter.

9. *Allium sativum Linn.* **(Liliaceae)**

   - *Common names:* Eng.: Garlic, Hindi: Lahsan, Beng.: Rasun.

   - *Distribution:* Native of central asia.

   - *Parts used:* Bulbs.

   - *Pharmacological activities:* Bulb extracts responded ecobolic in mice and rats[21], bulb extract in other experiment show oestrogenic activity in female albino rats[22].

   - *Chemical constituents:* See Anti-inflammatory chapter.

10. *Aloe barbadensis Mill.*

Syn. A. vera (L.) Burm. f. (Liliaceae)

- *Common names:* Eng.: Barbados aloe, Hindi: Ghikanvar, Guar-pata, Beng.: Ghritakumari.

- *Distribution:* A stoloniferous succulent shrubs, native to West Indies, now naturalized in India, also grown as ornamental in W. Bengal, Bihar and some other states, A salt resistant species is useful for side landscaping.

- *Parts used:* Leaves, roots.

- *Pharmacological activities:* Leaf extracts responded antifertility - activity in mice and rats[7], also showed oestrogenic activity in female albino rats[22], aqueous extracts show anti-implantations and antiovulatory activity in rats and rabbits[23]. Leaves and roots show antifertility activity in albino mice and rats[14]. In another study chloroform extract of the leaves responded significant reduction in fertility in female rats[24].

- *Chemical constituents:* See Anti-diabetic chapter.

11. *Aloe indica Royle* **(Liliaceae)**

- *Common name:* Eng.: Aloe.

- *Distribution:* Plains of Bengal, a herb with sword shaped leaves.

- *Parts used:* Leaves.

- *Pharmacological activities:* Leaf extracts show oestrogenic activity in female albino rats[22]. A significant increase in the fertility rate of experimental rabbits receiving 60 mg/kg more for aloe[25].

- *Chemical constituents:* Aloin is the principal active constituents of Aloes which is a mixture of glycoside. Barbalin is the main glucoside in aloin which is water soluble, besides this aloin contains isobarbaloin, (3-barbaloin, aloe-emodin resins etc. The percentage of barbaloin in Indian aloes extracted from Aloe vera var. offici shows that Indian species contained less quantity (3.8%) as compared to curaco aloe which contain 22.1%.

12. *Anagallis arvensis Linn.* **(Primulaceae)**

- *Common names:* Hindi: Jonkmari, Guj.: Anagalide.
- *Distribution:* An annual herb, bearing small red or white flowers occur in plains of India.
- *Parts used:* Whole plant.
- *Pharmacological activities:* Whole plant shows uterine stimulant activity on isolated uterus of guinea pig[26], uterotonic activity on isolated uterine strips of rat, humans and dog uterus in situ[3].
- *Chemical constituents:* An acetyl saponin isolated from the plant. Isolation and identification of curcurbitacins B, D, E, I, L and R curcurbitacin glucosides-arvenin I, II, III and IV- isolated and their structures were established.

13. *Ananas comosus Linn. Merill.*

   Syn. A. saf/VusSchull.f. (Bromeliaceae)

- *Common names:* Eng.: Pine apple, Hindi: Ananas, Mai.: Kazhudhachakha.
- *Distribution:* A biennial herb, native to S. America, now cultivated mostly in Tamil Nadu, coastal Andhra Pradesh, Assam, Kerala, Karnataka, West Bengal, Tripura, Orissa.
- *Parts used:* Unripe fruit, leaves, rhizomes.
- *Pharmacological activities:* Unripe fruits showing weak activity in pregnancy tests of rats[6], also anti-implantation activity in albino rats[27], rhizomes responded antifertility activity in albino rats and mice[14], roots have antifertility in mice and rats[7], estrogenic activity in rats[28] have been observed with wax from wastes.
- *Chemical constituents:* Ripe fruits contain vitamin C (63 mg/100g). Ergosterol peroxide, 5-stigmastene-3p, 7a-diol isolated from leaves besides (3-sitosterol, campesterol, stigmastanol and campestanol. Ergosterol peroxide, 5-stigmastene - 30, 7a-diol isolated from leaves besides (3-sitosterol, campesterol, stigmastanol and campestanol; 5-hydroxytryptamine from leaves of crown of pineapple fruit method for isolation of biologically active (anti-inflammatory, haemolytic) peptides from roots and juice.

14. *Anisomeles malabarica R.Br.* **(Lamiaceae)**

- *Common names:* Hindi: Kalabhangra, Eng.: Malabar catmint.
- *Distribution:* A woody herb or undershrubs found throughout India.
- *Parts used:* Plant without root.
- *Pharmacological activities:* Plants excluding roots show spermicidal activity in human and rat semen[19], saponin rom plant (without root) responded spermicidal in human simen[20].
- *Chemical constituents:* Ovatodiolide and anisomelic acid (anisbmelolide) were isolated. New macrocyclic diterpenes-malabaric' acid, 2-acetoxymalabaric acid anisomelyl acetate and anisomellol- along with anisomelolide and ovatodiolide isolated and their structures were determined.

15. *Ardisia nerifolia Wall* **(Myrsinaceae)**

- *Common name:* Hindi: Kadna Banjam.
- *Distribution:* Ornamental shrub found in North India and some other places in plains of India.
- *Parts used:* Plants excluding roots.
- *Pharmacological activities:* Plant extracts excluding roots showed spermicidal activity in human and rat semen[19].

16. *Areca catechu Linn.* **(Arecaceae).**

- *Common names:* Eng.: Betelnut palm, Aricanut, Hindi: Supari, Beng.: Supari.
- *Distribution:* An erect palm native of Malaysia now grown along the coasts of Karnataka, Kerala, Tamil Nadu, West Bengal, Assam and Maharashtra.
- *Parts used:* Nuts.
- *Pharmacological activities:* Petroleum ether extract, alcoholic and aqueous extract show anti-implantation activity in albino rats, extract also shows abortifacient activity in albino rats[29] also shows antifertility activity in rats[30], Nut-oil also shows antifertility activity in female albino rats[31].

- *Chemical constituents:* The nut contains arecain(0.1%), arecoline (0.07-0.1%) arecaieline, guvacoline, guvacine and choline occur only in traces. Leucocyanidin (acetate, m.p. 123°) from nut was isolated. Nitrogenous substances "Avenacines" A and B (saponin) are obtained from leaves, stems and flowers.

17. *Aristolochia indica Linn.* (Aristolochiaceae)

- *Common names:* Eng.: Indian birthwort, Hindi: Isharmul, Beng.: Isarmul.

- *Distribution:* A shrub found throughout the country mainly in the plains and lower hilly regions.

- *Parts used:* Roots.

- *Pharmacological activities:* Aristolic acid isolated from roots shows anti-implantation activity in mice[32]. Oral administration of p-coumaric acid isolated from roots at 50 mg/kg dose level produced 100 per cent interceptive activity in mice[33]. Methyl ester of aristolic acid extracts from roots show 100 per cent abortifacient activity in female mice[34] also roots extracts containing Aristolic acid showed marked antifertility activity in female albino rats[35]. A sesquiterpene isolated from the roots showed anti-implantation and anti-oestrogenic activities in female mice[36].

- *Chemical constituents:* A sesquiterpene, Ishwarene, a sesquiterpene ketone Ishwarone and sesquiterpene alcohol Ishwarol have been isolated from the plant. The root contains a bitter yellow compound named as isoaristochic acid ($C_{17}H_{(1}O_7N$). An alkaloid aristolochine ($C_{17}H_{19}O_3N$ crystalline powder, m.p. 215° centigrade) was isolated from the plant.

18. *Artabotrys odorautissimus R.Br.* (Annonaceae)

- *Common names:* Eng.: Climbing ylang-ylang, Hindi: Harichampa, Beng.: Katchampa.

- *Distribution:* A large, scandent shrub with greenish-yellow, fragrant flowers, often grows in gardens.

- *Parts used:* Leaves.

- *Pharmacological activities:* Leaf extracts show antifertility in albino rats. The drug is safe and its effect is of long duration[37]. The drug also showed anti-estrogenic activity in rats[38], significant anti-Implantation activity in female albino rats[39].

19. *Azadirachta indica A. Juss*

Syn. Melia azadirachta Linn. (Maliaceae)

- *Common names:* Eng.: Margosa tree, Hindi: Nim, Beng.: Nim.

- *Distribution:* A common tree in the plains of West Bengal and other regions in the plains of India.

- *Parts used:* Barks, leaves.

- *Pharmacological activities:* Aqueous extracts of bark causes immobilization of human and bovine spermatozo[40]. Application of sodium nimbinate from the seed oil shows strong spermicidal activity in rats[41] and humans[42].

- *Chemical constituents:* See Antidiabetic chapter.

20. *Bombax malabaricum DC* (Bombacaceae)

- *Common names:* Eng.: Red silk cotton, Hindi: Simul, Semur, Beng.: Simul.

- *Distribution:* A tall tree one of the finest trees in India, distributed throughout the country, most abundant in Assam, Andaman and West Bengal.

- *Parts used:* Roots.

- *Pharmacological activities:* Uterotonic activity on isolated uterus of rats, guinea pig and rabbit, dog and human[43].

- *Chemical constituents:* Hydrolysis of gum yielded arabinose, galactose, galacturonic acid and traces of rhamnose. Partial hydrolysis gave 6-0- (B-D-galactopyranosyluronic acid)-D-galactopyranose. 2,3,4,6-tetra, 2,6-di and 2,4-di-O-methyl-O-D-galactose and 2,3,5-tri and 2,5-di-0-methyl-L-arabinose identified as hydrolytic products of methylated gum.

21. *Bridelia retusa Spreng* **(Euphorbiaceae)**

   - *Common names:* Hindi: Khaja, Beng.: Geio, Sans.: Asana.
   - *Distribution:* Distributed throughout India.
   - *Parts used:* Bark.
   - *Pharmacological activities:* A mixture is made with pounded bark of the tree with gum of Sterculia urens Roxb, prescribed orally for 2-3 days after menstruation for complete infertility[44].
   - *Chemical constituents:* Bark contains tannin (16-40%).

22. *Butea monosperma* **(Lam.) Kuntze.**

   Syn. B. frondosa (Papilionaceae)

   - *Common names:* Eng.: Flame of the forest, Hindi: Dhak, Beng.: Palas.
   - *Distribution:* A small deciduous tree occurring throughout India, bears bright orange-red flowers.
   - *Parts used:* Leaves, flowers and seeds.
   - *Pharmacological activities:* Leaves responded chronic toxicity in dogs, rats and rabbits[45], pet ether extract shows negative antifertility activity in rats[46]. Flower extracts responded anti-estrogenic activity in mice[47], anti-implantation activity in rats[48], flower extract in another experiments show no anti-implantation activity in albino rats[27] and in female rats[49], insignificant estrogenic activity in female albino rats[1].
   - Alcoholic extract of seeds responded significant antifertility activity in female rats but pet ether extract shows no significant antifertility activity in female rats[46]. Alcoholic extract of seeds show anti-implantation activity in rats and anti-ovulatory activity in mice, higher doses responded toxicity[50].
   - *Chemical constituents:* Seeds contain 18% of a fixed oil called moodooga oil, small quantity of resin and large quantity of a water soluble albuminoids. Two new glycosides-monospermoside and isomonospermoside isolated together with butrin, isobutrin, coreopsin, isocoreopsin and sulfurein.

23. *Caesalpinia bonducella Flem.*

Syn. C. Crista Linn. (Caesalpiniaceae)

- *Common names:* Eng.: Molucca bean, Hindi: Karanju, Naktamala, Beng.: Nata Karanja.
- *Distribution:* A shrub distributed throughout the hotter parts of India, often grown as hedge plant.
- *Parts used:* Seeds.
- *Pharmacological activities:* Seeds have anti-estrogenic activity in mice and rabbits and antifertility action in mice and rats was found[51].
- *Chemical constituents:* Seeds contain, besides starchy matter 25.13% of an oil, 1.925% of a bitter principle, 6.83% sugar 3.791% salt. oc-Caesalpin, m.p. 187°, p-caesalpin, m.p. 243°, y-caesalpin and 8-caesalpine were isolated from seeds.

24. *Calamintha umbrosa Fisch. & Mey* **(Lamiaceae)**

- *Common names:* Sans.: Karidorna, Mai.: Karimthuma.
- *Parts used:* Whole plant.
- *Pharmacological activities:* Extracts of whole plant respondedspermicidal activity in rat semen[19].
- *Chemical constituents:* Leaves yield an essential oil.

25. *Calendula officinalis Linn. (Asteraceae)*

- *Common names:* Eng.: Pot-marigold, Hindi: Zergul.
- *Distribution:* An ornamental with bright orange yellow coloured heads.
- *Parts used:* Whole plant.
- *Pharmacological activities:* Extract whole plant showed spermicidal activity in rat semen[20].
- *Chemical constituents:* p-carotene, lycopene, violaxathin, rubixanthin, hentriacontane, and two phytosterol were isolated. Calenduloside A, m.p. 260° isolated and identified as galactosyl-glucoside of oleanic acid. Ceryl alcohol stigmasterol, faradiol, m.p. 196° and calender. m.p. 153° were isolated.

26. *Caltha palustris Linn.* **(Ranunculaceae)**

- *Common name:* Punjab: Mumiri.

- *Distribution:* Punjab and other parts of India.

- *Parts used:* Whole plant.

- *Pharmacological activities:* Extract whole plant show spermicidal activity in human and rat semen[19], saponin from whole plant show spermicidal activity in human semen[20].

- *Chemical constituents:* Saponin, heueborin and veratrin.

27. *Canscora decussata* **(Roxb.)** *J. A. Schult & J.H. Schult.* **(Gentianaceae)**

- *Common names:* Hindi: Sankhaphuli, Beng.: Dankuni.

- *Distribution:* A herb occurring throughout India.

- *Parts used:* Whole plant.

- *Pharmacological activities:* Extracts fraction I & II showed spermicidal activity in human semen and rat sperm suspension[52].

- *Chemical constituents:* Compounds I and II were isolated from whole plants. Gluanone, canscoradione, friedelin, friedelan-3b-ol, p-amyrin, sitosterol, stigmasterol and campesterol isolated from aerial parts; new xanthones-1,3,6,7-tetrahydroxyxanthone (I), 1,3,5,6-tetrahydroxyxanthone - 2C - glucoside (II) and 1,5,6- trihydroxy-3-methoxy-xanthone (III) isolated and characterised ; new xanthones - xanthone A, xanthone B and xanthone C isolated and characterised; structures of three xanthones revised to 1-hydroxy-3,5,6,7-tetramethoxy,   1,7-dihydroxy-3,5,6-tri-methoxy and 1,6,7 trihydroxy-3,6-dimethoxyxanthone isolated and characterised; (-) loliolide isolated; 1-methoxy-3, 5-dihydroxyxanthone (IV) and its 3-0-rutinosyl derivative (V) isolated from aerial parts; two new xanthone glucosides and two free xanthones isolated and identified as 1-glucosyloxy-3-hydroxy-5-methoxy-(VI), 7-glucosyloxy-1, 6-dihydroxy-3,5-dimethoxy-(VII), 1,5,6-trihydroxy-3,7-dimethoxy-(VIII)   and   1,5,7-trihy-droxy-3, 6-dimethoxy-xanthones (IX); structures of the two previously reported xanthone-4 and xanthone-12 ressigned as 1,3,5-trihydroxy-6,7-dimethoxy-(IX) and 1,5-dihydroxy-3,6,7-trimethoxy xanthones (XI) respectively.

28. *Capsella bursa-pastoris Linn.* **Medik (Brassicaceae)**

- *Common name:* Eng.: Shepherd's Purse.

- *Distribution:* A common weed of West Bengal, also some other regions of India.

- *Parts used:* Leaves, dry powdered plant.

- *Pharmacological activity:* Dry powdered plant impeded ovulation developed temporary infertility in adult female and male mice when fed at 40% level in diet[53].

- *Chemical constituents:* Contains an alkaloid bursin. The seeds yield a fatty oil (35%). A newflavonoid-luleolin-7-rutinoside, m.p. 184°, luteolin-7-galactoside, m.p. 228° and quercetin-3-rutinoside were isolated from bark.

29. *Carica papaya Linn.* **(Caricaceae)**

- *Common names:* Eng.: Papaw, Papaya, Hindi: Papita, Beng.: Pepe.

- *Distribution:* A small tree native to the West Indies and C. America, cultivated chiefly in Assam, Bihar, U.P, Gujrat and West Bengal.

- *Parts used:* Latex of green fruit, unripe fruit pulp, oil from pulp of unripe fruit, seeds.

- *Pharmacological activities:* Pet ether extract and alcoholic extract of unripe fruit pulp responded 60% anti-implantation activity in albino rats, alcoholic and aqueous extracts are abortifacient in albino rats[29], also pet ether extract showed significant antifertility activity in female albino rats[30], the oil from the pulp of unripe fruit responded antifertility activity in female albino rats[54], seeds extract also showed a decrease in fertility in albino mice but found to be highly toxic[55].

- *Chemical constituents:* Analysis of the fruit gave, moisture 89.6%, proteins 0.5%, carbohydrate 9.5%. The fresh fruit pulp contains sucrose, invert sugar, a resinous substance, papain, malic acid and salts of tar-taric and citric acids 1.2%. Identification of carotinoidsphytoene, phytofulene, p-carotine, cis-p-carotene, pigment X, 5,6-monoepony-p-carotene were isolated.

30. *Cedrus deodara* **(Roxb. ex D.Don) G. Don.**

Syn. C. libani Barrel var. deodara (Roxb. ex D. Don) Hook.f. (Pinaceae)

- *Common names:* Eng.: Himalayan cedar, Deodar, Hindi: Deodar, Beng.: Debdaru.
- *Distribution:* A tall evergreen tree distributed in N-W. Himalayan from Kashmir to Garhwal. Forest of deodar occur in Kulu, Kashmir, Chamba, Tehri-Garhwal, Almore, Simla, Chakrata and Mussoorie hill station.
- *Parts used:* Stems.
- *Pharmacological activities:* Stem show antifertility activity in femalerats[56].
- *Chemical constituents:* See Anti-inflammatory chapter.

31. *Celsia coromandeliana Vahl.*

Syn. Verbascum chinensis (L.) Sant (Scrophularjaceae)

- *Common names:* Hindi: Gadartambaku, Beng.: Kukshima.
- *Distribution:* A weed commonly found in West Bengal.
- *Parts used:* Whole plant.
- *Pharmacological activities:* Spermicidal activity in rat semen has been noted[19].
- *Chemical constituents:* A new sterol-celsianol, mp.166° isolated and its structure established as stigmasta 5,9 (11)-dien-3 p-ol; a constant melting sterol, mp.164° (celsianol) shown to be mixture of 5,6 hydrostigmasterol and alfa-spinasterol; three new saponins celsiosides A, B and C isolated which yielded on hydrolysis celsiogenins A, B and C respectively; the sugars obtained in each case were glucose, fucose and arabinose in molar ratios 1:1:1,1:1:1 and 2:1:1 respectively; structure of celsiogenin C determined as olean-11,13(18)-dien-3(3, 22P, 23, 28-tetrol, whereas celsiogenins A and B identified as olean-12,17(18)-dien-3p, 23-diol and olean-11,13(18)-dien-3p, 23, 28-triol respectively.

32. *Centratherum anthelminticum* **(L.) Kuntze**

Syn. Vemonia anthelmintica Willd. (Asteraceae)

- *Common names:* Hindi: Somraj, Beng.: Somraj, Kali-ziri.
- *Distribution:* A herb distributed throughout India.
- *Parts used:* Seeds.
- *Pharmacological activities:* Spermicidal activity in rat semen has been noted[19].
- *Chemical constituents:* Contain a fixed oil. 7(Z)24(28)-stigmastadienol (I), stigmasterol, 5-stigmasten-3p-ol and 7,22-stigmastadienol isolated from seeds; 8, 14, (Z)24(28)-stigmastatrienol acetate (II) isolated from seeds; a new clemanolide-vernodalol, mp.133° isolated from seeds; amino acid composition of seeds determined.

33. *Cicer arietimum Linn.* **(Papilionaceae)**

- *Common names:* Eng.: Gram, chick-pea, Hindi: Ghana, Beng.: chola.
- *Distribution:* A much branched herb cultivated in UP., Punjab, Haryana, Rajasthan, Bihar, M.P. as pulsecrop.
- *Pharmacological activities:* Seed oil of gram seeds showed some oestrogenic activity in albino rats[57] also oestrogenic activity of seeds in albino rats[58] & seeds responded ecbolic property in mice and rats[21].
- *Chemical constituents:* Contain a higher percentage of oil (4-5%). Isoliquiritigenin, isoliquiritigenin-4'-glucoside, 3',4',7-trihyddroxyflavone, daidzein, pratensein, p-coumaric acid, garbenzol and biochanin 7-glucoside from seedlings. Biochanin A content in plant 8.0 mg/kg; formononetin also detected; vanillic and p-hydroxy-benzoic acids from leaves.

34. *Cichorium intybus Linn.* **(Asteraceae)**

- *Common names:* Eng.: Cuicory, Wild endive, Hindi: Kasni, kasani.
- *Distribution:* North-West part of India. The cuicory is native of Europe, found in India, cultivated elsewhere.
- *Parts used:* Whole plant.

- *Pharmacological activities:* Resortive activity (84%) has been noted in female albino rats[6].
- *Chemical constituents:* See Antidiabetic chapter.

35. *Clerodendrum serratum Linn.* **Moon (Verbenaceae)**

- *Common name:* Hindi: Barangi.
- *Distribution:* Subhimalyantract and outer ranges, ascending to 5,000ft. Assam, West Bengal, Singbhum valley, shady slopeo not common.
- *Parts used:* Except root, whole plant and saponin from plant excluding root.
- *Pharmacological activities:* Plants excluding roots showed spermacidal activity in human and rat semen[19] also spermicidal activity in human semen[20] has been observed with saponin from the plant excluding roots,
- *Chemical constituents:* Glucose and D- (-) mannitol from root bark hydrolysis of crude saponin from bark yielded oleanolic acid, queretaroic acid and new serratagenic acid.

36. *Conium maculatum Linn.* **(Apiaceae)**

- *Common name:* Eng.: Poison hemlock.
- *Distribution:* South Africa, very poisonous biennial, stem dotted red.
- *Parts used:* Whole plant.
- *Pharmacological activities:* Tincture of the plant controls and inhibits the estrous cycle in white albino female rats[59].
- *Chemical constituents:* The plant contains alkaloid coniine.

37. *Corchorus olitorius Linn.* **(Tiliaceae)**

- *Common names:* Eng.: Jute, Hindi: Pat. Beng.: Mithapat, desipat.
- *Distribution:* A shrub grown in West Bengal, Bihar, Assam and U.P.
- *Parts used:* Seeds.
- *Pharmacological activities:* In mice and rats[21] seeds responded ecbolic property.

- *Chemical constituents:* Structure of olitoriside from seeds elucidated as strophanthidin-3-p-D-boirinosido-p-D-glucoside, a new cardiac glycoside-corchorside A from seeds; seeds contained aglycones-strophanthidin and corchorgenin; glycosides-corchsularin, olitoriside and corchorsides A and B; corchoralic acid, p-sitosterol and a saponin; glycosides determined colorimetrically and main components of glycoside mixture olitoriside and corchorside A separated TLC; veticoside, mp. 168° from seeds.

38. *Costus speciosus (Koening.)* **Sm. (Zingiberaceae)**

- *Common names:* Hindi: Keu. Beng.: Keu, Sans.: Kemuka.

- *Distribution:* An ornamental herb widely distributed in Assam, North Bengal Khasi, Jaientia Hills, Sub-Himalayan parts of U.P. and H.P. and West Bengal.

- *Parts used:* Rhizomes.

- *Pharmacological activities:* Administration of rhizome to albino rats[60] showed estrogenic activity and also antifertility activity due to abortifacient properties in albino rats[61]. Also, have shown strong ecbolic property in rats, guinea pigs[64] and saponin fraction showed abortifacient in rabbits[63].

- *Chemical constituents:* Tigogenin and diosgenin from rhizomes and stems; saponin A, mp. 305°, saponin B, mp. 232°, saponin C, mp. 301° and (3-sitosterol glucoside from rhizomes; rhizomes contained diosgenin (2.6%); cc-amyrin stearate, (3-amyrin and lupeol palmitates from leaves; effect of rhizome diameter (5.0 cm to 15.0 cm) on sapogenin content determined; thinnest group contained largest amount of sapogenin (2.7%).

39. *Cucumis melo Linn.* **(Cucurbitaceae)**

- *Common names:* Eng.: Musk melon, Hindi: Kharbuza, Beng.: Kharmuj.

- *Distribution:* A creeping annual, nature to Africa and is now commonly cultivated throughout India particularly in hot and dry climate for its fruits which are eaten.

- *Parts used:* Fruits.

- *Pharmacological activities:* In mice and rats ecbolic property was found[21].

- *Chemical constituents:* Meloside A (6C-diglucosyl-apigenin), meloside L (6C-diglucosylluteolin) and their caffeoyl esters isolated from leaves, six carotenes isolated, three of which identified as αc-carotene (1.82),(β-carotene (94.33) and γ-carotene (2.30%).

40. *Cucumis trigonus Roxb.*

Syn. *C. callosus* (Rottl.) Cogn. (Cucurbitaceae)

- *Common names:* Hindi: Bhakura, Beng.: Gomuk, Sans.: Vishala.

- *Distribution:* An annual or perennial climber, not cultivated, distributed in West Bengal and some other regions of India.

- *Parts used:* Fruits.

- *Pharmacological activities:* On isolated Guinea pig uterus stimulant activity has been noted[64] on application of fruits.

- *Chemical constituents:* The plants yield a fatty oil. Stigmast-7-en-3(3-ol, its p-D-glucoside, alnusenone and alnusenol isolated.

41. *Cuminum cyminum Linn.* (Apiaceae)

- *Common names:* Eng.: Cumin, Hindi: Jira, Beng.: Jira.

- *Distribution:* A herb native to the Mediterranean region and is now commonly grown in Punjab and U.P. for aromatic fruits which used as spices and for flavoring purposes.

- *Parts used:* Seeds.

- *Pharmacological activities:* In female albino rats 100 per cent antifertility effect has been shown[65] on application of seeds.

- *Chemical constituents:* Fruits yield an essential oil and also a fixed oil. A-pigenin-7-O-glucoside and luteolin-7-O-glucoside isolated from fruits.

42. *Curcuma domestica Valeton.*

Syn. C. longa Koe. (Zingiberaceae)

- *Common names:* Eng.: Turmeric, Hindi: Haldi, Beng.: Halud.

- *Distribution:* A perennial herb cultivated mainly in Tamilnadu, Abdhra Pradesh, Maharashtra, Bihar, Kerala and Orissa.

- *Parts used:* Rhizomes.

- *Pharmacological activities:* 100 per cent antifertility in female albino rats and no anti-ovulatory activity in rabbits[66], also antifertility activity in albino rats Petroleum ether extract showed resorption of the implants[67].

- *Chemical constituents:* Analysis of Indian turmeric gave the following values: moisture 13.1, Protein 6.3, fat 5.1, mineral matter 3.5 fiber 2.6, - carbohydrates 69.4 to and carotene calculated vitamin 4, 50 I.U./100 gms. A crystalline coloring matter curcumin ($C_{21}H_{20}O_6$, m.p. 180-183°) is also obtained from turmeric.

43. *Cuscuta reflexa Roxb.* **(Convolvulaceae)**

- *Common names:* Eng.: Dodder. Hindi: Akasbel, Beng.: Swarnalata.

- *Distribution:* A turning whitish yellow leafless thread-like parasitic herb growing in West Bengal and in some other states.

- *Parts used:* Whole plant.

- *Pharmacological activities:* On isolated guinea pig uterus stimulant activity has been noted[64].

- *Chemical constituents:* Dulcitol, luteolin, quercetin and a glycoside of luteolin, mp., 318 degree, isolated from stem.

44. *Cyperus esculentus Linn.* **(Cyperaceae)**

- *Common names:* Eng.: Earth almond, Hindi: Chichoda.

- *Distribution:* A perennial grass like sedge, indigenous to W. Asia and N. Africa but occurring commonly in U.P. Punjab and S. India. Corns are eaten as food and chufa oil obtained from corns is used for cooking.

- *Parts used:* Whole plant.
- *Pharmacological activities:* In mice and rats ecbolic property has been noted[21].
- *Chemical constituents:* p-sitosterol from tubers was isolated.

45. *Cyperus rotundus Linn.* **(Cyperaceae)**
    - *Common names:* Eng.: Nut grass. Hindi: Motha. Beng.: Muthaghas.
    - *Distribution:* A perennial sedge distributed throughout India.
    - *Parts used:* Rhizomes.
    - *Pharmacological activities:* In female rats anti-estrogenic property has been noted[68].
    - *Chemical constituents:* See Anti-inflammatory chapter.

46. *Daucus carota Linn.* **(Apiaceae)**
    - *Common names:* Eng.: Carrot, Hindi: Gajar, Beng.: Gajar.
    - *Distribution:* An annual or biennial much branched herb native to Europe and Mediterranean region and is extensively cultivated inPunjab, Haryana, U.P. and M.P. for its fleshy tap roots which are eaten raw cooked boiled.
    - *Parts used:* Seeds.
    - *Pharmacological activities:* Seeds have anti-implantation activity in mice[69] and chloroform fraction of petroleum ether extract of seeds responded marked inhibitory effect on oxytocin induced contractions on isolated rat uterus, along with inhibited the spontaneous activity of isolated rat uterus[70], good antifertility activity in female albino rats[71], showed anti-implantation activity in female rats[72], antiprogestational activity in rats[73] also showed anti-estrogenic, antifertility and antiprogestational activity[74] showed inhibitory effect on spontaneous uterine motility and oxytocin induced contractions[70] antifertility activity is significant in female albino rats[75], aqueous extract of seeds produced inhibition of implantation in rats[76], petroleum ether extract of seeds inhibited implantation in

albino rats[77], treatment of alcoholic extract of seeds in rats showed significant antifertility activity[78].

- *Chemical constituents:* Volatile oil, an aldehyde, mp. 112° and a compound mp. 230° isolated from fruits; a new sesquiterpene- daucene, bp. 96° /4 mm from essential oil; analysis of oil showed presence of a-pinene, nopinene, sabinene, dipentene, p-thymol, linalool, geraniol, bergamottin, p-bisabolene a sesquiterpene alcohol, mp. 119° from essential oil of wild carrot, linalool, geraniol, geranyl acetate, a and (3-pinene, sabinene, limonene, bergamotene, bisabolsene, daucene, carotol, daucol, p-thymol,.- a-carcumene asarone and elemiein from essential oil of fruits of wild carrot growing in Northern Caucasus; farnesene and p-elemene also isolated; structure of daucol; choline and a quaternary base isolated from seeds; a diglycoside of cyanidin isolated from var sativa DC.

47. *Deeringia amaranthoides Merrill*

Syn. D. celosioides R-Br. (Amaranthaceae)

- *Common names:* Hindi: Latman, Beng.: Golamohani, Assam: Monbir.
- *Distribution:* Bihar, Tirhut, N.Bengal, C.Bengal.
- *Parts used:* Whole plant excluding root.
- *Pharmacological activities:* Spermacidal activity has been noted in human and rat semen[19].

48. *Dimeria gracilis Nees* (Poaceae)

- *Distribution:* S.E. Asia, Indoma, Australia.
- *Parts used:* Whole plant.
- *Pharmacological activities:* Whole plant extract showed spermicidal activity in human and rat semen[19], saponin from whole plant showed spermicidal activity in human semen[20].

49. *Dryopteris filix-mas (I.) Schott*

Syn. Aspidium filix-max SW. (Aspidiaceae)

- *Common name:* Beng.: Dhenki sak.
- *Distribution:* West Bengal and other parts of India.

- *Parts used:* Rhizomes.

- *Pharmacological activities:* Rhizome extracts in mice showed decreased fertility, the drug had some toxic effects[79].

- *Chemical constituents:* Filicin, mp. 92°, cc-flavaspidic acid, mp. 93°, albaspidin, mp. 145° and filixic acid, mp. 168° from rhizomes; syntheris of filicinic acid; five acids identified in fronds- hesadeca- 7,10,13-trienoic, octadeca-9, 12,15-trienoic, eicosa-8,11,14-trienoic, eicosa-5,8,11,14-tetraenoic and eicosa-5,8,11,14,17-pentaenoic acids.

50. *Embelia ribes Burm.f.* (Myrsinaceae)

- *Common names:* Hindi: Baberang, Beng.: Biranga, Sans.: videnga.

- *Distribution:* A large climbing shrub with greenish yellow flower distributed in Sikkim Himalaya foot hills ascending to 4,000ft, Assam, Manipur 3-5000ft, hills of Western peninsula with flowering in Nov-Feb.

- *Parts used:* Berry fruits, seeds, roots.

- *Pharmacological activities:* Aqueous extract of fruit female rats showed anti-implantation activity, no toxic effects[80], anti-estrogenic activity in women and female albino rats, seed extract markedly inhibited estrogen induced alkaline phosphatase activity in the endometrium of immature rabbits[81], no antifertility shown in mice[82], also 66.6 per cent activity on late pregnancy in female albino rats[6], application of embelin showed anti-implantation activity in albino rats[83], treatment of embelin showed 100 per cent anti-implantation in female albino rats, anti-ovulatory activity in rabbits, no estrogenic or anti-estrogenic activity in rat[84], mixture with ingredient of Piper longum, Ferula assafoetida and Embelia ribes along with borax exhibited contraceptive effect[85], extracts of berry fruit showed oestrogenic activity in female albino rats[86], antifertility activity in female rats[87], root has significant antifertility activity in female albino rats[75] treatment with embelin showed slight prolongation of the estrus phase of the vaginal cycle in rats and guinea pigs[88].

- *Chemical constituents:* A new compound vilangin (0.06%) mp. 264°, identified as methylenebis- (2,5-dihydroxy-4-undecyl-3,6-benzoquinone) isolated from berries. Embelin was isolated.

51. *Ensete superbum* **(Roxb.)** *Cheesman Syn. Musa superba Roxb.* **(Musaceae)**

    - *Common name:* Eng.: Chowani.

    - *Distribution:* Distributed from Bombay to Western Ghats to Travancore hills and ravine slopes and in Assam. Tropical Acrica, Madagascar, S.China, S.E.Asia, Indomal.

    - *Parts used:* Seeds.

    - *Pharmacological activities:* Showed antifertility in female albino rats[89]. Antifertility effect of VIDR-2GD fraction of seed extract in mice and rats. Incomplete inhibitory effect of pregnancy in rabbits[90].

52. *Euphorbia dracunculoides Lamk.* **(Euphorbiaceae)**

    - *Common names:* Hindi: Chagulputputi, Beng.: Jychee, Punjab: Kangi.

    - *Distribution:* Sub tropical and warm temperature regions.

    - *Parts used:* Whole plant.

    - *Pharmacological activities:* On uteri Guinea pig, rat and rabbits cholinergic effect was demonstrated, on isolated human uterine strips, short lived spasms were encountered[91].

    - *Chemical constituents:* Euphorbol, mp. 90° and a flavone glycoside isolated from plant. Leaves and stalk contain a glyco-alkaloid, euphorbine, and the seeds, a phenolic substance besides a high percentage of fined drying oil.

53. *Euphorbia tirucalli Linn.* **(Euphorbiaceae)**

    - *Common names:* Eng.: Milk bush, Hindi: Kanpal sehund, Nevli, Beng.: Lanka sij.

    - *Distribution:* A native of Africa, naturalized in Bengal and Western Peninsula, chiefly as a large hedge plant.

    - *Parts used:* Latex.

    - *Pharmacological activities:* On isolated non-gravid guinea pig uterus oxytocic activity was shown[92].

- *Chemical constituents:* Hentriacontane, hentriacontanol, p-sitosterol, taraxerol, 3,3'-di-0-methylellagic acid and ellagic acid isolated stems.

54. *Ferula alliacea Boiss.* (Apiaceae)

- *Parts used:* Fruits.

- *Pharmacological activities:* Fruit extract complete inhibition of human chorionic gonadotrophin[93]. Comarin from fruit blocked the uterotropic responses of exogenous oestrogen. There was no effect on progesterone response of uterus. Irregularity of oestrus cycle, delay in mating, significant decrease in both fertile mating and in the number of offspring, influenced the sexual maturity of immature female rats[94]. Suppressed the action of the hormone in human chorionic gonadotrophin (HGG)[95], coumarin from fruit also completely annuls the biological potency of HGG[96].

- *Chemical constituents:* Coumarin.

55. *Ferula assafoetida Linn.*

Syn. F. foetida Regel (Apiaceae)

- *Common names:* Eng.: Asafoetida, Hindi: Hing, Beng.: Hing, Sans.: Balhika.

- *Distribution:* A perennial herb, commonly grown in Punjab and Kashmir.

- *Parts used:* Fruits.

- *Pharmacological activities:* Estrogen induced alkaline phosphatase activity in the endometrium of immature rabbits could be inhibited by simultaneous administration of the plant extract[97], mixture of ingredients of Embelia ribes, Piper longum, Ferula assafoetida and borax showed contraceptive effect[85].

- *Chemical constituents:* The plants yield an essential oil, oleum Asea Foetidae. Luteolin and luteolin-7-O-p-D-glucopyranoside from fruits.

56. *Glycyrrhiza glabra Linn.* (Papilionaceae)

- *Common names:* Eng.: Liquorice, Beng.: Jashtimadhu, Hindi: Mulhatti.

- *Distribution:* A perennial herbs, native to the Meditenanean region and is now grown in Punjab, Jammu & Kashmir and South India.
- *Parts used:* Roots.
- *Pharmacological activities:* Estrogenic effect in rats have been observed[98].
- *Chemical constituents:* See Antiulcer chapter.

57. *Gossypium herbaceum Linn.*

Syn. G. obtusifolium Roxb. (Malvaceae)

- *Common name:* Eng.: Levant cotton.
- *Distribution:* A shrub commonly cultivated for cotton.
- *Parts used:* Stem, stem bark, root, seeds.
- *Pharmacological activities:* No anti-implantation activity in albino rats have been recorded[27]. Gossypol, a phenolic compound extracted from plant, reduces sperm density to less than 4 million/mL 99.9% of men and impairs sperm motility. Normal sperm density is restored within several months of discontinuation of the drug.

58. *Grewia asiatica Linn.* (Tiliaceae)

- *Common name:* Beng.: Phalsa.
- *Distribution:* Commonly planted fruit tree, grown in West Bengal and some other regions.
- *Parts used:* Seeds.
- *Pharmacological activities:* Significant antifertility activity in female albino rats have been noted[31], when treated with seed oil. Petroleum ether extract, alcoholic and aqueous extract of seeds responded anti-implantation activity in albino rats[29].
- *Chemical constituents:* Taraxasterol, (3-sitosterol and erythrodiol isolated from bark, p-amyrin and betulin from bark; lupeol, lupenone, betulin andfriedelin isolated from plant; p-sitosterol, quercetin, its 3-0-glucoside, haringenin and its 7-0-glucoside isolated from flowers; a new lactone-3-21,24-trimethyl-5,7-dihydroxyhentriaeontanoic acid 8-lactone isolated from flowers and grewinol isolated from flowers and identified as tetratriacontan-22-ol-13-one.

59. *Gypsophila cerastioides D.Don* **(Caryophyllaceae)**
    - *Common name:* Eng.: Werbaceous annual.
    - *Distribution:* Egypt, Australia, New Zealand.
    - *Parts used:* Whole plant.
    - *Pharmacological activities:* Extracts whole plant showed spermicidal activity in human and rat semen[19] treatment with saponin from whole plant showed spermicidal activity in human semen[20].
    - *Chemical constituents:* Saponin.

60. *Hagenia abyssinica* **(Bruce) J.F. Gmelin**

    Syn. Brayera anthiemintica Kunth. (Rosaceae)
    - *Common name:* Eng.: Kousso.
    - *Distribution:* Abyssinia to Malawi.
    - *Parts used:* Flowers.
    - *Pharmacological activities:* Flower extracts responded decreased fertility in female mice but was highly toxic[55].
    - *Chemical constituents:* Four phloroglucinol derivatives - kosins K, mp.167°, K$_2$, mp.110°, K$_3$, mp.177° and K$_4$, mp. 174° isolated as mixtures of isobutyryl, isovaleryl and 2-methyl isobutyryl esters; structure of kosin K, elucidated.

61. *Hibiscus rosa-sinensis Linn.* **(Malvaceae)**
    - *Common names:* Eng.: Chine-rose, Shoe flower, Beng.: Jaba.
    - *Distribution:* Throughout India.
    - *Parts used:* Flowers.
    - *Pharmacological activities:* Alcoholic extract of flowers has significant effect on testis in albino rats[99], benzene extract showed antifertility activity in albino rats[100], alcoholic and benzene extract suppressed the oestrone induced gain in uterine weight in immature albino rats[101], showed anti-implantation activity in women[102], benzene extract disrupted the oestrus cycle rats, reduction in ovarian uterine and pituitary weights[103], responded post-coital antifertility activity in female albino rats. Tubules spermatagenes arrested at early spermated stage

in male rats[104], extract of flowers also responded 80% per cent antifertility activity in female rats[105], benzene extract of flowers failed to show estrogenic progestrogenic activity and also androgenic activities[106].

- *Chemical constituents:* Quercetin-3-diglucoside, 3-7-diglucoside, cyanidin-3, 5-diglucoside and cyanidin-3-sophoroside-5-glucoside isolated from deep yellow flowers; all above compounds and kaempferol-3-xylosyl-glucoside isolated from ivory white flowers.

62. *Hippophae salicifolia D.Don* **(Elaeagnaceae)**

- *Common names:* Hindi: Chuma, Kalabis.

- *Distribution:* Europe, Asia, North America. A small deciduous tree occurring in temperate Himalayas.

- *Parts used:* Bark.

- *Pharmacological activities:* Degenerative changes in semniferous epithelium of young male rats have been noted. Inhibition of testosterone stimulated development of seminal vesicals in castrated rats has been observed[107].

- *Chemical constituents:* Asterol glycoside, two phytosterols, three waxy compounds and a compound, mp. 222°, isolated from bark.

63. *Hodrocotyl javanica Thunb.* **(Apiaceae)**

- *Common names:* Mar.: Karinga, Tarn.: Vallarei, Tel.: Saraswataku.

- *Distribution:* Herb distributed in the Himalaya from Kashmir and Khasi Hills at 600 to 2000m, also on mountains of Western Ghats, Nilgiris and Palnis.

- *Parts used:* Whole plant.

- *Pharmacological activity:* Produced spermicidal activity in rat semen[19].

64. *Hyptis suaveolens Poit.* **(Lamiaceae)**

- *Common names:* Hindi: Vilayati tulsi, Beng.: Bilati tulsi, Oriya: Banga tulsi.

- *Distribution:* Throughout India.

- *Parts used:* Leaves.

- *Pharmacological activities:* In female albino rats 100 per cent antifertility have been noted[65].
- *Chemical constituents:* Isolation and structure determination of two new diterpenes- suaveolic acid and suaveolol. Plant yields essential oil containing l-sabinene, d-limonene and azulenic sesquiterpenes. Anti-A hemagglutinin from seeds.

65. *Impatiens duthiei Hook.f.* **(Balsaminaceae)**
- *Parts used:* Whole plant.
- *Pharmacological activities:* Spermicidal activity in rat semen has been noted[19].
- *Chemical constituent:* The plant contains active constituent 2-methoxy-1,4-naphthoquinone.

66. *Jatropha curcas Linn.* **(Euphorbiaceae)**
- *Common names:* Eng.: Physic nut, Hindi: Bagbherenda, Beng.: Erandagacti.
- *Parts used:* Fruits and seeds.
- *Pharmacological activities:* Application of dry fruits or seeds (2.3%) showed no sign of pregnancy in female rats but recorded full reproduction efficiency when fed with normal diet only[109].
- *Chemical constituents:* Ash of seeds (4.38%) contained Ca, Mg, Na, K and traces of P; presence of oleic, linoleic, mynstic, palmitic, steric, arachidic acids and sitosterol; detection of glucose, arabinose, xylose and rhamnose in seeds by PC.

67. *Lithospermum officinale Linn.* **(Boraginaceae)**
- *Common name:* Eng.: Gromwell.
- *Distribution:* Herb distributed Kashmir and Kumaon at 1500-2700m alt.
- *Parts used:* Whole plant.
- *Pharmacological activities:* Reversible inhibition of estrus in mice noted when aqueous extract was employed[109].
- *Chemical constituents:* Non-saponifiable matter from root of Japanese var erithorhizon contained valeric and isovaleric acids; isolation of an octadeca- 4,8,12,15-

tetraenoic acid from fruits; isolation of scyllitol from plant and caffeic, chlorogenic and ellagic acids and amino acids from leaves; rutin (0.54%) isolated.

68. *Lithospermum ruderale Dougl. ex. Lehm.* **(Boraginaceae)**

  • *Parts used:* Roots.

  • *Pharmacological activities:* Treatment of root extract on adult female mice with regular cycles had prolonged diestrus[110,111], cold water infusion of roots induce sterility when taken daily for a period of 6 months[112]. Follicular atresis of ovaries and mild uterine atrophy were shown when roots are given to virgin mice for one year[113], roots reduce ovarian stimuli in female mice[114], also antiestrus effect in rats have been noted[115]. The aqueous extract precipitated with alcohol has been effective variously influences growth retardation, adrenal hypertrophthymus involution and atrophy of the sex organs along with cessation of estrus, effective in normal and adrenelectomised rats, indicating that the action is not mediated through adrenals[116].

69. *Madhuca butyracea* **(Roxb.) Macbr.**

  Syn. Aisandra butyracea (Roxb) Bachni (Sapotaceae)

  • *Common names:* Hindi: Phalware, Kumaun: Bhalel.

  • *Distribution:* Distributed in U.P. and Bihar.

  • *Parts used:* Seeds.

  • *Pharmacological activities:* Spermicidal activity in human and rat semen has been noted[19], saponin from seeds induce spermicidal activity in human semens[20].

  • *Chemical constituents:* A sterol glucoside, mp. 276° and a flavonoid, mp. 222° from nuts; proanthocyanins consisting of leucocyanidin and oligosa-ccharide units (R-0-xylose-arabinose-rhamnose-glucose) isolated; a-spinasterol and beta-sitosterol-(3-D-glucoside, a- and p-amyrin acetates from bark and fruit pulp.

70. *Maesa indica* **(Roxb.) DC.**

  Syn. M. dub/a (Wall.) DC. (Myrsinaceae)

  • *Common names:* Beng.: Ramjani, Assam: Awnapat, Mar.: Atki.

- *Distribution:* India and Nepal.

- *Parts used:* Whole plant excluding root.

- *Pharmacological activities:* Spermicidal activity in rat semen has beennoted[19].

- *Chemical constituents:* Sitosterol and quercetin-3-rhamnoside isolated from leaves.

71. *Mallotus philippiensis (Lam.) Muell, Arg. (Euphorbiaceae)*

- *Common names:* Eng.: Kamalatree, Hindi: Kamala, Beng.: Kamala.

- *Distribution:* India and Nepal.

- *Parts used:* Seeds, gland and hairs of the capsule of fruit.

- *Pharmacological activities:* Whole plant showed antifertility activity in rats[117], seeds have no antifertility activity in albino rats and mice[118], glands and hairs from the capsular fruits have some effect to produces in fertility in mice, the oestrus cycle was so disturbed that animals fail to mate[82], antifertility effect of the active substance was due to counteraction of the effect of chorionic gonadotrophin[119] also reduced the fertily of male and female rats and guineapigs[120].

- *Chemical constituents:* Betulin-3-acetate, lupeol, lupeol acetate, sitosterol and bergenin isolated from heartwood; acetylaleuritolic acid, a-amyrin, sitosterol and bergenin isolated from bark. Rottbrin and acetyl rottbrin from the plant extract.

72. *Medicago sativa Linn.* **(Fabaceae)**

- *Common names:* Eng.: Alfalfa, Hindi: Lasunghas, Punjab: Lusan.

- *Distribution:* A perennial herb of temperate Europe, Asia and North Africa widely cultivated as fodder for live Hock.

- *Parts used:* Whole plant.

- *Pharmacological activities:* Coumesterol from plant increases the age of maturity and depresses the egg production in white leghorn pullet[121].

- *Chemical constituents:* A highly toxic saponin (I) isolated and characterised as triglucoside of medicagenic acid; detection of monogalactosyl (3.2), digalactosyl (7.7) and sulfoquinovosyl (0.8%) diglycerides in glyceroglyco lipids from leaves by GC; a saponin isolated from roots yielded on hydrolysis hederagenin, glucose and arabinose; myrcene, limonene and linalool isolated from flowers; a new isoflavon-sativin, mp. 125° isolated from leaves; medicarpin-p-D-glucoside isolated from roots; coumesterol isolated; benzoyl mesotartaric acid and benzoyl (s) (-) malic acid isolated; a-tocopherol found predominant tocopherol isomer in alfalfa concentrate.

73. *Mentha arvensis Linn.* (Lamiaeceae)

- *Common names:* Eng.: Field mint, Hindi: Podina, Beng.: Pudina.

- *Distribution:* West Bengal and other parts of India.

- *Parts used:* Leaves.

- *Pharmacological activities:* Significant antifertility activity in female albino rats has been noted[122], and no post-coital antifertility activity in other experiments[123]. Alcoholic extract showed 80-100% anti-implantation activity in female rats[124] experiment on rabbits showed anti-ovulatory activity[125]. Aqueous extract responded 60% anti-implantation activity whereas petroleum ether extract has abortifacient activity and alcoholic extract responded 80 per cent anti-implantation activity in female albino rats[126].

- *Chemical constituents:* The plants yield an essential oil. Acacetin, apigenin, diosmetin, eriodictyol, hesperitin and luteolin isolated from aerial parts.

74. *Michelia champaca L* (Magnoliaceae)

- *Common names:* Hindi: Champa, Beng.: Champa.

- *Distribution:* Wild in the Eastern Himalayas and North-East India up to 900m, Western ghats and South India, widely cultivated in various regions of India.

- *Parts used:* Bark.

- *Pharmacological activities:* Bark is employed as an abrotifacient for 2-3 months old pregnancy. A root paste (roots 6-8mm long) with black paper (21 fruits) is employed as an oral contraceptive given for 3 days after menstruction[15].

75. *Momordica charantia Linn.* (Cucurbitaceae)

- *Common names:* Eng.: Bitter gourd, Hindi: Karela, Beng.: Karala.

- *Distribution:* A climbing herb found throughout India, often cultivated for fruits which are used as vegetables.

- *Parts used:* Roots, leaves.

- *Pharmacological activities:* Roots showing uterine stimulant activity on isolated guinea pig uterus[64]. Aqueous extract of leaves shows no significant antifertility and estragenic activity in pregnant rats[127].

- *Chemical constituents:* Fruits contain stigmast-5, 25-diene-3(3-0-glucoside, (3-sitosterol gluscoside, and a hypoglycemic substance charantin m.p. 266°. A glycoalkaloid-vicine, was obtained from seeds.

76. *Moringa oleifera Lam.*

Syn. M. pterigosperma Gaertns.(Moringaceae).

- *Common names:* Beng.: Sojna; Hind: Shajnah, Sans.: Shobhajana.

- *Distribution:* Throughout India.

- *Parts used:* Root, Stem-bark.

- *Pharmacological activities:* Roots have effect in antifertility activity on late pregnancy in rats[6], stembark has little oxitoxic activity on isolated guinea pig uterus[92], but no antifertility activity in albino mice and rats[118].

- *Chemical constituents:* One antibiotic named ptergos-permin was isolated form plant root. It is reddish brown oil and is must active at pH of 5 and activity decreases as the pH approaches 8.

77. *Morus alba Linn.* (Moraceae)

- *Common names:* Eng.: White Mulberry, Hindi: Tut, Beng.: Toot.

- *Distribution:* Cultivated throughout the plain parts of India.

- *Parts used:* Leaves.

- *Pharmacological activities:* Leaves have ecbolic property in mice and rats[69].

- *Chemical constituents:* Mulberrin, mp. 153°, mulberro-chromene, mp. 232° cyclomulberrin, cyclomulberro-chromene, mp. 233°, characterised from stems, roots and bark.

78. *Ocimum americanum Linn.*

Syn. Ocanum Sims (Lamiaceae)

- *Common names:* Eng.: Hoary Basil, Hindi: Kalatulsi, Sans.: Ajaka.

- *Distribution:* Throughout the tropical regions of the world.

- *Parts used:* Seeds.

- *Pharmacological activities:* In women 90 per cent antifertility activity (along with Actinopteris radiata) has been noted[11].

- *Chemical constituents:* Polysaccharide contained xylose, arabinose, rhamnose and galactose, galacturonic acid and glucuronic acid detected by PC.

79. *Ocimum sanctum Linn.* **(Lamiaceae)**

- *Common names:* Eng.: Sacred Basil, Hindi: Tulsi, Beng.: Tulsi.

- *Distribution:* A strongly scented shrub. It is cultivated throughout India, and also considered a sacred plant to the Hindus. These plants are of two types, one is purple type, called Krishna tulsi and another is green type called sri tulsi.

- *Parts used:* Leaves.

- *Pharmacological activities:* Benzene extract of leaves responded 80% antifertility activity in female rats, but petroleum ether extract responded 60% antifertility activity in female rats[105], also anti-implantation activity in albino rats has been noted[128].

- *Chemical constituents:* See Hepatoprotective chapter.

80. *Ougeinia dalbergioides Benth.*

   Syn. O. Oojeinensis (Roxb) Hochr. (Fabaceae)

   - *Common names:* Eng.: Sandan, Hindi: Sandan, Beng.: Tinis.
   - *Distribution:* Throughout India and Nepal.
   - *Parts used:* Stem bark.
   - *Pharmacological activities:* Stem Bark extract responded spermicidal activity in rat semen[19].
   - *Chemical constituents:* Bark contains tannin (7%). The heartwood contains homoferreirin (0.4%) and a new isoflavanone, ougenin.

81. *Oxalis corniculata Linn.* **(Oxalidaceae)**

   - *Common names:* Eng.: Indian sorrel, Hindi: Amrul sak, Beng.: Amrul sak.
   - *Distribution:* Throughout India and Nepal.
   - *Parts used:* Whole plant.
   - *Pharmacological activities:* Crude drug extract showed estrogenic activity in female albino rats[1].

82. *Paeonia emod/Wall. ex Royle.* **(Poeoniaceae)**

   - *Common names:* Eng.: Himalayan Peony, Hindi: Ud-salap, Punjab: Mamekh.
   - *Distribution:* Bihar, Punjab, Kashmir.
   - *Parts used:* Tubers.
   - *Pharmacological activities:* Tubers have marked uterotonic activity in isolated uteri of rat, guineapig, rabbit and dog in situ[3].
   - *Chemical constituents:* Starch (9.5), sucrose (5.4), malic acid (0.47), oxalic acid (0.36), tartaric acid (0.34%) and benzoic acid present in roots.

83. *Petroselinum hortense Hoffm. Syn. P. crispum* **(Apiaceae)**

   - *Common names:* Eng.: Parsley, Kan Achu mooda.
   - *Distribution:* A herb, native of Europe, now cultivated throughout India.
   - *Parts used:* Whole plant.

- *Pharmacological activities:* Ecbolic property in mice and rats have been noted[21].

- *Chemical constituents:* Apiole (1-allyl-2, 5-dimethoxy-3, 4-methylenedioxybenzene), allyltetramethoxybenzene, myristicine, a mixture of flavone glycosides and a compound, mp. 145°, from seeds; 1 -allyl-2,3,4,5-tetra-methoxybenzene, apigenin-7-apioglucoside and luteolin-7-apioglucoside from fruits; a new synthesis of apigenin, mp. 346°.

84. *Pimpinella anisum Linn.* **(Apiaceae)**

- *Common names:* Eng.: Aniseed, Hindi: Saunf, Beng.: Muhuri, mithajira.

- *Distribution:* Africa, North America, South America.

- *Parts used:* Seeds and roots.

- *Pharmacological activities:* Oil extracted from seeds and roots has oestrogenic activity in rats[129].

- *Chemical constituents:* An aliphatic alcohol, mp.74°, an essential oil, a fixed oil and mannitol from seeds; myricanol and mannitol from roots.

85. *Pimpinella diversifolia DC.* **(Apiaceae)**

- *Distribution:* Decan.

- *Parts used:* Whole plant.

- *Pharmacological activities:* Plant extract responded spermicidal activity in rat semen[19].

- *Chemical constituents:* Ammirin (isoangenomalin) and oxypeucedanin isolated from aerial parts.

86. *Piper aurantiacum Wall. ex.Hook. f*

Syn. P. WaW/e/H/Nand, Mazz. (Piperaceae)

- *Common names:* Hindi: Shambhaluka bui, Beng.: Renuk.

- *Distribution:* West Bengal.

- *Parts used:* Fruits.

- *Pharmacological activities:* Oxytocic activity has been observed by alkaloidal fraction. The defatted tannic free alcoholic extract has shown parasympathomimetic activity[90].

- *Chemical constituents:* Piperine, piperettine, sylvatine and p-sitosterol isolated from fruits. A new amide-aurantiamide and its acetate isolated from seeds. Stearic and linoleic acids, triacontane, cholesterol, cholestanol also isolated from fruits.

87. *Piper belle Linn.* (Piperaceae)

- *Common names:* Eng.: Betel, Beng.: Pan, Hindi: Tambul.
- *Distribution:* West Bengal, Orissa, U.P., Bihar, Assam.
- *Parts used:* Root.
- *Pharmacological activities:* Roots extract have[61] antifertility activity.
- *Chemical constituents:* p-sitosterol from the root and also from the leaf. Leaves contain starch, sugars, tannin, diastases (0.8 to 1.8%) and essential oil (Betel oil) to the extents of eveb 4.2% in some leaves. The essential oil is a light-yellow liquid of aromatic odor and sharp burning taste. The specific gravity varies from 0.958 to 1.057.

88. *Piper chaba Hunter.*

Syn. P. retrofractum vahl (Piperaceae)

- *Common names:* Eng.: Java long pepper, Hindi: Chab, Beng.: Chai.
- *Distribution:* North-East Himalaya.
- *Parts used:* Fruits.
- *Pharmacological activities:* Fruits have antifertility activity[130].
- *Chemical constituents:* A new amide-N-butyl-tridea-p (3,4 methylenedixyphenyl) 2,4,12 trienamide isolated from frutis. Filfiline (N-isobutyldocosa-transe-2, transe-4 CIS-10 trienamide) also isolated from fruit.

89. *Piper longum Linn.* (Piperaceae)

- *Common names:* Eng.: Long pepper, Hindi: Pipal, Beng.: Piplamor.
- *Distribution:* Cultivated in West Bengal, Karnataka and Tamil Nadu.
- *Parts used:* Roots, leaves and fruits.

- *Pharmacological activities:* Mixtures of roots and leaves along with ingredients of Embelia ribes and Ferula assafoetida responded contraceptive responses[131], frutis of P.longum have inhibitory activity in fertile female rats[132], estrogen induced alkaline phosphatase activity in the endometrium of immature rabbits was inhibited by treatment of the drug from fruits and roots[81] also extracts showed antifertility activity in rats[133].

- *Chemical constituents:* Piperlongumine, piperlonguminine piperine, sisamine, methyl 3,4,5 trimethoxycinnamate isolated from roots.

90. *Pisum sativum Linn.*

Syn. *P. arvense Linn.* (Fabaceae)

- *Common names:* Eng.: Pea, Hindi: Matar, Beng.: Matar.
- *Distribution:* W.Bengal, Bihar, U.P. and some other states.
- *Parts used:* Seeds and seed oil.
- *Pharmacological activities:* Seeds have contraceptive action in albino rats[134,135,136] and only meta-xyto-hydro-quinine (not its isomers) interfered with progesterone level in blood[137], single dose (0.1 mg) of the active principle responded abortion, reabortion but the substance did not prevent nidation[138] ecbolic property in mice and rats[21], has been observed application-of meta-xylo-hydroquinone to mature female rats control condition, before mating and during first trimester of gestation, failed to delay mating also prevent implantation[139], seed oil showed temporary sterility produced in both sexes of rats[140].

- *Chemical constituents:* D-Galacturonyl-L-rhamnose isolated from hydrolysate of an acidic polysaciharide isolated from seeds. A cerebroside isolated from seeds which on hydrolysis yielded hydroxytricosanoic acid, sphingoxine loase and glucose.

91. *Pittosporum nilghirense W.& A.* **(Pittosporaceae)**

- *Distribution:* Eastern and Western Ghats of South India.
- *Parts used:* Plants excluding root.

- *Pharmacological activities:* Responded spermicidal activity in human & rat semen[19].

92. *Plumbago indica Linn.*

Syn. *P. rosea Linn.* (Plumbaginaceae)

- *Common names:* Hindi: Chitra, Beng.: Lal-chitra, Sans.: Chitraka.
- *Distribution:* Throughout India. Parts used: Roots.
- *Pharmacological activities:* Responded weak antifertility activity in late pregnancy in rats[6], also showed oxytoxic action on isolated uterus of rat, guinea pig and human[141].
- *Chemical constituents:* The root bark contains on orange-yellow pigment plumbagin (2-methyl-5 hydroxy-1,4 napthoquinone, C_6H_2O, m.p. 77-78°) a sitosterol glycoside ($C_MH_{56}O_6$ m.p.259-60°), a sitosterol, a fatty alcohol, probably arachidyl alcohol, tannin and amorphous brown pigment. The flowers contain 3-rhamnosides of pelargonidin, cyanidin, delphinidin and kaempferol.

93. *Plumbago zeylanica Linn.* **(Plumbaginaceae)**

- *Common names:* Hindi: Chita, Beng.: Chita, Sans.: Chitraka.
- *Distribution:* Gangitic plains of India.
- *Parts used:* Root and fruits.
- *Pharmacological activity:* Alcoholic extract (50 per cent) responded 100 per cent anti-implantation activity in rats but no anti-implantation activity on rabbits[24].
- *Chemical constituents:* Plumbagin, 3-chloroplumbagin and a new substance 3,3' biphobagin, a new leinapthaguinone-chitranone-together with zeylinone, isozeylinone, euiptinone and droserone isolated from roots.

94. *Plumeria acutifolia Poir.*

Syn. P. acuminata Ait. (Apocynaceae)

- *Common names:* Eng.: Temple tree, Hindi: Golainchi, Beng.: Dalan phul
- *Distribution:* Throughout India.
- *Parts used:* Bark.

- *Pharmacological activities:* Responded uterine stimulation on isolated guinea pig uterus[28].

- *Chemical constituents:* Fulvoplumierin, mp. 147°, plumericin, mp. 211° and three new compounds-isoplumericin, mp. 200°, p-dihydroplumericin, mp. 191° and p-dihydroplumericinic acids, mp. 189° from roots; fulvopulmierin, (3-sitosterol, lupeol and plumieride from stem bark.

95. *Polygonum hydropiper Lm.*

Syn. *P. flaccidum* Meissn (Polygonaceae)

- *Common names:* Eng.: Smart weed, Beng.: Packur-mul, pani-maricha.

- *Distribution:* Throughout India, ascending to an altitude of 7000 ft in the Himalayas.

- *Parts used:* Roots, leaves, whole plant.

- *Pharmacological activities:* Roots responded sterility in female guinea pig, no evidence of estrogenic or androgenic activity[142]. In other experiments 66.6% anti-fertility activity on early pregnancy in rats[143], petroleum ether extract responded anti-ovulatory activity in rabbits[125] and anti-implantation in albino rats[128] leaves have no significant antifertility activity in rats[144] but the whole plant impaired the fertility of male and female mice and produced temporary sterility in guinea pig[142].

- *Chemical constituents:* The herb contains formic acid, acetic acid and baldrianic acid, much tanin and small amount of essential oil, the root contains oxymethyl-anthraquinones.

96. *Psoralea corylifolia Linn.* (Fabaceae)

- *Common names:* Eng.: Bakuchi, Hindi: Babchi, Beng.: Bavachi, Sans.: Bakuchi.

- *Distribution:* Throughout India.

- *Parts used:* Seeds.

- *Pharmacological activities:* Fertility of adult female rats was impaired by seed extract[145].

- *Chemical constituents:* See Anti-inflammatory chapter.

97. *Pterolobium indicum A. Rich.* **(Fabaceae)**

- *Parts used:* Plant excluding root.

- *Pharmacological activities:* Saponin from plant (excluding root) responded spermicidal activity in human semen[20], plant excluding roots responded spermicidal activity in human and rat semen[19].

98. *Punica granatum Linn.* **(Punicaceae)**

- *Common names:* Eng.: Pomegranate, Hindi: Anar, Beng.: Dalim.

- *Distribution:* Small tree generally cultivated throughout India, Gujrat and other regions.

- *Parts used:* Fruit skin.

- *Pharmacological activities:* Fertility of female rats and guinea pigs was reduced[120].

- *Chemical constituents:* The plants contain iso-pelletierine. Sitosterol and ursolic acid isolated; two tannins-punicalagin and punicalin isolated from peels and their structures determined, hydrolysis of punicalagin yielded ellagic acid and punicalin, the latter yielded glucose and a tetralactone; pectin isolated from fruits contained mannose, galactose, rhamnose, arabinose and glucose in ratio of 1:1.3:2.1:4.4:6.2; principal sugar acid was galacturonic acid.

99. *Randia dumetorum Poir.*

Syn. *R. spinosa* Poir. (Rubiaceae)

- *Common names:* Eng.: Common emetic nut, Hindi: Mainphal, Beng.: Mainphal.

- *Distribution:* India and Nepal.

- *Parts used:* Fruits, seeds and pulp.

- *Pharmacological activities:* Ethanolic extract of fruits and seeds shows no anti-implantation activity in rats but anti-ovulatory effect in rabbits has been observed[144], pulp showed uterine stimulant activity on isolated guinea pig uterus[64], Anti-implantation activity in albino rats has been observed with the treatment of oleanolic acid 3-p glucoside isolated from seeds[147].

- *Chemical constituents:* Oleanolic acid 3-p glucoside.

100. *Rauvolfia serpentina Benth.ex.Kurz.* **(Apocynaceae)**

- *Common names:* Eng.: Serpentina root, Hindi: Chandrabhaga, Beng.: Chandra, Sarpa-gandha.

- *Distribution:* A small shrub found from Himalayas southwards to Peninsula of India.

- *Parts used:* Roots.

- *Pharmacological activities:* Roots responded decreased reproduction capacity in rats[114] and release of pituitary gonadotrophin (hence ovulation) backed in rats and mice[148] has been observed.

- *Chemical constituents:* Roots contain reserpine. Structure elucidation of reserpine and deserpidine essential oil (0.22%) from roots yielded chief terpene constituent-serpoterpine, bp. 131°; isolation of reserpine, mp. 360°, ajmaline, mp. 158°, serpentine, mp. 155°, serpentinine, mp. 265° and ajmalieine (d-yohimbine), mp. 250°, from roots; reserpine, serpajmaline (mixture of serpentine, serpentinine, ajmaline and 2 unknown compounds, free of reserpine), resajmaline (mixture of serposterol and unsaturated higher alcohols), rescinnamine and ajmalexin (mixture of reserpine and rescinnamine) were isolated from roots; detection of reserpine, reserpinine, yohimbine, ajmaline, serpentine and serpentine by PC; serpentinine characterised as 3-hydroxyserpentine; absolute stereo-chemistry of ajmaline and isoajmaline; raugalline isolated and identified as ajmaline; detection of raunatine in root extract by PC; stereochemical studies in structure elucidation of yohimbine and reserpine.

101. *Rubus ellipticus Sm.* **(Rosaceae)**

- *Common names:* Hindi: Hinsalu, anchhu.

- *Distribution:* From Punjab to Assam extending South-wards in the Western Ghats.

- *Parts used:* Plant excluding roots.

- *Pharmacological activity:* Alcoholic extract responded anti-implantation activity in rats but no anti-ovulatory activity in rabbits has been observed[149].

102. *Salix babylonica Linn.* (Salicaceae)

- *Common names:* Eng.: Weeping willow, Tel: Attuppali, Punjab: Bisa.
- *Distribution:* Throughout the temperate regions of the world. Native of Central China, now cultivated in northern parts of India.
- *Parts used:* Plant excluding root.
- *Pharmacological activities:* Anti-implantation in rats has been shown by alcoholic extract but no anti-ovulatory activity has been noted in rabbits[149].
- *Chemical constituents:* Bark and leaves are reported to contain 3-9% and 4.9% tannin. Leaves contain delphidinin and cynidin, Fragilin, salicin salicortin, salidroside, tremuloidin, triandrin and vimalin.

103. *Salix tetrasperma Roxb.* (Salicaceae)

- *Common names:* Eng.: Indian willow, Hindi: Bod, Jalmala, Oriya: Baisi. Beng.: Panijana, Boishakhi.
- *Distribution:* Throughout the temperate regions of the world.
- *Parts used:* Stem bark.
- *Pharmacological activities:* Alcoholic extract of stem bark responded anti-implantation activity in rats but failed to respond anti-ovulatory activity in rabbits[151].
- *Chemical constituents:* Bark is reported to contain 6.5% tannin. Analysis of sun-dried nature leaves gave ash, 10.05; Calcium, 2.71; Carbon, 45.06; and nitrogen, 2.07%.

104. *Samanea saman Merrill*

Syn. Pithecolobium saman (Mimosaceae)

- *Distribution:* Chhotonagpur.
- *Parts used:* Plant excluding root.
- *Pharmacological activities:* Saponin from whole plant (excluding root) responded spermicidal activity in human semen[20], also whole plant (excluding root) has spermicidal activity in human and rat semen[19].

- *Chemical constituents:* Octacosanoic acid, lupeol, oo-spinasterol, cc-spinasterone and lupenone isolated from bark; a new saponin-samanin B- shown to be constituted of acacic acid and glucose arabinose, xylose and rhamnose present in molar ratio of 4:2:1:1; another new saponin-samanin C, mp. 146° isolated from wood and found to contain acacic acid along with glucose, arabinose, xylose, fucose and rhamnose in molar ratio of 6:1:2:3:4; a new saponin-samanin D isolated from flowers con-. tained acacic acid along with glucose, arabinose, xylose and rhamnose in ratio of 5:4:3:1.

105. *Sapindus mukorossi Gaertn.* (Sapindaceae)

- *Common names:* Hindi: Ritha, Beng.: Ritha, Sans.: Urista, phenila.

- *Distribution:* Decan. Soap nut tree of N. India.

- *Parts used:* Fruit.

- *Pharmacological activities:* Saponin from fruit responded spermicidal activity in human semen[20], fruit responded spermicidal activity in human and rat semen[19].

- *Chemical constituents:* Two saponins - sapindoside A, mp.214° and sapindoside B, mp.276° isolated and characterised as hederagenin-3 (a-L-arabinopyranosyl-2 a-L-rhamnopyranoside) and hederagenin-3-(a-L-arabino-pyranosyl-2 a-L-rhamnopyranosyl-3 p-D-xylopyranoside) respectively; isolation and characterisation of sapindoside C, mp. 235° isolation and structure of sapindoside D; isolation and structure of sapindoside E; quercetin and kaempferol identified; stigmasterol, its glucopyranoside, 28-norolean-12-en-3|3, 17p-diol and 2,23-ethylidene-hederagenin isolated from pericarp of fruits; lauric, palmitic, oleic, stearic and arachic (arachidic) acids also detected.

106. *Sapindus trifoliatus Linn.*

Syn. S. laurifolius Vahl. (Sapindaceae)

- *Common names:* Eng.: Soap nut-tree, Hindi: Reetha, Beng.: Bararitha.

- *Distribution:* Decan.

- *Parts used:* Pulp and seeds.
- *Pharmacological activity:* Pulp and seeds have uterine stimulant activity on isolated guinea pig uterus (24), seeds have anti-implantation activity in female rats[124].
- *Chemical constituents:* Fruit possess emetic, tonic, astringent & anthelmintic properties. Dried fruit contains 11.5% saponin. A new saponin emerginatoside (C^H^O,) m.p. 210-12° has been isolated from the aqueous extract of fruits. Kernels contain 45.4% oil. The oil has the following fatty acid composition; Palmitic 5.4; stearic, 8.5; arachidic, 20.7; behenic, 2.1; oleic, 55.1; and linoleic 8.2%.

107. *Schefflera capitata* (W.& A.) Harms.

Syn. Brassaia capitata (W.& A.) Clarke (Araliaceae)

- *Distribution:* Nilgiri Hills. Tropical & Sub-tropical regions of the world.
- *Parts used:* Whole plant excluding root.
- *Pharmacological activities:* Saponin from plant showed spermicidal activity[150], treatment with whole plant (excluding root) also responded spermicidal activity in human and rats[19], saponin from plant (excluding root) showed spermicidal activity in human semen[20].
- *Chemical constituents:* A new saponin - scheffleraside isolated which on hydrolysis yielded echinocystic acid, fucose, galactose and glucuronic acid in equimolar ratio.

108. *Semecarpus anacardium L.f.* (Anacardiaceae)

- *Common names:* Hindi & Beng.: Bhela, Tel: Bhallataki.
- *Distribution:* Throughout hotter parts of India, also in the foot hills of the Himalayas up to 1100m.
- *Parts used:* Fruit (nut).
- *Pharmacological activities:* See Anti-inflammatory chapter.

109. *Sesamum indicum Linn.*

Syn. S. orientate Linn. (Pedaliaceae)

- *Common names:* Eng.: Sesame, Hindi: Til, Sans.: Tila.
- *Distribution:* Cultivated throughout India.
- *Parts used:* Seeds.

- *Pharmacological activities:* Estrogenic effect in female albino rats has been noted[151].

- *Chemical constituents:* A flavonoid glucoside- pedaliin (0.3%), mp. 254° isolated from leaves.

110. *Sesbania sesban (L.) Marr.*

Syn. *S. aegyptiaca* (Poir.) Pers. (Fabaceae)

- *Common names:* Eng.: Egyptian Rattle Pod, Hindi: Jainti, Beng.: Jainti.

- *Distribution:* Throughout India.

- *Parts used:* Flowers, leaves.

- *Pharmacological activities:* Leaves have no antifertility activity in albino rats and mice[118], Flowers have variety effects, it causes antifertility effect in mice and rats[7] and abortifacient in mice[124], also antifertility response in albino rats and mice has been observed[118].

- *Chemical constituents:* Determination of fatty acid composition of seed oil. Leaves contain good amounts of Protein, Calcium & Phosphorus. At least six flavonols, magnesium and traces of Iron are present. Vitamin C content of seeds is reported to be 89.4 mg/100 mg. Seed extract (with petroleum ether) yields an oil. Oil contains palmitic, 9.0; stearic 17.5; lignoseric, 1.9; oleic, 24.4; Linoleic, 36.3; Linolenic 10.9: acids.

111. *Solatium khasianum C.B. Clarke, emend. Sen Gupta*

Syn. *S. viarum* Dunal (Solanaceae)

- *Common name:* Beng.: Bon-Begun.

- *Distribution:* North-east Himalaya.

- *Parts used:* Whole plant.

- *Pharmacological activities:* Anti-ovulatory effect in rabbits has been observed when treated with alcoholic extract[152].

- *Chemical constituents:* Solasonine, mp. 276°, isolated solasodine and solakhasianin, mp. 251°, isolated from berries.

112. *Solarium xanthocarpum Schrad. & Wendl.*

Syn. *S. surattense* Burm.f.(Solanaceae)

- *Common names:* Eng.: Yellow Berried Nightshade, Hindi: Kateli Kantakari.

- *Distribution:* Throughout W. Bengal.

- *Parts used:* Fruits, stems, leaves, whole plant.

- *Pharmacological activities:* Whole plant responded spermicidal activity in rat semen[19], stem, leaves have no antifertility effect in rats and guinea pigs[120], fruits also have no antifertility activity[153].

- *Chemical constituents:* Contains 1% of alkaloids, can form a source for cordicortisone and sex hormone preparation. A new sterol-carpesterol characterised as (22R) 22- hydroxy-6-oxo-4 cc-methyl-5a-stigmast-7-en-3-p-yl benzoate; scopoletin, esculin and esculetin isolated; solasodine, solasonine, solamargine and p-solamargine in fruits of Nepalese plant; two new sterols-norcarpesterol (22-hydroxy-6-oxo-4-cc-methyl-24-methylcholest-7-en-3-p-yl benzoate) and 4-cc- methyl - 24 -methylcholest-7-en-3-p, 22-diol (I) isolated; dry fruits contained acids and caffeic acids (0.035%); quercetin-3-O-p-D-glucopyranosyl (1-4)-mannopyranoside isolated together with apigenin and sitosterol.

113. *Solidago virgaurea Linn.* **(Asteraceae)**

- *Common name:* Eng.: Woundwort.

- *Distribution:* Plains and Himalayan tracts of Bengal.

- *Parts used:* Whole plant, saponin from whole plant.

- *Pharmacological activity:* Whole plant responded spermicidal activity in human and rat semen[19]. Saponin from whole plant showed spermicidal activity in human semen[20].

- *Chemical constituents:* Quercitrin, rutin, isoquercitrin, astragulin and kaempferol rhamnoghecoside isolated.

114. *Spondias cytherea Sonn.*

Syn. *S. dulcis Soland.* ex. Forst.f. (Anacardiaceae)

- *Common names:* Eng.: Great Hog-plum, Golden apple, Beng.: Bilati Amra.

- *Distribution:* Common in West Bengal. Parts used: Bark.

- *Pharmacological activities:* Bark showed antifertility effect on mice and pigs[154].

- *Chemical constituents:* Analysis of fruits (from the Philippines) gave: moisture, 59.65; protein, 0.80; fat 1.79; sucrose, 8.05; crude fibre, 3.60; and ash 0.65%. Content of carotene in the fruit is 0.26 mg/100g vitamin C. Fruits are also good sources of Iron. Tree exudes a gum composed of d-galactose, l-arabinose, d-xylose, a mono-0-methyl glucuronic acid and traces of l-rhamnose and l-fucose.

115. *Stephania hernaudiifolia* (Willd.) Walp.

Syn. *S. Japonica Miers* (Menispermaceae)

- *Common names:* Eng.: Tape-vine, Beng.: Akanadi, Sans.: Vanatiktika.

- *Distribution:* West Bengal, Orissa, Assam. Parts used: Rhizomes.

- *Pharmacological activities:* Rhizomes have fertility promoting as well as antifertility properties in mice and rats[7]. In other experiments antifertility effect in albino mice and rats[118] have been observed.

- *Chemical constituents:* Alkaloid aknadine. Steponine isolated; protostephanine, mp. 72°, obtained chemically from bromoprotoste-phanine; fangchinoline, mp. 238°, dl-tetrandrine, mp. 257°, d-tetrandrine, mp. 217° and d-isochondrodendrine, mp. 309° isolated from roots; an amorphous alkaloid as 0-acetyl derivative, mp. 113°, from aerial parts; a new alkaloid hernandoline (aknadinine) from herb; new alkaloids aknadine, mp. 133° aknadinine, mp. 70°, aknadicine, mp. 156° and a compound mp. 66° from roots and rhizomes; estimation of aknadine in roots and rhizomes by TLC; isolation and structure elucidation of new alkaloid-4-demethylhasubanonine (aknadinine) from roots; crystal structure of aknadinine determined.

116. *Symplocos gardneriana Wight.* (Symplocaceae)

- *Distribution:* Throughout Bengal.

- *Parts used:* Plant excluding roots.

- *Pharmacological activities:* Spermicidal activity in rat semen has been observed[19].

117. *Taxus baccata Linn. (Taxaceae)*

- *Common names:* Eng.: Common yew, Hindi: Thuno, Beng.: Burmie.

- *Distribution:* W.Bengal, Bihar, U.P., Kashmir.

- *Parts used:* Leaves, Drug mixed with red ochre.

- *Pharmacological activities:* Leaves have various effects on reproductive cycle. It responds anti-implantation activity in albino rats[155], aqueous extract shows anti-implantation activity in albino rats[156] also anti-ovulatory activity in rabbits[157], no uterine stimulant activity in isolated guinea pig uterus[64], the same effect in rats and Guinea pigs[120]: When the drug mixed with red ochre female albino rats showed some antifertility effects[67].

- *Chemical constituents:* Chemical studies on taxine, isolated from leaves; a flavonoid mp. 294°, isolated from leaves, similar in many respects to sciadopitysin; two new biflavones- isomers of sciadopitysin (I) and sotetsuflavone (II) mp. 212° and 300°, respectively isolated from leaves; both compounds yielded same demethyl derivative; rhodoxanthin and eschscholtzxanthone from fruits; (3-sitosterol a methoxytriterpene (baceatine), mp. 219°, and a compound D, mp. 161°, from root bark; p-sitosterol also isolated from wood, bark and leaves.

118. *Terminalia arjuna Wight & Arn.* **(Combretaceae)**

- *Common names:* Eng.: Arjun, Beng.: Arjun, Hindi: Maruthu, Kahu, Arjun.

- *Distribution:* Throughout West Bengal and some other regions in India.

- *Parts used:* Bark.

- *Pharmacological activity:* In female rats' antifertility effect has been observed

- *Chemical constituents:* Arjunolic acid, tomentosic acid, p-sitosterol, jellagic acid, (+) leucodelphinidin and a saponin, mp. 216°, isolated along with an ester, mp. 87°;

saponin on hydrolysis yielded arjunoiic acid and glucose; structure of arjunoiic acid confirmed by synthesis.

119. *Terminalia bellirica Roxb.* **(Combretaceae)**

- *Common names:* Eng.: Belleric myrobalan, Hindi: Bahera, Beng.: Bhairah.
- *Distribution:* Throughout India.
- *Parts used:* Fruits.
- *Pharmacological activities:* Fruits have spermicidal activity in rat semen[19] saponin from fruit showed spermicidal activity in human semen[20].
- *Chemical constituents:* A new cardiac glycoside-bellericanin isolated which yielded glucose and gaiactose. Heartwood, bark and fruits contain ellagic acid and the seed-coat of the fruit contains gallic acid.

120. *Trifolium alexandrinum Linn.* **(Fabaceae)**

- *Common names:* Hindi: Berseem, Eng.: Egyptian clover, Barseem.
- *Distribution:* An important forage crop in Punjab, Kangra in H.P. and Western U.P., also cultivated in small scale in M.P., Bihar, Maharashtra, Tamil Nadu and Karnataka.
- *Parts used:* Seeds.
- *Pharmacological activities:* In rats estrogenic activity has been observed[98].
- *Chemical constituents:* l-Ascorbic acid and reducing sugar content during growth and successive cuttings. Biochanin A (0.013), genistein (0.025%) and formononetin found in plant; coumesterol also isolated.

121. *Trigonella foenum-graecum Linn.* **(Fabaceae)**

- *Common names:* Eng.: Fenugreek, Hindi: Methi, Beng.: Methi.
- *Distribution:* Throughout India.
- *Parts used:* Seeds, saponin from seeds.
- *Pharmacological activities:* Causes ecbolic effect in mice and rats[21], in other experiments aqueous extract causes immobilization of human and bovine spermafozoa[40] and

spermicidal activity in human and rat semen[19] has been observed saponin from seed showed spermicidal activity in human semen[19].

- *Chemical constituents:* Two flavonoid glycosides, quercetin and luteolin, and two steroidal saponins from seeds identified by PC.

122. *Uraria lagopodioides* (L.) Desv.

Syn. U. lagopoides D.C. (Fabaceae)

- *Common names:* Hindi: Petwan, Beng.: Golak Chakulia, Tel.:Kolaponna.

- *Distribution:* W. Bengal, Bihar, Maharashtra and Pulni Hills.

- *Parts used:* Whole plant.

- *Pharmacological activities:* Aqueous extract of the plant showed anti-implantation activity in albino rats[156].

123. *Vitex negundo Linn.* (Verbenaceae)

- *Common names:* Hindi: Sambhalu, Beng.: Nisinda, Sans.: Nirgundi.

- *Distribution:* Throughout India.

- *Parts used:* Roots and seeds.

- *Pharmacological activities:* Roots have less antifertility activity in rats, but seeds have significant anti-ovulatory activity in rats[158].

- *Chemical constituents:* n-Tritriacontane, n-hentriacontane, n-nonacosane, (3-sitosterol, P-hydroxybenzoic acid and 5-oxyisophthalic acid from seeds; 3, 4 dihydroxybenzoic acid also isolated; vanillic and p-hydroxybenzoic acids and luteolin isolated from bark; two new leuco-anthocyanidins isolated from stem bark and their structures determined as 6, 8-di-O-methyllecodelphinidin and 3', 4'-di-0-methylleucocyanidin-7-0 rhamnoglucoside.

124. *Withania somnifera Dunal.* (Solanaceae)

- *Common names:* Eng.: Ashvaganda, Hindi: Asgand, Beng.: Ashvaganda.

- *Distribution:* Under shrub, found in drier parts of India.

- *Parts used:* Roots and tuber roots.

- *Pharmacological activities:* Roots have infertility in mice and did not completely abolish oestrus or mating but it delayed the processes. Roots -have also affect to produce infertile mating and caused a decrease in litter size[82], tuber roots have no uterine stimulant activity on isolated guinea pig uterus.

- *Chemical constituents:* The water-soluble extract of root contains black resin which contained hentriacontane, $C_{31}H_{64}$, a phytosterol, $C_{27}H_{46}0$ (mp 135-36°), a mixture of fatty acids consisting of palmitic, stearic, cerotic, oleie acids etc. A C-28 steroid lactone isolated from roots and identified as, 5, 20a-dihydro-6a, 7a-cpoxy-1-oxowitha-2,24-dienolide (withanolide); nine new steroidal lactones-withanolides E, F, G, H, H, I, J, K, L and M-isolated from leaves; seven of these characterised as 20 hydroxy-1-oxo-20R, 22R-witha-2,5,8(14), 24-tetraenolide (Withanolide G), 20,27-dihydroxy-1-oxo-20R, 22R-witha-2, 5, 8(14),24-tetraeno-lide (Withanolide H), 20-hydroxy-1-oxo-20R, 22R-witha, 3, 5, 8(14), 24-tetraenolide (withanolide I), 17,20-dihydroxy-1-oxo-20S,20R-witha2,5, 8(14),24-tetra-enolide (withanolide J),17,20-dihydroxy-1-oxo-20S, 22R-witha-3,5,8(14),24-tetraenolide (withanolide K), 17,20-dihydroxy-1-oxo-20S, 22R-witha-2, 5,14, 24-tetraenolide (withanolide L) and 17, 20-dihydroxy-1-oxo-14,15a-epoxy 205, 22R-witha 2, 5, 24-trienolide (withanolide M); another withanolide-WS-1 isolated from seeds.

125. *Woodfordia fruticosa Kurz*

Syn. W. floribunda Salisb. (Lythraceae)

- *Common names:* Eng.: Fire-Flame Bush, Hindi: Dawi, Beng.: Dhai.

- *Distribution:* Throughout India.

- *Parts used:* Flowers.

- *Pharmacological activity:* Abortifacient effect in mice has been observed[2].

- *Chemical constituents:* Ellagic acid, polystachoside, myricetin-3-galactoside and pelargonidin-3, 5-diglucoside isolated from leaves and flowers. Cyanidin-3, 5-diglucoside isolated from flowers; octacosanol, p-sitosterol and chrysophanol-8-O-p-D-glucopyranoside isolated from flowers.

References

1. Tewari, P.V., Mapa, H.C & Chaturvedi, C., *J.Res. Indian Med. Yoga & Homeop.*, (1976), 11(4), 7.

2. Pakrashi, A., Basak, B. & Mookherjee, N., *Indian J. Med.Res.*, (1975), 63, 378.

3. Mishra, M.B., Tiwari, J.P. & Mishra, S.S, *Indian J. Physiol. Pharmacol.*, (1966), 10, 3.

4. Desai, R.V. & Rupawala, E.N., *Indian J.Pharm..* (1967), 29, 235.

5. Das, P.C., Brit. 10, 25, 372, April 6, 1966, *Chem Abstr.*, (1966), 64, 19328h.

6. Prakash, A.O. & Mathur, R, *Indian J. Exp* Bio/., (1976), 14, 623.

7. Bhaduri, B., Ghosh, C.R., Bose, A.M., Moza, B.K. & Basu, U.P., *Indian J. Phartn.*, (1967), 29, 346.

8. Desai, V.B. & Sirsi, M., Curt. Set., (1964), 33, 585.

9. Desai, R.V. & Rupawala, E.N., Indian J. Pharma., (1966), 28, 344.

10. Pakrashi, A. & Bhattacharya, N, Indian J. Exp. Biol., (1977), 15(10), 856.

11. Dixit, S.K. & Bhatt, G.K., J. Res. Indian Med., (1975), 10, 77.

12. Gupta, O.P., Anand, K.K., Ghatak, B. J & Atal, C.K., Indian J. Exp. Biol., (1978), 16(10), 1075.

13. Gupta, O.P., Sharma, Ml., Anand, K.K., Ghatak, B.J.R. & Atal, C.K., Indian J. Pharm.,(1976), 38,169,Abstr. C. 53.

14. Bhaduri, B., Ghosh, C.R., Bose, A.M., Moza, B.K. & Basu, U.P., Indian J. Exp. Biol.,(1968), 6(4), 252.

15. Setty, B.S., Kamboj, V.P.& Khanna, N.M., Indian J. Exp. Biol., (1977), 15, 231.

16. Setty, B.S., Kamboj, V.P., Garg, H.S & Khanna, N.M., Contraception, (1976), 14, 571.

17. Vohora, S.B. & Khan, M., S.Y., Indian J. Pharm, (1974), 36, 77.

18. Dhar, Ml., Dharm, M.M., Dhawan, B.N., Mehrotra, B.N. & Ray.C., Indian J. Exp.Biol., (1968), 6(4), 232.

19. Setty, B.S., Kamboj, V.P. & Khanna, N.M., Indian J. Exp. Biol, (1977), 15, 231.

20. Setty, B.S., Kamboj, V.P., Garg, H.S. & Khanna, N.M., Contraception, (1976), 14, 571.

21. Sharaf, A., Qua/if. Plant. Mat. Veg., (1969), 17, 153.

22. Tewari, P.V., Mapa, H.C. & Chaturvedi, C., J. Res. Indian Med. Yoga & Homeop.,(1976), 11(4), 7.

23. Gupta, Ml., Gupta, T.K. & Bhargava, K.P., J. Res. Indian Med., (1971), 6(2), 112.

24. Goswami, C.S. & Bokadia, M.M., *Indian Drugs,* (1979), 16(6), 124.

25. Sharma, S.C., Chadha, H. & Burjorjee, M.N., The effect of Aloe Mica on the fertilityof female rabbits. Proc. XVI All India Obstetric & Gynaecological Congren, New Delhi, 1972.

26. lamwal, K.S. & Anand, K.K., Indian J. Pharm., (1962), 24(9), 231.

27. Garg, S.K., Saksena, S.K. & Choudhury, R.R., Indian J. Med. Res., (1970), 58,1285.

28. Feurt, S.D. & Fox, I.E., Science, (1955), 121, 42.

29. Garg, S.K & Garg, G.P., Indian J. Med. Res., (1970), 59, 302.

30. Garg, S.K. & Garg, G.P., Indian J. Pharmacol., (1971), 3, 23.

31. Garg, S.K., Planta Med., (1974), 26, 391.

32. Pakrashi, A. & Chakrabarty, B. Indian J. Exp. BioL, (1978), 16(12), 1283.

33. Pakrashi, A. & Pakrasi, P., Indian J. Exp. BioL, (1978), 16(12), 1285.

34. Pakrashi, A. & Shaha, C, Experentia, (1978), 34(9), 1192.

35. Pakrashi, A. & Chakrabarty, B., Experentia, (1978), 34(10), 1377.

36. Pakrashi, A. & Shaha, C., Indian J. Exp. Biol., (1977), 15, 1197.

37. Chakrabarty, B., Choudhuri, A. & Choudhury, P.R., J. Indian Med. Ass., (1968), 51, 227.

38. Prakash, A.O., Indian J. Exp. Biol., (1978), 16(11), 1214.

39. Prakash, A.O. & Mathur, R., Probe, (1977), 16,115.

40. Rath, R.K. & Mohanty, B.N., J. Res. Bhubanewar, (1972), 1,177.

41. Sharma, V.N., & Saksena, K. P., Indian J. Med. Res., (1959), 47, 322.

42. Sharma, V.N., & Saksena, K.P., Man J. Med. Sci., (1959), 13, 1038.

43. Mishra, M.B, Tiwari, J. P. & Misra, S.S., Indian J. Physiol. Pharmacol., (1966), 10, 3.

44. Jain, S.K. & Pal, D.C. Cultivation & Utilization of Medicinal Plants, Reg. Res. Lab. Jammu -7am, C.S.I.R. ed C.K. Atal & B.M. Kapur, (1982), 543, 550, 552.

45. Sachdev, K.S., Roy, P.B., Vasudeva, S.A., Dave, K.C. & Jaseph, A.D., Indian J. Pharma., (1965), 28, 253.

46. Khanna, U. Handa, S. & Choudhury, R.R., Indian J. Pharm., (1966), 28, 343.

47. Laumas, K.R. & Uniyal, J.P., Indian J. Exp, Biol., (1966), 4, 246.

48. Khanna, U, & Choudhury, R.R., Indian J. Med, Res., (1968), 56, 1575.

49. Lai, B., Srivastava, R.N. & Udupa, K.N., Indian Med. Yoga Homeop., (1976), 11,112.

50. Khanna, U. & Choudhury, R.R., Indian J. Med, Res., (1968), 56,1575.

51. Bhide, M.B., Nikam, S.T. & Chavan, S.R., 16th Annual Conference Ass. Physiol, Pharmacol., India, 28.

52. Madan, B.R., Arch. int. Pharmacodyn, (1960), 124, 358.

53. East, J., J. Endocrinol., (1955), 12, 267.

54. Garg, S.K., Planta Med., (1974), 26,391.

55. Sareen, K., Mishra, N., Verma, D.R., Amma, M.K.P. & Gujral, Ml., Indian J. Physiol.Pharmacol., (1961), 5, 125.

56. Dhar, Ml., Dharm, M.M., Dhawan, B.N., Mehrotra, B.N. & Ray, C., Indian J. Exp.Biol., (1968), 6(4), 232.

57. Bose, J. L. & Chandran, K, J. Sci. Industr. Res., (1955), 14C, 128.

58. Bose, Jl. & Chandran, K., J. Industr. Res., (1954), 13B, 88.

59. Deb, C., Biswas, N.M. & Paul, B., Hohnemannian Gleanings, (1977), 44, 177.

60. Shamer Singh, Sanyal, A.K., Bhattacharya, S.K. & Pandey, V.B., Indian J. Med. Res.,(1972), 60,287.

61. Tewari, P.V., Chaturvedi, C. & Pandey, V.B., Indian J. Pharm., (1973), 35,114.

62. Tewari, P.V., Sharma, P.V., Prasad, D.N. & Pandey, V.B., J.Res. Indian Med., (1972), 7, 14.

63. Tewari, P.V., Sharma, P.V., Prasad, D.N., Pandey, V.B. & Chaturvedi, C., Med. Surg.Baroda, (1972), 12, 17.

64. Jamwal, K. S. & Anand, K. K., Indian J. Pharm., (1962), 24(9), 231.

65. Garg, S.K., Planta Med. Res., (2976), 64, 1133.

66. Garg, S.K, Planta Med., (1974), 26, 225.

67. Garg, S.K, Bull. Postgraduate Inst. Med. Education & Res., Chandigarh, (1971), 5,178.

68. Indira, M, Sirsi, M, Radomir, S. & Dev, S., J. Sci. Industr. Res., (1956), 15C, 202.

69. Sharma, M.M., Gopal Lai & Jacob, D, Indian J. Exp. Biol., (1976), 14, 506.

70. Dhar, V.J, Mathur, V.S. & Garg, S.K, Planta Med., (1975), 28, 12.

71. Dhar, J, Mathur V.S. & Garg, S.K, Indian J. Pharmacol., (1973), 5, 259.

72. Garg, S.K, Indian J. Pharmacol., (1973), 5, 272.

73. Garg, R.P, Farooq, A, Sharma, R.C, Gupta, S.P. & Arora, R.B., Indian J. Pharmacol., (1973), 5, 282.

74. Gupta, S.P, Ghatale, N, Farooq, A. & Arora, R.B., Indian J. Pharmacol., (1972), 4, 101.

75. Garg, S.K, Mathur, V.S, Choudhury, R.R, Indian J. Exp. Biol., (1978), 16, 1077.

76. Khan, R, Asif, M. & Tariq, M, Nagarjun, (1977), 21(4), 8.

77. Kaliwal, B.B. & Appaswamy Rao, M, J. Karnatak Univ. (ScL), (1977), 12, 167.

78. Lai, B, Udupa, K.N. & Singh, R.H., J. Res. Indian Med. yoga Homeop, (1979), 14(1), 128.

79. Olarto, J., Mora, M.V., Velencia, D., Guaqueta, M., Prjuella, M., Moya, M., Gonzalex,C. & Forero, I.C. Abstract paper presented at 24th meeting of the International Congress for Research on Medicinal plants, Munich, Section A, 6-10, Sept. 1976.

80. Arora, R.B., Gharak, N. & Gupta, S.P., J. Res. Indian Med., (1971), 6, 107.

81. Chakravarty, H.S., Indian J. Med. Res., (1961), 57, 322.

82. Parasar, G.C., Thesis for M.V. Sc (Pharmacology) Degree, Vikram Univ. Ujjain, 1963.

83. Radhakrishnan, N. & Muzaffer Alam., Indian J. Exp. Bio!., (1975), 13, 70.

84. Rathinam, K., Santhakumari, G. & Ramiah, N., J. Res. Indian Med. Yoga Homoep., (1976), 11,84.

85. Das, P.C., Brit. 10, 25, 372, April 6, 1966., Chem. Abstr., (1966), 64, 19328h.

86. Prakash, A.O., Planta Med., (1979), 35(4), 370.

87. Kholkute, S.D, Kekare, M.B., Jathar, V.S. & Munshi, S.R., Indian J. Exp. Biol., (1978), 16(10), 1035.

88. Raman, G, Munshi, S.R. & Rao, S.S, Indian J. Med. Res., (1976), 64, 959.

89. Amonkar, A.J., Trivedi, G.K. & Bhattacharya, S.C., Indian J. Chem., (1978), 16B(1), 12.

90. Banerjee, S.P. & Damdiya, P.O., Indian J. Physiol. Pharmacol., (1966), 10, 7.

91. Prasad, D.N., Gode, K.D., Sinha, P.S. & Das, P.K., Indian J. Physiol. Pharmacol., (1966), 10, 9.

92. Saha, J.C., Savini, E.G. & Kashinathan, S., Indian J. Med. Res., (1961), 49(1), 130.

93. Pakrashi, A., Ann. Biochem. Exp. Med, (1963), 23, 73.

94. Pakrashi, A., Indian J. Exp. Biol., (1967), 5, 75.

95. Pakrashi, A., Indian J. Exp. Biol., (1967), 5, 167.

96. Pakrashi, A., Ann. Biochem, Exp, Med., (1963), 23, 357.

97. Chakravarty, H. S., Indian J. Med. Res., (1961), 57, 322.

98. Sharaf, A. & Gomaa, N., Qualit. Plant. Mat. Veg., (1971), 20, 271.

99. Kholkute, S.D., Chatterjee, S., Srivastava, D.N. & Udapa, K.N., J. Res. Indian Med., (1972), 7, 72.

100. Kholkute, S.D. & Udupa, K.N., Planta Med., (1976), 29, 321.

101. Kholkute, S.D. & Udapa, K.N., Indian J. Exp. Biol., (1976), 14, 175.

102. Tiwari, P.V., J. Res. Indian Med., (1974), 9, 96.

103. Kholkute, S.D., Chatterjee, S. & Udupa, K.N., Indian J. Exp. Biol., (1976), 14, 703.

104. Kholkute, S.D. & Udupa, K.N., J. Res. Indian Med., (1974), 9, 99.

105. Batta, S.K. & Santhakumari, G., Indian J. Med. Res., (1971), 59, 777.

106. Kholkute, S.D. & Udupa, K.N., J. Res. Indian Med. Yoga Homeop., (1978), 13(3), 107.

107. Joshi, M.S., Ambaye, R.Y. & Panse, T.B., Indian J. Exp. Biol., (1965), 3, 206.

108. Mameesh, M.S., El-Hakim, LM. & Hassan, A., Planta Med., (1963), 11, 98.

109. Wiesner, B.P. & Yudhin, J. Nature, Lond., (1952), 170, 274.

110. Cranston, E.M., J. Pharmacol. Exp. Therap., (1945), 83, 130.

111. Drasher, Ml. & Zahl, P.A., Proc. Soc. Exp. Biol. Med., (1946), 63, 66.

112. United States Department of Agriculture - A Treatise on Medicinal Uses of Plants., used by Indian Tribes of Niveda, 1951.

113. Zahl, P.A., Proc. Soc. Exp. Biol. Med., (1948), 67, 405.

114. Cranston, E.M. & Robinson, G.A., Proc. Soc. Exp. Biol. Med., (1949), 70, 66.

115. Plundett, E.R., Calpitts, R.V. & Noble, R.L, Proc. Soc. Exp. Biol. Med., (1950), 73, 311.

116. Sketton, F.R. & Grant, G.A., Amer. J. Physiol., (1951), 167, 372.

117. Gujrat, Ml., Verma, D.R., Sareen, K.N. & Roy, A.K., Indian J. Med. Res., (1960), 48, 52.

118. Bhaduri, B., Ghosh, C.R., Bose, A.N., Moza, B.K. and Basu, U.P., Indian J. Exp. Biol., (1968), 6(4), 252.

119. Verma, D.R., Sareen, K.N., Roy, A.K. & Gujral, Ml., Indian J. Physiol. Pharmacol., (1959), 3, 246.

120. Gujral, Ml., Verma, D.R. & Sareen, K.N, Indian J. Med. Res., (1960), 48, 46.

121. Mohsin, M. & Paul, A.K, Indian J. Exp. Biol., (1977), 15, 76.

122. Garg, S.K, Mathur, V.S, Choudhury, R.R., Indian J. Exp. Biol., (1978), 16, 1077.

123. Kholkute, S.D, Mudgal, V. & Deshpande, P.J., Planta Med., (1976), 29(2), 151.

124. Bodhankar, S.L, Garg, S.K. & Mathur, V.S, Indian J. Med. Res., (1974), 62(6), 831.

125. Kapoor, M, Garg, S.K. & Mathur, V.S, Indian J. Med. Res., (1974), 62, 1225.

126. Bodhankar, S.L, Garg, S.K. & Mathur, V.S, Bull. Postgrauate Inst. Med. Education & Res., Chandigarh, (1971), 5, 66.

127. Saksena, S.K, Indian J. Physiol. Pharmacol., (1971), 15, 79.

128. Vohora, S.B, Garg, S.K. & Choudhury, R.R, Indian J. Med. Res., (1969), 57(5), 893.

129. Sharaf, A. & Gomaa, N, Quas//f. Plant. Mat. Veg., (1971), 20, 271.

130. Tewari, J.P., Datta, K.C. & Mishra, S.S, Labdev, (1964), 2, 117.

131. Das, P.C, Brit. 10, 25, 372, April 6, 1966, Chem. Abstr., (1966), 64, 19328h.

132. Kholkute, S.D., Kekare M.B., & Munshi, S.R., Indian J. Exp. Biol., (1979), 17(3), 289.

133. Chandhoke, N., Gupta, S. & Dhar, S., Indian J. Pharm, Sci., (1978), 40(4), 113.

134. Sanyal, S.N., Calcutta Med. J., (1950), 47, 313.

135. Sanyal, S.N., Calcutta Med. J., (1951), 48, 399.

136. Sanyal, S.N., Calcutta Med. J., (1952), 49, 353.

137. Noble, R.L & Grahani, R.C.B., Canad. Med. Ass. J., (1953), 69, 576.

138. Batra, K.B. & Hakim, S., J. Endocrinol., (1956), 14, 228.

139. Thiersch, J.B., Acta Endocrinol. Copenhagen. Suppl., (1956), 28, 46.

140. Sanyal, S.N., Sci. & Cult., (1949), 15,159.

141. Mishra, M.B., Tiwari, JP. & Bapat, S.K., Labdev, (1966), 4, 55.

142. East, J., J. Endocrinol., (1955), 12, 252.

143. Prakash, A.O. & Mathur, R., Indian J. Exp. Biol., (1976), 14, 623.

144. Barnes, C.S., Price, J.R. & Hughes, R.L., Uoydia, (1975), 38(2), 135.

145. East, J., J. Endocrinol., (1955), 12, 261.

146. Vohra, S.B., Khan, M.S.Y., & Afaq, S.H., Indian J. Pharm., (1970), 32, 164.

147. Pillai, N.R., Alam, M.& Purushothaman, K.K., J. Res. Indian Med. Yogo & Homoep, (1977), 12(3), 26.

148. Purshottam, V., Amer. J. Obstet. Gynec., (1962), 83, 1405.

149. Gupta, Ml., Gupta, IK. & Bharganva, K.P., J. Res. Indian Med., (1971), 6(2), 112.

150. Jain, G.K., Sar, J.P.S & Khanna, N.M., Indian J. Pharm., (1976), 38, 158, abstr. B33.

151. Tewari, P.V., Mapa, H.C. & Chaturvedi. C., J. Res. IndianMed. Yoga. Homoep., (1976), 11 (4), 7.

152. Kohli, R.P., Singh, N. & Srivastava, R.K., J. Res. Indian Med., (1971), 6, 125.

153. Dhar, Ml., Dharm, M.M., Dhawan, B.N., Mehrotra, B.N. & Ray, C., Indian J. Exp.Biol., (1968), 6(4), 232.

154. Olarto, J., Mora, M.V., Valencia, D., Guaqueta, M. Orijuella, M. Moya, M., Gonzalex, C. & Forero, I.C. Abstract of papers presented at 24th Meeting of the International Congress for Research on Medicinal Plants, Munich, Section A, 6-10 Sept, 1976.

155. Garg, S.K., Indian. J.Med. Res., (1972), 60,159.

156. Khanna, U., Garg, S.K., Vohora, S.B., Walia, H.B. & Choudhury, R.R., Indian J. Med.Res., (1969), 57(2), 237.

157. Choudhury, A.R., Saksena, S.K. & Garg, S.K., J. Reprod. Fertil., (1970), 22, 151.

158. Vohra, S.B., Khan, M.S.Y. & Afaq, S.H., Indian J. Pharm., (1973), 35(3), 100.3

4 Medicinal Plants with Hepato-Protective Properties

The liver is perhaps the most impressive organ in the body in size and in the diversity of its activities. As with several other vital organs, such as the kidneys or lungs, the amount of tissue in the liver seems to be superabundant. If need be, we can lose three quarters of our liver cells without a perceptible failure of function.

The liver of a healthy young adult weighs about four times as much as his heart or two kidneys. It is enclosed in a smooth membrane line a capsule and is flat, with a rounded dome which fits against the curved diaphragm. Human liver has about the same appearance as beef liver. Since it stores many substances, and converts them into modified forms as well, its size varies with nutrition and age.

The liver lies in the upper right quarter of the abdominal cavity and is covered for the most part by the lower ribs. Its left lobe, which is not a clear division, overlies part of the stomach and the duodenum. The right adrenal gland and the upper pole of the kidney lie against the underside of its right lobe. The gallbladder is partly embedded in its mid-lower expanse near the hilum, where the great vascular trunks enter, and the bile duct drain the liver.

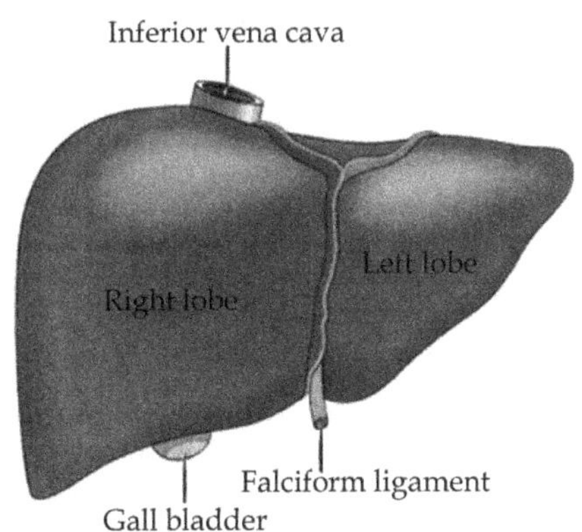

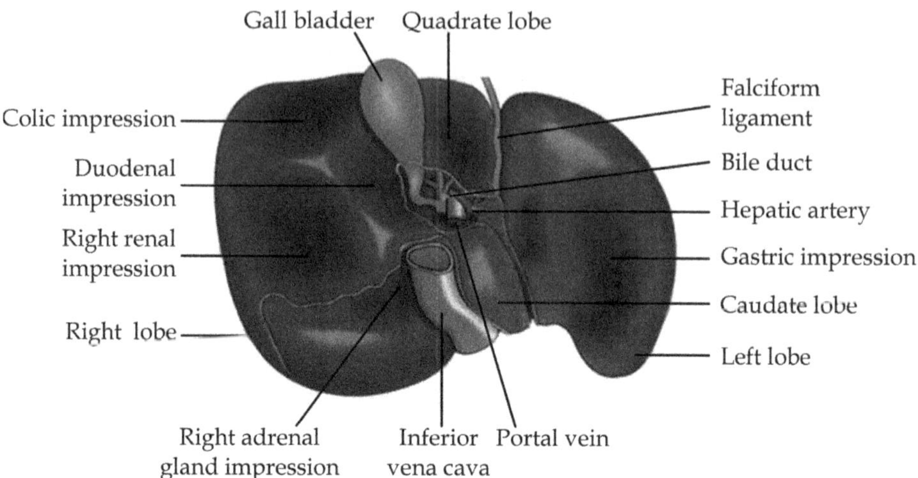

Fig. 4.1 Liver, a. Anterior and b. Posterior.

There are various ways of describing the structure of the liver, but its pattern is most easily explained in relation to its unique blood supply. The portal venous system, which contributes the greatest quantity of blood to the liver, is a shuttle from the gastrointestinal tract and the spleen and pancreas directly to the liver. All other venous blood in the body returns to the right side of the heart, by way of the venae cavae. The portal blood, carrying products of absorption from the intestine, and iron from the breakdown of blood in the spleen, supplies the liver with a full measure of metabolites for its many duties of synthesis, degradation, and storage. But this blood, being venous, is not sufficiently oxygenated and must be joined by blood flowing from the aorta by way of the hepatic artery. These large blood vessels - the portal vein and the hepatic artery - branch through the liver side by side, but as they divide into their finest ramifications their two types of blood mix. Thus, the ultimate functioning unit, the cord of liver cells, stretches along a delicate walled sinus, or channel, which contains the richest blood in the body. A series of these sinuses and liver cords converge toward a central lobular vein which, as its name suggests, can be regarded as the center of a functioning group, or lobule. A single lobule of the human liver is about the size of the head of a pin. Its periphery is ill-defined and merges with the borders of adjacent lobules.

Anatomy of Liver

On histological examination the liver appears to be comprised of radical columns of cells arranged in lobules around a central efferent vein. At the periphery of the lobules lie portal tracts, each having a small branch of the hepatic artery and of the portal vein and a small bile duct. Between the columns of liver cells are sinusoids lined with cells of the reticulo-endothelial system known as Kupffer cells. Small bile canaliculi lie between the liver cells, forming a network which opens ultimately into the interlobular ducts situated in the portal tracts.

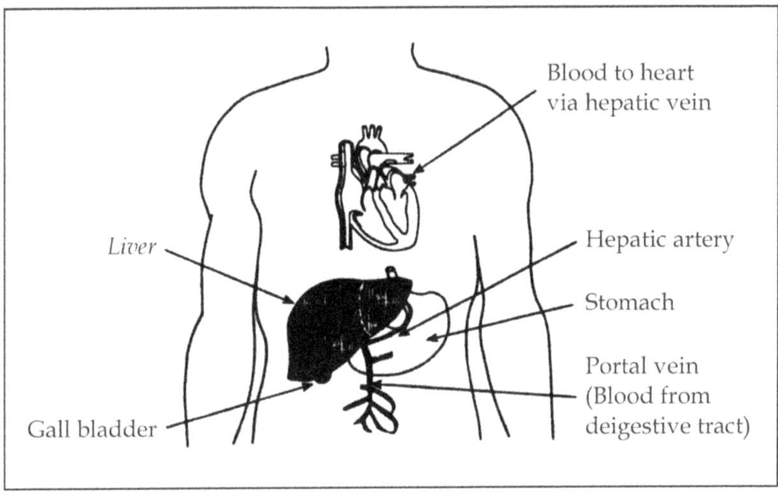

Fig. 4.2 Blood to heart via hepatic vein.

From the portal vein and from the hepatic artery in the portal tract, blood passes into the sinusoids and reaches the central vein, which drains into the hepatic veins. Mixing of portal venous and hepatic arterial blood appears to take place in the sinusoids. When the usual architecture of the liver, including presinusoidal sphincters on the arterioles, is spoiled by disease, direct transmission of the high arterial pressure to the portal system may be hardly responsible for the portal venous hypertension found in such circumstances.

Bile, secreted by the liver cells, passes, in opposite direction to the blood flow, through canaliculi to the periphery of the lobule. There, the bile ducts are lined with cuboidal epithelium and progressively become larger as they advance to the porta hepatis. Finally, the common hepatic duct is formed by the union of the ducts from the right and left lobes of the liver, and this, with the cystic duct from the gallbladder, forms the common bile duct. This usually traverses the substance of the head of the pancreas, where it is connected, in the majority of cases, by the pancreatic duct. The united ducts then open into the second part of the duodenum through the ampulla of Vater, the opening being controlled by the sphincter of Oddi.

Blood Supply

The liver is unique in that the greater part of the blood flowing to it is venous and comes via the portal vein which drains the large and small intestine, stomach, pancreas and spleen. The total blood flow through the adult human liver averages 1,500 ml/minute. This often becomes considerably reduced in chronic hepatic disease. Though the hepatic artery supplies only about 20 per cent of the blood to the liver, it carries up to 50 per cent of the oxygen used by the organ. The large supply of venous blood results in an oxygen supply that is probably always dangerous, so that the liver is susceptible to chronic hypoxia. In chronic passive congestion, for instance, there is degeneration and sometimes necrosis of the cells furthest from the entry of well-aerated blood, i.e. in the center of lobule. Contrilobilar necrosis is found also in thyrotoxicosis, in which the oxygen demand by the liver cells is increased. In addition, in the majority of acute toxic or infective liver diseases, in which there is neither hypoxia nor excessive oxygen utilization, necrosis in this zone is generally found. Damage to the parenchymal cells in these circumstances may be aggravated by the relative oxygen shortage in the center of the lobule.

The blood supply to the liver through the portal vein is believed to follow two main streams, one from the stomach, spleen and descending colon to the left, and other from the small intestine and ascending colon to the right lobe. This distribution of blood does not conform strictly to the anatomical lobes of the liver. Acute massive necrosis, which may in part, at least, be due to dietary deficiency, may show damage predominantly in the left lobe, presumably because essential dietary constituents are especially deficient in blood draining the stomach, spleen, and descending colon. Similarly, abscesses from an infected appendix occur mainly in the right lobe.

Activities of the Liver

The manner in which blood gains deep-rooted contact with hepatic cells facilitates the speedy transfer of metabolites. Apart from the Kupffer cells of the reticuloendothelial system, all the cells of the liver are similar and appear capable of performing the many functions of the liver. It plays an important role in the sustenance of internal environment through its multiple diverse functions. It involved in the intermediary metabolism of proteins, fats and carbohydrates[1] and in the synthesis of number of plasma proteins. Such as albumin, fibrinogen and clotting factors in the production of varies enzymes and development and excretion of bile.

1. **Metabolism of Carbohydrate**

   The liver is the important organ in the body for the maintenance of a normal concentration of blood glucose. It is able to convert glucose, fructose, galactose, glycerol, certain amino acid residues, and 2-and 3-carbon compound (e.g. lactate, pyruvate and oxalo-acetate) to glycogen. In hypoglycemia it hydrolyses stored glycogen to glucose. These mechanisms are inherent functions of the organ, but they are influenced by many extrahepatic factors, e.g. insulin, adrenaline, thy-roxin, cortisol and glucagon.

2. **Metabolism of Protein**

   The liver is the most important site of deamination of amino acids, as a introductory step in their interconversion and oxidation. Urea synthesis from the amino groups made available by this method occurs solely in the organ. Plasma albumin, prothrombin, fibrinogen and the other clotting factors, V, VII, IX and X are synthesized perhaps solely in the parenchymal cells of the liver, alfa and beta globulin are mainly formed in the liver, while gamma globulin is formed by cells of the reticulo-endothelial system. As a result of these synthesis, the protein pattern of the plasma is to a large extent determined by liver function.

3. **Metabolism of Lipid**

   The liver plays an important part in fat metabolisms. Fats are oxidized in the liver insofar as the four-carbon chain stage (ketone bodies). The amount of this oxidation depends, inter alia, upon the availability of carbohydrate and is severely increased when sugar is absent as in fasting or when there is difficulty in its use as in diabetes mellitus. The ketone bodies themselves do not appear to be oxidized in the liver and are released into the blood stream for peripheral oxidation. Triglycerides are created in the liver and synthesis of phospholipid from fatty acid, glycerol, phosphate and a nitrogenous base, e.g. choline, also occurs largely in the liver. Cholesterol is synthesized in the liver and is also esterified there. Cholesterol and triglycerides circulate in the blood as lipoproteins; not only is the liver and important source of these complexes which maintain lipid in colloidal solution, but also it contains an enzyme which can break the lipid-protein bond. Bile salts, the breakdown products of cholesterol, are synthesized in the liver cells and in turn assist the excretion of cholesterol in the bile.

4. Metabolism of Vitamins

The liver is directly or indirectly concerned with the metabolism of many vitamins. Fat-soluble vitamins rely to some extent for their absorption upon a normal biliary secretion. Vitamin K is required by the hepatic cells for the production of prothrombin and factor VII. The liver contains enzymes and prosthetic groups. The phosphorylation of thiamin, which is a necessary prior to its function as a coenzyme, the methylation of nicotinic acid and the 25-hydroxylation of vitamin D also occur in the liver.

5. Hormones Inactivation

Estrogen, corticosteroids and other steroid hormones are conjugated in the liver with glucuronic acid and excreted in the urine, though other forms of inactivation also occur. Thyroxin and vasopressin are probably inactivated in the liver, but the mechanisms are unknown.

6. Drugs Detoxification

The liver plays a critical role in the detoxification of drugs as well as endogenous hormones. This is accomplished by enzyme systems of broad specificity located on the endoplasmic reticulum (microsomal enzymes). At these sites the drugs are rendered more water soluble and can then be excreted in the bile and urine. Alkaloids such as morphine or atropine are partially destroyed in the liver, ammonia is converted to urea, barbiturates suffer oxidation of their side chain and are rendered pharmacologically inert. Conjugation with glucuronic acid occurs with salicylates, morphine and chloral hydrate, and these conjugates are less active than their precursors. Acetylation of sulphonamides also occurs though this method makes these drugs less soluble and potentially more harmful.

The duration and power of action of many drugs are largely determined by the speed at which they are metabolized by these microsomal enzymes of the liver. The activity of the enzymes can be modified by dietary and nutritional factors or alterations in hormonal balance. The activities of the enzymes may also be markedly increased by the simultaneous administration of drugs. This increase in activity appears to symbolize an increased concentration of enzyme protein; it is referred to as enzyme induction and may be of great importance in man because of the consequent alteration in duration and intensity of drug action. This enzyme induction may have important therapeutic implications, e.g. a decreased response to coumarin anticoagulants whilst taking barbiturates followed by a considerably diminished dose requirement on withdrawal of the barbiturate. Besides, some drugs can stimulate their own metabolism, an effect which may explain the increased tolerance for alcohol of the alcoholic.

7. Bile Production

Bile is produced by the liver and passes through the intrahepatic biliary channels to the common hepatic duct and then to the gall-bladder. The principal constituents, apart from water and inorganic salts, are bilirubin, bile acids, cholesterol, alkaline phosphatase and mucin.

(a) *Bilirubin:* Hemoglobin is broken-down by reticulo-endothelial cells chiefly in the spleen, liver and bone marrow. The bile pigment, bilirubin, is derived from the non-iron-containing residue of hemoglobin after the detachment from globin. A small amount of bilirubin is derived from other haem-containing compounds like hemoglobin precursors in the bone marrow, myoglobin and the cytochromes. In the blood this unconjugated bilirubin (prehepatic bilirubin) is bound to plasma albumin and, therefore, does not pass readily through the glomerulus of the kidney into the urine. Unconjugated bilirubin is actively transported from the blood to the bile by the liver cells and during its passage it is detached from its protein and is conjugated with glucuronic acid. Conjugation occurs in the microcosms of the liver cells by the activity of glucuronyl transferase and renders the pigment water-soluble so that it becomes capable of being more easily excreted in the urine. This compound is called conjugated bilirubin. In patients with unconjugated hyperbilirubinaemia the level of bilirubin in the plasma can be lowered by the administration of barbiturates which excite microsomal enzyme action.

In the small intestine conjugated bilirubin is metabolized by bacteria to a number of isomers of stercobilinogen which on oxidation form the main fecal pigment stercobilin. The majority of these pigments is excreted in the stool (250 mg/day) but some is reabsorbed from the gut. Most of this is excreted by the liver cells into the intestine and a small part is excreted in the urine (2-4 mg/day) where it is called urobilinogen. Urobilinogen and its oxidation product urobilin are chemically analogous with stercobilinogen and stercobilin, respectively.

(b) *Excretion of bile acids and cholesterol excretion:* Bile acids are the breakdown products of cholesterol. They are synthesized in the liver and conjugated with glycine and taurine to form bile salts which are secreted straightway into the bile. Here they may form micelles when in ample concentration and these micelles, which also contain phospholipid, permit the solubilization of cholesterol although its biliary concentration far exceeds its aqueous solubility in a simple solution. An alteration of these solutes in bile is now accepted as a major factor in the precipitation of cholesterol and provides the nidus for gall-stone formation.

In the lumen of the proximal small intestine bile salts are indispensable for the solubilization of the products of fat digestion. Lack of this detergent property of bile explains the steatorrhea which, although often latent, is a well acknowledged feature of hepatobiliary disease. In addition to dietary glycerides there can be malabsorption of fat-soluble vitamins leading to a bleeding tendency (vitamin K), osteomalacia (vitamin D) and night blindness (vitamin A). About 90 per cent of the bile salts are reabsorbed from the distal ileum and return to be re-excreted by the liver. This very efficient enterohepatic circulation preserves the small total body pool of bile salts which may recycle two to three times per meal. Only a small quantity (300 mg) of bile salts escapes daily into the colon. When there is disease, resection or bypass of the terminal ileum there is an exorbitant loss of bile salts in the faces. In the colon the bile salts have a cathartic action due to intervention with the resorption of electrolytes and water. In addition to a troublesome diarrhea there is also steatorrhea since the liver cannot make up for the increased loss of bile salt and the concentration of bile salts in the duodenum is insufficient to form micelles. In patients with an overgrowth of bacteria in the small bowel (blind loop syndrome, there may be malabsorption of various nutrients and steatorrhea is often a characteristic. The malabsorption of lipid is believed to be the outcome of bacterial alteration of the bile salt molecule (deconjugation and dehydroxylation) so that the effective concentration of bile salts in the gut lumen is critically reduced. Similar alterations in the structure of bile salts may also happen in patients with cholangitis. Whilst in pruritus there may be raised levels of bile salts in the skin and plasma a definite relationship between bile salts and pruritus has not yet been established.

(c) *Enzymes excretion:* The serum alkaline phosphatase is derived mainly from the intrahepatic biliary system and the level tends to increase when there is obstruction to biliary excretion. An isoenzyme produced by the osteoblasts accounts for a variable proportion of alkaline phosphatase activity in growing children and in disease of bone. In about 50 per cent of healthy individuals there is in the serum a small amount of alkaline phosphatase which is formed by the intestinal mucosa. Yet another isoenzyme is produced by the placenta and accounts for some of the serum alkaline phosphatase activity in pregnancy. Various malignant tumours, e.g. of lungs and pancreas, have been shown to produce alkaline phosphatase which has comparable physico-chemical properties to the placental isoenzyme. The different isoenzymes can be identified by starch gel electrophoresis and studies of enzyme susceptibleness to heat inactivation.

Hence, any injury to liver or impairment of its function has grave implication for the health of the affected person. Every year about 18,000 people are reported to die due to liver cirrhosis caused by hepatitis[1,2]. Although viral infection is one of the main causes of hepatic injury, xenobiotics, extreme drug therapy, environmental pollutants and chronic alcohol ingestion can also cause severe liver injury since it plays a central role in processing, metabolizing and disposition of foreign chemicals it is susceptible to their harmful effect.

Though liver diseases are among the important diseases affecting mankind, no treatment is available to majority of them at present. However, number of medicinal preparations have been recommended in traditional systems of medicine, especially in Ayurveda, for treating liver disorder. Their usage is in practice since centuries and are quite often claimed to offer significant relief. In addition, usage of many folklore remedies, mainly plant products, is also quite widespread throughout India. Despite such extensive use interest in hepatoprotective activity kindled, especially outside India, only after the publication of the report[3,4] on isolation of silymiran, a flavonolignan, from silybum marianum and its effectiveness as a hepato-protective agent. This discovery drew the focus of research workers throughout the world towards medicinal plants to search for hepatoprotective agents among them. The search was further simplified by the description of in vitro technique involving evaluating test drugs against carbon tetrachloride induced cytotoxicity in cultured hepatocyte by Hikino and coworkers [5,6] which enables the research workers to screen large number of test drugs by adopting this program as a primary screen.

There is scarcity[7] of reviews on medicinal plants possessing hepatoprotective activity. Hence it was thought worth-while to collect and enumerate reports on medicinal plants possessing hepatoprotective activity so that it could serve as a source of information to furnish an idea about the current trends in research on plants possessing hepato-protective activity.

Medicinal Plants with Hepatoprotective Properties

1. *Acacia catechu* (L.f.) **Wild (Mimosaceae)**

   - *Common names:* Eng.: Black catechu, Hindi: Katha, Beng.: Khair.

   - *Distribution:* A small tree widely distributed in drier regions of India, Punjab, M.P., U.P., Bihar, A.P, Orissa & Rajasthan.

   - *Parts used:* Heart wood of 20-30 years old plants.

   - *Pharmacological activities:* Hepatoprotective activity against CCI_4 induced hepatic injury was found [7].

   - *Chemical constituents:* Cyanidanol (+) has been isolated from the plant.

2. *Allium sativum I.* **(Liliaceae)**

   - *Common names:* Eng.: Garlic, Hindi: Lahsan, Beng: Rasoon.

   - *Distribution:* Native to central India, grown in several places in India.

   - *Parts used:* Bulbs.

   - *Pharmacological activities:* Mechanism of action of hepatoprotection has been reported. The hepatoprotective activity is due to antioxidative property of S-allyl-mercaptocysteine and S-methylmercaptocysteine inhibiting CCI_4 induced free radical formation measured by the electron spin resonance (ESR) and lipid peroxidation [8].

   - *Chemical constituents:* See Anti-inflammatory chapter.

3. *Andrographis paniculata* **(Burm. f.) wall. ex.Nees (Acanthaceae).**

   - *Common names:* Eng- King of bitters; Hindi: Kiryat, Kalmegh, Beng: Kalmegh.

- *Distribution*: A branched annual herb occurring through-out India mainlyin the plains.

- *Parts used:* Leaves.

- *Pharmacological activities:* The active compound andro-grapholide and neoandrographolide possess hepato-protective activity which has been reported to be effective in preventives liver damage caused by *Plasmodium berghei*[9].

- *Chemical constituents:* Andragraphdide has been isolated from the plant. Stereostructure of a diterpene glucoside neoandrographolide was also isolated. Andrographin, panicolin, apigenin 4,7-dimethyl ether and mono-0-methyl within were isolated from roots. Caffeic, chlorogenic and dicaffeylquinic acids were isolated from leaves.

4. *Artemisia capillaries Linn.* **(Asteraceae)**

- *Distribution*: North-East Himalaya.

- *Parts used:* Bulbs.

- *Pharmacological activities:* The active compounds from buds of the plant studied against CCl_4 and Gal-N induced cytotoxicity in primary cultured hepatocytes [10].

- *Chemical constituents:* Capillarism, axcapillin, quercetin and isorhamnetin isolated from buds.

5. *Baccharies trimera Linn.* **(Asteraceae)**

- *Parts used:* Whole plant.

- *Pharmacological activities:* The active compound phalloidin isolated from the plant possesses hepatoprotective activity (unpublished work).

- *Chemical constituents:* Phalloidin, a flavonoid compound has been isolated.

6. *Boerhaavia diffusa L*

   Syn. *B. repensL.* (Nyctaginaceae).

- *Common names:* Eng.: Horse-purslane, Hogweed, Hindi: Punarnava, Beng.: Punarnava.

- *Distribution:* A herb distributed throughout India.

- *Parts used:* Roots and aerial parts.

- *Pharmacological activities:* Chloroform and methanolic extracts of the root and aerial parts of the plant showed hepatoprotective activity against CCl₄ induced liver injury[11].

- *Chemical constituents:* The active compounds retenoid, steroid, a flavone isolated from chromatographic fractionation. Another active principle punarnavin has been isolated. Hentriacontane, p-sitosterol and ursolie acid isolated from roots; a polysacchararide isolated which on hydrolysis yielded glucose, xylose, glucuronic acid, galactose, a-arabinose and cc-rhamnose, a glycoprotein with molecular weight of 16,000-20,000 deltons isolated from roots.

7. *Boerhavia repanda Linn.* **(Nyctaginaceae)**

   - *Distribution:* Himalayan tracts of Bengal.

   - *Parts used:* Roots.

   - *Pharmacological activities:* Extracts of root of the plant[12] responded hepatoprotective activity in rats against hepatotoxicity induced by CCl₄, galactsamine (Gal-N) and paracetamol. Petroleum ether, chloroform and methanolic extracts showed significant activity against CCl₄ induced liver injury chloroform and methanolic extracts showed response against Gal-N induced hepatotoxicity. Both the extracts failed to inhibit paracetamol induced liver injury. None of the extracts of the aerial parts exhibited any hepatoprotective activity against CCl₄ induced liver damage.

8. *Butea monosperma (Lam.) Kuntze Syn. B. frondosa* **(Papilionaceae)**

   - *Common names:* Eng.: Flame of the forest, Bengal kemo, Hindi: Dhak, Beng.: Palas.

   - *Distribution:* A deciduous tree occurring throughout India. Bears bright orange red flowers.

   - *Parts used:* Fresh juice and Gum from the stem.

   - *Pharmacological activities:* Hepatoprotective effect has been reported in isobutrin (3,4,2',4'-tetrahydroxychalcone

3,4'-diglucoside), butrin (7,3',4'-trihydroxy flavonone, 7,3'-diglucoside) and two flavonoids isolated from flower extract of the plant (13) along with the other studies in 20(S)-ginsenoside -RH$_2$, 20(R)- ginsenoside RG$_3$ and 20(S)-ginsenoside-RS against CCl$_4$ induced cytotoxity[14].

- *Chemical constituents:* Isobutrin (3,4,2', 4'-tetrahydroxy-chalcone 3, 4'-diglucoside), butrin (7, 3', 4'-trihydoxy flavonone, 7, 3'-diglucoside) and two flavonoids have been isolated from the plant. A nitrogenous acidic compound along with palasonin isolated from seeds; two new glucoside-monospermoside and isomonospermoside-isolated together with butrin, isobutrin, coreopsin, isocoreopsin and sulfurein and structures of mono-spermoside and isomonospermoside determined isolation and structure of jalaric ester I, II and laccijalaric ester III, IV form soft resin a-amyrin, p-sitosterol, its glucoside sucrose isolated from seeds; isolation and structure of a new lactone n-heneicosaroic acid-d-lactone mp. 70" from seeds.

9. *Calotropis gigantea (Linn.) R.Br. Ait.* **(Asclepiadaceae)**

- *Common names:* Eng.: Madai, Hindi: AK, Lal madar, Beng.: Sweet Akanda.

- *Distribution:* A perennial undershrub distributed throughout India. It is an erect perennial shrub growing chiefly in waste lands. It ascends to an altitude of 300ft on Himalaya, extend from Punjab to south India, Assam, Ceylon and Singapur and is distributed to Malaya Islands and south China.

- *Parts used:* Flowers.

- *Pharmacological activities:* Hepatoprotective activity[15] against CCl$_4$ induced liver damage has been found in the ethanolic extracts of the flower of the plant.

- *Chemical constituents:* The latex which is present in all part of the plant contains water soluble matter 860-95.5% and caoutchoue 0.6-1.0%. The coagulum consists of caoutchoue 5.1-18.6%, resins 73.6-87.8% - and insoluble matters 4.5-13.8%. Latex contains oc-calotropeol (C$_{30}$H$_{50}$0, m.p. 204.5°) and p-calotropeol (m.p. 216-217°) mainly in ester combination with acetic and isocaleric acids and p-amyrin.

10. *Canarium album (Lour) Raeusch.* **(Burseraceae)**

   - *Pharmacological activities:* Brevifolin, hyperin, allagic acid and 3'-di-0 methyl-allagic acid isolated from the plant were found to be effective hepatoprotective compounds which has been ascribed due to their antioxidative effects[16].

   - *Chemical constituents:* Brevifolin, hyperin, allagic acid and 3'-di-0 methyl-allagic acid have been isolated from the plant.

11. *Canarium bengalense Roxb,* **(Burseraceae)**

   - *Common names:* Eng.: East Indian copal, Assam: Nerebi, Sylhet: Dhuna.

   - *Distribution:* A tree occurring in Assam and North Bengal.

   - *Parts used:* Leaves.

   - *Pharmacological activities:* Leaves possess hepato-protective activity (unpublished work).

12. *Canscora decussata Schult* **(Gentianaceae)**

   - *Common names:* Hindi: Shankaphuli, Beng: Dankuni, Sans: Sankhapushpi.

   - *Distribution:* A herb occurring throughout India.

   - *Parts used:* Whole plants.

   - *Pharmacological activities:* Mangiferin isolated from the plant protected rats against CCl_4 induced liver injury[17].

   - *Chemical constituents:* Mangiferin, a xanthone has been isolated from the plant. Gluanone, Canscoradione, friedeline, friedelan-3p-ol, (3-angrin, sitosterol, stigma-sterol and campesterol was isolated from aerial parts.

13. *Cichorium intybus Linn.* **(Asteraceae)**

   - *Common names:* Eng.: Chicory, Wild eudive, Hindi: Kasani.

   - *Distribution:* The Chicory is native to Europe, found in India, cultivated at elsewhere.

- *Parts used:* Root.

- *Pharmacological activities:* Dried root is used in homoeopathy for liver diseases (unpublished report).

- *Chemical constituents:* The plants contain quercitrin, apigeninm, hyperin, luteolin-7-p-D-glucopyranoside, caffeic, dicaffeoylter acids, apigenin-7-O-L-arabinoside, chlorogen and neochlorogenic and inflorescense contains umbelliferne, 6,7-dihydroxy coumarin and esculin.

14. *Curcuma domestica Val.*

    Syn. *C. longa* Linn (Zingiberaceae)

    - *Common names:* Eng.: Turmeric, Hindi: Haldi, Beng.: Halud.

    - *Distribution:* A perennial herb cultivated mainly in Tamil Nadu, Andhra Pradesh, Maharashtra, Bihar, Kerala and Orissa.

    - *Parts used:* Rhizomes.

    - *Pharmacological activities:* Hepatoprotective activity against CCl_4 induced liver damage has been observed in ethanolic extract of the rhizomee of the plant

    - *Chemical constituents:* See Antifertility chapter.

15. *Cynara scolymus Linn.* **(Asteraceae).**

    - *Common names:* Eng.: Globe, Hindi: Hathichak. Beng.: Hathichoke.

    - *Distribution:* Bihar and W. Bengal.

    - *Parts used:* Whole plant.

    - *Pharmacological activities:* Hepatoprotective activity in Cymarune, a polyphenolic compound against CCl_4 and Gal-N induced cytotoxicity in cultured rat hepatocytes have been observed (unpublished work).

    - *Chemical constituents:* Cymarine, a polyphenolic compound has been isolated from the plant. Cynaropicrin and grosheimin isolated from Italian plant; cynaropicrin and dehydrocynaropicrin isolated from polish plant; absolute stereochemistry of cynaropicrin, dehydro-cynaropicrin and grosheimin; hydroxymethylacrylic acid isolated from leaves. Cynaropicrin isolated from leaves and structure elucidated; taraxasterol, p-sitosterol, stigmasterol and cynarogenin from receptacles; cynarin, m.p. 235°, from leaves; cynarotrioside, mp. 274°, from leaves; cynarolide, mp. 126°, from leaves, caffeic acid, 1-,3, 4- and 5-caffeoyl 1,4-dicaffeoyl - quinic acids, luteolin-7-3-D-glucoside and 7- [3-rutinoside from leaves.

16. *Dianthus superbus varcalamus L (Caryophyllaceae)*

   - *Pharmacological activities*: D-lanoside 'H', 'A', 'F, 'E' and 'D' isolated from the plant showed hepatoprotective activity (unpublished report).

   - *Chemical constituents*: D-Lanoside 'H', 'A','F','E' and 'D' isolated from the plant.

17. *Emblica officinalis* **Gaertn.**

   Syn. *Phyllanthus emblica* L. (Euphorbiaceae)

   - *Common names*: Eng.: Emblic, Indian goose berry, Hindi: Amla, Beng.: Amlaki.

   - *Distribution:* Amoderate sized deciduous tree native to S.E. Asia and is now distributed throughout India.

   - *Parts used:* Fruits.

   - *Pharmacological activities:* Raw fruits are used medicinally as diuretic and laxative and dried form in diarrhoea and dysentery. Phyllembin obtained from fruit pulp has been found to have mild depressant action on central nervous system. Fruit is considered to be good liver tonic. Aqueous extract of the fruit of the plant can prevent toxic effect of lead nitrate [$Pb(NO_3)_2$] and alluminium sulphate [$Al_2(SO_4)_3]_3$, $18H_2O$ on liver parenchyma cells (unpublished work).

   - *Chemical constituents:* Phyllembin obtained from fruit pulp. Seed fat contained linoleic acid (64.8%) and closely resembled linseed oil. Ellagic acid and lupeol was isolated from roots. Trigalloylglucose, terchebin, corilagin, ellagic acid from fruits.

18. *Euphorbia nematocypha Forst. F.* **(Euphorbiaceae)**

   - *Parts used:* Whole plant.

- *Pharmacological activities:* Significant hepatoprotective activity has been found due to presence of brevifolin, hyperin, ellagic acid and 3,3'-di-0 methyl-ellagic acid in the plant. The hepatoproteciive activity of these compounds has been ascribed to their antioxidative effects[16].

- *Chemical constituents:* Brevifolm, hyperin, ellagic acid and 3, 3'-di-Omethyl-ellagic acid have been isolated from the plant.

19. *Fructuss chizandrac L*

- *Parts used:* Kernel.

- *Pharmacological activity:* Significant hepatoprotective activity has been reported from the Kernals of the plant[17,18].

- *Chemical constituents:* Lignans belonging to dibenzocylo octeno group isolated from the alcoholic extract of the Kernals of the plant.

20. *Garcinia kola Hechel.* **(Clusiaceae)**

- *Distribution:* Tropical, Asia, Africa.

- *Pharmacological activities:* Kolaviron isolated from the plant was found to produce significant hepatoprotective effect against CCl_4 induced liver injury[19]. Later studies showed that Kolaviron, a mixture of bioflavonoids and Kolaflavanone isolated from the plant against thioacetamide induced liver toxicity in rats which was measured by thiopental sleeping time indicating significant hepatoprotective activity. Besides, they were also found to alter serum microsomal enzyme levels.

- *Chemical constituents:* Kolaviron, a mixture of bio-flavonoids and Kolaflavanone has been isolated from the plant. Beta-sitosterol isolated from seeds; lipid from seed consisted of unsaturated and saturated and saturated acids; stearic, palmitic, myristic and oleic acids identified.

21. *Garcinia mangostana L.* **(Clusiaceae).**

- *Common names:* Eng.: Mangosteen, Hindi: Mangustan, Beng.: Mangustan.

- *Distribution:* Tree native to Malaysia. Mangosteen fruits are chiefly imported into India from Singapore and the strait settlements, though to some extent it is cultivated in Madras.

- *Parts used:* Fruits.

- *Pharmacological activities:* Fruit is used in chronic diarrhoea and dysentery. It also possesses hepato-protective activity (unpublished work).

- *Chemical constituents:* Three new xanthones gartanin, 8-deoxygartamin and normangostin was isolated from isolated from fruits. Mangostin was isolated and its structure was chemical.

22. *Glycyrrhiza glabra Linn.* (Fabaceae).

- *Common names:* Eng.: Liqnorice, Beng.:Jashtimadhu, Hindi: Mul.

- *Distribution:* Persian gulf, Asia minor, Turkestan, Siberia, China, Prance,Germany, Italy.

- *Parts used:* Roots.

- *Pharmacological activities:* The plant showed hepato-protectiveactivity glycyrrhizin analogues (Glycyrrhizin glycyrrhetinic acid) have beenisolated from the plant[20].

- *Chemical constituents:* See Antifertility chapter.

23. *Gymnosporia montana* (Roth) Benth.

Syn. *G. spinosa* (Celastraceae)

- *Common names:* Hindi: Vingar, Beng.: Vaichigacnha. Sans.: Vikankata.

- *Distribution:* Tropical, subtropical and Africa.

- *Parts used:* Leaves.

- *Pharmacological activities:* Leaf extract of the plant showed hepatoprotective activity. Primary screening was carried out in mice by noting the effects on CCl_4 induced prolongation of pentobarbitone sleep. Extract found effective in the primary test, was further evaluated in rats by noting their effect on CCl_4 induced alterations in morphological, biochemical and histopathological parameters. Methanolic extract of defaulted leaf (ME) of the plant produced significant reversal of majority of the altered biochemical parameters studied and histo-pathological studies confirmed the presence of significant hepatoprotective activity in the extract[21].

- *Chemical constituents:* Tingenone, 3-0-acetyloleanolic acid, hexacosane, betulin, p-amyrin, hexacosanol and p-sitosterol isolated from stem bark, root bark and leaves.

24. *Hypoestes triflora L* (Acanthaceae)

- *Parts used:* Leaves.

- *Pharmacological activities:* Treatment with aqueous extract of the leaves prevented CCl_4 induced prolongation of duration of barbiturate sleep indicating presence of hepatoprotective activity in it. The active principle responsible for the hepatoprotective activity is reported to be benzoic acid. It prevented CCl_4 induced elevation in transaminase activity in mice[22].

- *Chemical constituents:* Benzoic acid.

25. *Indigofera tinctoria Baker, Syn. /. sumatrana* (Fabaceae)

- *Common names:* Hindi: Neel, Beng.: Neel, Tarn.: Nils.

- *Distribution:* Available in W. Bengal, Bihar, Tamil Nadu, Karnataka.

- *Parts used:* Aerial parts.

- *Pharmacological activities:* A detailed investigation of the alcoholic extract of the aerial part of the plant[23,24] has been done. The extract was found to afford significant protection to mice, rats and rabbits against' CCl_4 induced hepatic injury. Parameters measured were pentobarbitone sleeping time, prothrombin time and bromo sulphaleine excretion. It was also found to increase liver weight and bile flow in rats indicating microsomal enzyme induction.

- *Chemical constituents:* Analysis of the leaves gave the following values (dry basis); Nitrogen (N), 5.11; Phosphoric acid (P_2O_5), 0.18; Potash (K), 1.67; and lime (CaO) 5.35%.

26. *Lawsonia alba* **Lam.**

Syn. *L. inermis* Linn. (Lythraceae)

- *Common names*: Eng.: Henna, Hindi: Mehandi, Beng.: Mehandi.

- *Distribution*: A much branched shrub or small tree native to Arabia and Parsia and is now cultivated in Haryana, Gujrat and to a small extent in M.P. and Rajasthan.

- *Parts used:* Barks.

- *Pharmacological activities:* Hepatoprotective activity has been reported[25] in ethanol water extract of the bark of the plant against CCI_4 induced liver toxicity[26]. The extract was effective in preventing CCI_4 induced prolongation of hexobarbitone induced sleep and alteration in biochemical parameters and BSP clearance.

- *Chemical constituents:* Two new xanthones- laxanthones I and II isolated and characterized as 1,3 dihydroxy 6, 7 dimethoxy-xanthone and 1-hydroxy-3, 6-diacetoxy-7-methoxyxanthone respectively. Laxanthone III isolated and characterized as 1-hydroxy-3,7-dimethoxy-6-acetoxy-xanthone.

27. *Liquidambar formosana Hance* **(Hamamelidaceae)**

- *Common name:* Eng.: Fragment maple.

- *Distribution:* A tree native to china, now reported to have been introduced in Lalbagh gardens, Bangalore.

- *Parts used:* Fruits.

- *Pharmacological activities:* Hepatoprotective activity has been reported in betulonic acid, an isolate from fruit of the plant[8].

- *Chemical constituents:* Betulonic acid has been isolated from fruit of the plant.

28. *Luffa echinata* **Roxb. (Cucurbitaceae)**

- *Common names:* Punjab: Bakru, U.P.: Taknoi, Kashmir: Tata bateri, Beng.: Bindal.

- *Distribution:* Hills of Kashmir, U.P. Kumaun.

- *Parts used:* Fruits.

- *Pharmacological activities:* Alcoholic and ether extracts of the plant was found to protect rats against CCl₄ induced injury[27,28] from the extract of the plant, echinatin, cucurbitacin B, a saponin glycoside of gypsogenin, a flavonoid-chrysoeriol, flavones epigenin and futeolin have been isolated by different workers, but which one of them is responsible for hepatoprotective activity remains to be determined.

- *Chemical constituents:* Echinatin, cucurbitacin B, a saponifying glycoside of gypsogenin, a flavonoid-chrysoeeriol, flavones epigenin and futeolin have been isolated from alcoholic and ether extracts of the plant. Cucurbitacin B (3.5), mp. 176°, cucurbitacin E (0.05%), mp. 234° and a bitter saponin composed of a triterpene acid, glucose arabinose and rhamnose, from fruits; cucurbitacin B, (3-sitosterol, two unidentified triterpene alcohols echinatol A; mp. 144° and echinatol B, mp. 167° from seeds; constitution of cucurbitacin B established; structures of cucurbitacins A and C proposed.

29. *Nymphaea stellata Willd.* **(Nymphaeaceae).**

    - *Common names:* Eng.: Indian blue water lily, Hindi: Nilpadma, Beng.: Nilshapla.

    - *Distribution:* Native of South East Asia, aquatic herb found in ponds and ditches.

    - *Parts used:* Whole plant.

    - *Pharmacological activities:* Petroleum ether extract of the plant provides significant protection to rats against CCl₄ induced functional, histopathological and morphological changes[29]. The extract was found to promote parenchymal tissue regeneration.

    - *Chemical constituents:* Analysis of the dried tubers gave the following values: moisture, 4.20; fat, 0.45; proteins, 14.56; carbohydrates, 67.49; fibre, 5.45 and ash, 7.85%.

30. *Ocimum sanctum Linn.* **(Lamiaceae).**

    - *Common names:* Eng.: Sacred basil, Hindi: Tulsi, Beng.: Tulsi.

- *Distribution:* A well-known sacred plant of India grown in gardens, temples, houses all over India.

- *Parts used:* Leaves.

- *Pharmacological activities:* Extracts protected rats against CCl_4 induced liver injury[30,31].

- *Chemical constituents:* It is reported to contain ursolic acid, apigenin, luteolin, apigenin-7-O-glucuronide, luteolin-7-0-glucuronide orientin and molludistin. However, no study has been made to evaluate hepato-protective activity of these compounds. Eugenol (70.5), its methyl ether (4.8), nerol (6.4), caryphyllene (7.5), terpinen-4-ol (0.4), decylaldehyde (0.2), y-selinene (0.4), p-pinene (0.4), camphene (2.0) and a-pinene (3.5%) identified in essential oil by GC.

31. *Paederia foetida Linn.* **(Rubiaceae).**

- *Common names:* Hindi: Ghandhali, Somraji, Beng.: Gandhal, Sans.: Prasarani.

- *Distribution:* Found in Central and Eastern Himalayas, extending to Calcutta.

- *Parts used:* Leaves.

- *Pharmacological activities:* Leaf extract of the plant responded hepatoprotective activity[32]. Primary screening was carried out in mice by noting the effects on CCl_4 induced prolongation of pentobarbitone sleep. Extracts effects were evaluated in rats by noting their effect onCCl_4 induced alterations in morphological, biochemical and histopathological parameters. Methanolic extract of the plant also showed reversal of some of the altered biochemical parameters. However, the extract did not prevent CCl_4 induced histopathological changes to significant extent.

- *Chemical constituents:* Asperuloside and four new iridoid glucosides-paederoside, mp.122°, paederosidic acid, scandoside, m.p. 139° anddeacetyl asperuloside were isolated and characterized. Hentriacontane, hentria-contanol, methyl mercaptan, ceryl alcohol, palmitic acid, sitosterol, stigmasterol, campesterol, ursolic acid and iridoid glycosides-aspcruloside, paederoside and scandoside isolated from leaves and stems.

32. *Peumus boldus Molina* **(Monimiaceae)**

- *Part used:* Whole plant.

- *Pharmacological activities:* It has been reported the presence of hepatoprotective activity in dried hydroalcoholic extract of the plant against tart – butyl hydroperoxide induced cytotoxicity in isolated rat hepatocytes. It also protected mice against CCI_4 toxication (*in vitro*). Boidine the main alkaloid of the plant has been implicated for the hepatoprotective activity.

- *Chemical constituents:* An alkaloid boldine has been isolated.

33. *Phyllanthus amarus (Euphorbiaceae)*

- *Distribution:* South India.

- *Parts used:* Whole plant.

- *Pharmacological activities:* In an interesting study, it has been reported hepatitis - B virus inactivating activity in the alcoholic extract of the plant in an in vitro test system (unpublished work).

34. *Phyllanthus fraternus* **Webster.**

Syn. P. m'rur/sensu Hook.f.(non-L.) (Euphorbiaceae)

- *Common names:* Sans.: Bhumyamalaki, Hindi: Jar-amla, Beng.: Bhui-amla,

- *Distribution:* Throughout the hotter parts of India from Punjab to Assam and Southwards to Travancore, ascending to the hills to 2000ft.

- *Parts used:* Whole plant.

- *Pharmacological activities:* The plant is used as remedy for jaundice (unpublished work).

- *Chemical constituents:* The plant contains the bitter substances phyllanthin and hypophyllanthin. The phyllanthin was characterised as (+) 3, 3', 4,4', 9,9' hexa-methoxy 8,8' butyrolignan. Three new lignans -niranthin; nirtetralin and phyltetralin isolated from leaves; detection of estradiol in bark and roots by TLC estradiol content

155-350 u.g/100g in plant samples; Kaempferol-4'-rhamnopyranoside and eridictyol-7-rhamnopyranoside isolated from roots; lup-20(29)-en-3p-ol and its acetate isolated from roots.

35. ***Picrorhiza Kurroa Royle ex Benth.* (Scrophulariaceae)**

- *Common names:* Hindi: Kuru, Beng.: Kutki, Sans.: Katuka.

- *Distribution:* The Himalayas from Kashmir to Sikkim.

- *Parts used:* Roots.

- *Pharmacological activities:* CDRI group through an elaborate study[33] employing a number of biochemical parameters, has evaluated hepatoprotective activity in Picoliv, a standardized fraction of the root of the plant containing about 60% of a mixture of picroside I and Kutkoside in the ratio of 1:1.5. The test drug significantly reversed alterations in number of biochemical parameters caused by CCl_4 administration. Noteworthy among these parameters is lipoprotein-X, which is found to be elevated markedly in the serum of rats' toxicity with CQ_4 and is not present in measurable quantity in normal rats. In the drug treated group it was lowered significantly and could not be measured. The overall hepatoprotective activity was evaluated by measuring 'PAV value, i.e percentage proportion of abnormal value, which was found to be significantly less in Picroliv treated group in comparison with CCl_4 control rats.

- *Chemical constituents:* Picroliv which is a mixture of picroside I and kutkoside in the ratio of 1:1.5 has been obtained from the root of the plant. A new iridoid glucoside -picroside II - isolated and characterized as 6-vanilloylcatalpol. Picroside III was isolated and characterized as 6'-(4-hydroxy-3-methoxy cinnamoyl) catalpol.

36. ***Piper longam Linn.* (Piperaceae)**

- *Common names:* Eng.: long pepper, Hindi: Pipal, Beng.: Piplamar.

- *Distribution:* Cultivated in West Bengal, Karnataka and Tamil Nadu, also in plains of Bengal.

- *Pharmacological activities:* Milk extract (decoction with milk) of the plant has been tested for hepatoprotective activity against CCl_4 induced hepatic injury[34]. The extract though ineffective in preventing acute changes, promoted regeneration process by restricting fibrosis. Chemical constituents: See Antifertility chapter.

37. *Quercus infectoria Olivier* **(Fagaceae).**

   - *Common names:* Hindi: Maza, Muphal, Beng.: Majuphal, Eng.: Gak oak.

   - *Distribution:* A shrub or small tree indigenous to Greece, Syria and Iran.

   - *Parts used:* Fruits.

   - *Pharmacological activities:* Some co-workers have[15] screened fruit of the plant for hepatoprotective activity against CCl_4 induced liver damage. Ethanolic extract of the fruit of the plant was found to afford significant protection.

   - *Chemical constituents:* Methyl betulate, methyl oleanolate sitosterol, syringic, gallic and ellagic acids were isolated from the plants.

38. *Ricinus communis Linn.* **(Euphorbiaceae)**

   - *Common names:* Eng.: Castorseed, castor, Castorbean, Castor oil plant. Hindi: Arandi, Beng.: Reri.

   - *Distribution:* A small tree cultivated chiefly in Andhra Pradesh, Maharashtra, Karnataka, Orissa, available in wild condition in W. Bengal. Parts used: Roots.

   - *Pharmacological activities:* Crude extract and its butanol soluble fraction of the plant have been reported to afford significant protection to rats against Gal-N induced hepatic damage[9].

   - *Chemical constituents:* Palmitic (1.2), Stearic (0.7), arachidic (0.3), hexadecenoic (0.2), oleic (3.2), linoleic (3.4), linolenic (0.2) ricinoleic (89.4%) and dihydroxystearic acid as Me-esters in castor oil was defected. Lupeol and 30-norlupan-3(3-o1 -20-one from coat of castor bean was reported.

39. *Salsola collina Linn.* **(Chenopodiaceae)**

- *Distribution:* North-East Himalaya.

- *Parts used:* Shoot.

- *Pharmacological activities:* Ethanolic extract of shoot (above ground part) was found to provide good protection against CCl$_4$ induced changes in metabolic functions and liver cytoarchitecture[35].

40. *Sambucus formosana Rehder* **(Caprifoliaceae).**

- *Common name:* Eng.: Elder.

- *Distribution:* Eastern Himalaya.

- *Parts used:* Whole plant.

- *Pharmacological activities:* Significant hepatoprotective activity has been observed against CCl$_4$ induced liver injury[36]. The hepatoprotective activity was due to sambuculin A isolated from the plant. From the same plant (3-amyrin and oleanolic acid were also isolated. A mixture of oc-amyrin and [3-amyrin palmitate exhibited strong hepatoprotective effect CCl$_4$ induced liver injury.

- *Chemical constituents:* Sambuculin A, p-amyrin and oleanolic acid have been isolated.

41. *Silybum marianum (L.) Gaertn.* **(Asteraceae)**

- *Common name:* Eng.: Milk thistle.

- *Distribution:* Widely distributed in S. American.

- *Parts used:* Seeds.

- *Pharmacological activities:* Reported to have hepato-protective activity (unpublished work).

- *Chemical constituents:* Optically active dehydro diconifenyl alcohol isolated from seeds; twelve polyacetylenes and one polyene detected in roots; structure of seven of these determined whereas other substances could only be partially characterised; and isomer of silymarin-silychristin-isolated from fruits and characterised; myristic, palmitic, stearic and oleic acids, taxifolin, silybin and silydianin, silibonol isolated from seeds; a new flavonohignan-2, 3-dehydrosilymarin and 2, 3-delyotro-silychristin isolated from seeds; silymonin and silanctrin isolated from fruits; tanins determined in flowers, leaves and stem.

42. *Solanum incanum Kuntze*

    Syn. **S. coagulans** Forsk. (Solanaceae)

    - *Common names:* Sans.: Congulus forsk, Punjab: Barimalehari.

    - *Pharmacological activities:* Hepatoprotective activity was assessed by CCl_4 induced pentobarbitone (PBN) sleep prolongation and elevation of transaminase activity. Aarpesterol an isolate, completely prevented PBN sleeping besides lowering transaminase activity to almost normal level (unpublished work).

    - *Chemical constituents:* Aarpesterol has been isolated from the plant, besides solasodene, solamargine and solasonine and wrsolic acid. Diosgenin and yamogenin were isolated in 1.2% yield from fruit.

43. *Tephrosia purpurea Pers* (Fabaceae)

    - *Common names:* Sans.: Sharapunkha, Hindi: Dhamasia, Beng.:Ban-nil-gachh.

    - *Distribution:* It is a sub-erect herbaceous perenirial found all over India, ascending to the Himalayas up to an altitude of 6000ft.

    - *Parts used:* Dried herb intact.

    - *Pharmacological activity:* Hepatoprotective activity has been observed (unpublished work).

    - *Chemical constituents:* The roots contain tephrosin, deguelin, isotephrosin, rotenon etc. The leaves contain about 2% a glycoside, osyritin. Caffeic acid isolated from dormant seeds; rutin, p-sitosterol and lupeol isolated from leaves; delphinidin chloride and cyanidin chloride isolated from flowers.

44. *Thujapsis dolabrata Bleb. & Zucc.* (Cupressaceae)

    - *Distribution:* Japan.

    - *Parts used:* Whole plants.

- *Pharmacological activities:* Hepatoprotective activity in desozyprodophyllotoxin isolated from the plant has been observed[4].

- *Chemical constituents:* Desozyprodophyllotoxin has been isolated from the plant.

45. *Tinospora cordifolia (Willd.) Miers ex hook. f. & Thorns* **(Menispermaceae)**

- *Common names:* Hindi: Gulancha, Giloe, Beng.: Gadancha, Sans.: Amrita.

- *Distribution:* A climbing shrub distribution throughout tropical India and Andamans.

- *Parts used:* Dry stems with bark.

- *Pharmacological activities:* Biochemical, morphological and histopathological parameters have been evaluated from the decoction of the plant[37] and hepatoprotective activity against CCl_4 induced hepatic injury has been tested.

- *Chemical constituents:* Two bitter substances, substances, substance A ($C_{22}H_{34}O_{10}$, $5H_2O$) m.p. 226°-228° substance B (m.w. 495 melts 186°-188°). Giloin, $C_{23}H_{32}O_{10}H_{20}$, a glycoside, m.p. 226-228°, Gilenin $C_{17}H_{,8}O_5$, a non-glycoside bitter m.p. 210-212° and Gilo sterol, $C_{28}H_{48}O$, m.p.192-93° were isolated.

46. *Vitex negundo I.* **(Verbenaceae)**

- *Common names:* Hindi: Sanbhalu, Beng.: Nishinda, Sans.: Nirgundi.

- *Distribution:* A shrub or smell tree found in W. Bengal.

- *Parts used:* Seeds.

- *Pharmacological activities:* Significant hepatoprotective activity in the alcoholic extract of the plants seed has been observed. The effect was found to be significantly reverse CCl_4 induced changes in morphological, biochemical and functional parameters studied.

- *Chemical constituents:* n-Tritriacontane, n-hentriacontane, n-pentatriacontane, n-nonacosane, beta-sitosterol, p-hydroxybenzoic acid and 5-oxyisophthalic acid from seeds; 3, 4-dihydroxybenzoic acid also isolated; vanillic and p-hydroxybenzoic acids and luteolin isolated from bark; two new leucoanthocyanidins isolated from stem bark and their structures determined as 6,8-di-O-methyl-leucodelphinidin and 3', 4'-di-0-methylleucocyanidin-7-0-rhamnoglucoside.

47. *Wedelia chinensis Merrill*

Syn. IV. *calendulaceae* Less. (Asteraceae)

- *Common name:* Hindi: Bhangra.
- *Distribution:* A herb found in U.P, Assam, Arunachal Pradesh and West Bengal.
- *Parts used:* leaves.
- *Pharmacological activities:* Hepatoprotective activity has been observed in the methanol extract of the plant. Extract tested against CCI_4 and Gal -N induced cytotoxicity in primary cultured hepatocytes[38].
- *Chemical constituents:* Isolation of wedelolactone.

48. *Withania frutiscens* (Solanceae)

- *Parts used:* Leaves.
- *Pharmacological activity:* Ethanolic extract of the leaves of plant has been reported to prevent CCI_4 induced alterations in pentobarbitone sleep, biochemical parameters studied and derangement of liver cytoarchitecture has been observed[39].

49. *Withania coagulans Dunal* (Solanaceae)

- *Common names:* Eng.: Vegetable rennel, Indian cheese maker, Hindi: Akri, Punir, Tel.: Panneru-gadda.
- *Distribution:* A small shrub found in Punjab.
- *Parts used:* Fruits.
- *Pharmacological activities:* Fruits are used in liver complaints. A withanolide, 3-(3-hydroxy-3, 3-dihydro withanolide F, isolated from the fruit of the plant also showed significant hepatoprotective activity against CCI_4 induced liver injury. The activity was assessed by measuring pentobarbitone sleeping time, serum transaminase acitvity and through histopathologicai studies[40].

- *Chemical constituents:* Different compounds (with milting points 125°, 90°, 81° and 128°) was isolated from the fruits. A new steroif-5, - 27- dihydroxy- 6cc, 7a-epoxy - 1-oxo-5a- witha - 2, 24 dienolide along with withaniol and withaferin A was isolated. A uithanolide, 3-p-hydroxy-3,3-dihydro uithanolide F was isolated from fruits of the plant.

50. *Withania somnifera Dunal* (Solanaceae)

- *Common names:* Eng.: Ashvaganda, Hindi: Asgand, Beng.: Ashvaganda.

- *Distribution:* This is an erect shrub found throughout the drier parts of India, Baluchistan and Ceylon.

- *Parts used:* Roots and tuber roots.

- *Pharmacological activities:* Alcoholic extract of the leaves of the plant was found to significantly inhibit CCl_4 induced alterations in transaminase activity and pentobarbitone sleeping time indicating presence of hepatoprotective activity. This was confirmed through histopathological studies[41].

- *Chemical constituents:* See Antifertility chapter.

References

1. Handa, S.S., *Pharmatimes*, (1991), 23(4), 13.

2. Vogel, G. in: New Natural Products and Plant Drugs with Pharmacological, Biologicalor Therapeutical Activity, (Wagner, H. and Wolff, S.P-ed) Springer-ver-lag, Berlin-Heldelberg-New York, (1977).

3. Vogel, G. Arznein-Forsch, Drug Research., (1968), 18, 1063.

4. Hikino, H.Sugai, I, Konno, C. Hashinota, L, Terasaki, S. and Hirino, I., Plants Med., (1979), 36,156.

5. Hikino, H., Kiso, Y., Wagner, H. and Fiebig, M.F., Planta Med.,.(1984), 50(3), 248.

6. Handa, S.S., Sharma, A. and Chakraborti, K.K., fitoferap/a.,(1986), 57(5), 307.

7. Rege, N., Dahanukar, S. and Karandikar, S.M., Indian Drugs, (1984), 21(12), 556.

8. Konno, C., Oshima, Y., Hikino, H., Yang, L.L. and Yen, K.Y., Planta Med., (1988), 54(5), 417.

9. Annual Report: Central Drug Research Institute, Lucknow, 1987-88.

10. Hikino, H., Tohkin, M., Kiso, Y, Namiki, I, Nishimura, S and Takeyama, K., PlantaMed, (1986), No.3, p-163.

11. Chakraborti, K.K. and Handa, S.S., Indian Drugs, (1989), 27(3), 161.

12. Chakraborti, K.K. and Handa, S.S., Indian Drugs, (1989), 27(1), 19.

13. Wagner, H., Geyer, B., Fiebig, M., Kiso, Y. and Hikino, H., Planta Med., (1986), No.2,p-77.

14. Hikino, H., Kiso, Y, Kinouchi, J., Sarada, S. and Shoji, J., Planta Med., (1985), No.1, p-62.

15. Patel, R.B., Raval, J.D., Gandhi, IP. and Chakravarty, B.K., Indian Drugs, (1988), 25(6), 224.

16. Ito (nee Someya), M., Shimura, H., Watanabe, N., Tamal, M., Handa, K., Takahashi,A., Tanaka, Y, Arai, I., Zhang, P.L., Chang, R., Chen, W.M., Yang, J.S., su.L. and Wang, Y.L, Chem, Pharm, Bull., (1990), 38(8), 2201.

17. Shankaranarayan, D., Gopalkrishnan, C., Kameswaran, L. and Arumugum, Mediscope, (1979), 22, 65.

18. Liu. G.T., Chinese Med J., (1989), 102(10), 740.

19. Braide, V.B., Phytotherapy Research, (1991), 5(1), 35.

20. Yoshinobu, K., Tohkin, M., Hikino, H., Hattari, M., Sujamoto, T. and Namba, I, PlantaMed (1984), 50, 298.

21. De, S., B. Ravishankar and Bhavsar, G.C., Indian Drugs, (1991), 29(3), 107.

22. Van Puyvelde, L, Kayonga, A., Brioen, P., Costa, J., Nadimubakunzil, A., de Kimpe,N. and Schamp, N., J. Ethnopharmac., (1989), 26(2), 121.

23. Anand, K.K., Dewanchand and Ray Gharak, B.J., Indian J. Exp. Biol., (1979), 17, 685.

24. Anand, K.K., Dewanchand, Ray Gatak, B.J. and An/a R.K. , Indian J. Exp. Biol., (1981), 19, 298.

25. Anand, K.K. Singh, B., Chand, D. and Chandan, B.K., Planta Med., (1992), 58(1), 22.

26. Chattopadhay, R.R., Sarkar, S.K., Ganguly, S., Medda, C. and Basu, T.K., Indian J.Pharmacol., (1992), 24, 163.

27. Lauria P., Sharma, V.N., Vanjani, S. and Sangal, B.C.: IVth Ann. Conf. Indian Pharmacol.Soc., March, 1972, Indian J. Pharmaccl., (1972), 4(2), 152.

28. Lauria, P., Sharma, V.N., Vanjani, S. and Sangal, B.C., Indian J. Pharmacol., (1976), 8, 129.

29. Singh, N., Nath, R., Singh, D.R., Gupta, Ml. and Kohli, R.P., Quart. J. Crude DrugRes., (1978), 16, 8.

30. Bhargava, K.P. and Singh, N., Indian J. Med. Res., (1981), 73, 443.

31. Seethalakshmi, B., Narasappa, A.P. and Kenchaveerappa, S.: Proc. Indian Pharmacol.

32. Soc. XIV Ann. Conf., Dec., 1981, Indian J. Pharmacol., (1982), 14, 63.32. De, S., Ravishankar and Bhavsar, G.C.: Proceedings of 41st Indian Pharmaceutical Congress, 1989, Indian J. Pharm. Sci., (1990), 52(1), 63.

33. Dwivedi, Y, Rastogi, R., Chander, R., Sharma, S.K., Kapoor, N.K., Garg, N.K. and Dhawan, B.N., Indian J. Med. Res., (1990), 92(B), 195.

34. Rege, N., Dahanukar, S. and Karandikar, S.M., Indian Drugs, (1984), 21(12), 569.

35. Vengerovsky, A.I., Chuchalin, V.S., Sedykh, I.M. and Saratkov, A.S., RastitelnyeResursy, (1989), 25(4), 575.

36. Li, C.N. and Tome, W.P., Plants Med., (1988), 54(3), 223.

37. Singh, I.D. in Text Book of Biochemistry and Human S/o/ogy(Talwar, G.P.-ed), PrenticeHall of India, New Delhi, 1980.

38. Yang, L.L., Yen, K.Y., Konno, C., Oshima. Y., Kiso, Y. and Hikino, H., Planta Med., (1986), No.6, p-499.

39. Montilla, M.P., Cabo, J., Navarro, M.C., Risco, S., Jimenez, J. and Aneiros, J., Phytotherapy Research, (1990), 4(6), 212.

40. Budhiraja, R.D., Garg, K.N., Sudhir, S. and Arora, B., Planta Med., (1986), No.1, p-28.

41. Sudhir, S., Budhiraja, R.D., Miglani, G.P., Arora, B., Gupta, L.C. and Garg, K.N., PlantaMed., (1986), No.1, p-61.

5 *Medicinal Plants with Anti-Inflammatory Properties*

......"For what avails
Valour or strength, though matchless, quelled with pain,
Which all subdues, and makes remiss the hands
Of mightiest? Sense of pleasure we may well
Spare out of life perhaps, and not repine,
But. live content - which is the calmest life;
But pain is perfect misery, the worst
Of evils, and, excessive, overturns
All patients". *

Subsequently ages it is well known that any form of injury to men or animals can elicit a series of chemical changes in the injured area. Consequently, inflammation can be described as tissue retort to injury. The term 'inflammation' is derived from Latin - inflammare or burn.

In the old ages, especially in the Greek and the Roman era, inflammation was contemplated as a single disease caused by disturbances of body fluids. However, William Harvey (1628) provided a more judicious explanation of inflammation. The modern concept of inflammation is based on the theory of John Hunter (1794) who considered inflammation to be a salubrious operation, resulting from some disturbance or disease. Nevertheless, a more deceiving explanation was put forward by Specter and Willoughby (1963) who defined inflammation as 'the response to injury of the living microcirculation of allied tissues'. Celsus (30BC - 30AD) described the cardinal signs of inflammation as calor, rubor, tumor and dolor - heat, redness, swelling and pain. Virchow (1858), consequently added the fifth sign, *functio laesa*, or loss of function. Thus, it may he referred to that inflammatory impetus results in events resembling to cardinal signs.

Inflammation customarily involves a sequence of changes which can be summed up as:

A. Acute Transient Phase

1. Alteration in vascular calibre and blood flow.

2. Enhanced vascular permeability resulting in the development of inflammatory exudate and local edema.

B. Delayed-Subacute Phase

1. Emigration of leukocytes and phagocytes from blood into the extravascular tissues.

C. Chronic-Proliferative Phase

1. Tissue degradation and fibrosis.

Inflammation can also be described based on the cardinal signs.

- *Calor:* Due to augmentation of blood flow at the site of tissue injury, there is an increase of the local temperature.

- *Rubor:* Involves distention of small blood vessels, arterioles, capillaries and venules within the injured area.

- *Tumor:* The dilation of blood vessels outcome in increased permeability of the vessels walls, thereby admitting protein rich fluid (containing high number of leukocytes) to exit into the tissues of the damaged area - leading to local edema formation.

- *Dolor:* Inflammation results in liberate of endogenous mediators, specially histamine, serotonin, bradykinin, prostaglandin (and prostaglandin derivatives). Such mediators evoke pain response even when released in minute quantities. Pain may also result from the increased tissue strain caused by inflammatory exudates (edema formation). Thus, discharging of pus from wounds, abscesses and boils may result in instantaneous lowering of pain.

- *Loss of function:* Pain may result in dropped muscular movement and such prerequisites of muscular movement is upset following edema or swelling in the inflamed area.

In order to comprehend the inflammatory process, it is fundamental to have a broad idea on the endogenous mediators which play a important role in this inflammatory process.

Histamines and serotonin (5 hydroxtryptamine - 5HT) play a prevailing role in acute inflammation. Thus, histamine antagonist has emerged as competent drugs in controlling urticarias and asthma.

Kinins are an assembly of peptides released in blood by kallikreins. The kinins generated locally, furnish in the acute and possibly chronic phase of inflammation thus producing vasodilatation, local edema and pain. Kinins also mediate leukocyte migration.

Ultimately prostaglandin (products of oxidative metabolism of arachidonic acid) play a dominant role in the complete inflammatory process. The arachidonic acid is metabolized by two pathways -cyclooxygenase (produce prostaglandin, thromboxanes - elicit inflammatory response) and lipooxygenase pathway (produces leukotrienes; leukotriene B4 in particular, is a highly potent inflammatory mediator). These products are hyperalgesic, potent vasodilators and also contribute in erythema, edema and pain. The recently accessible nonsteroidal anti-inflammatory drugs (NSAID's) are potential inhibitors of this cyclooxygenase pathway of arachidonic acid metabolism.

Platelet activating factor (Paf-acether) is one of the most currently reported mediator believed to be involved significantly in the inflammatory process. The mediator is a phospholipid, formed by different cells, such as eosinophils, macrophages, platelets and neutrophils. It is synthesized from membrane phospholipids with the help of phospholipase A2. Paf is also known to stimulate free arachidonic acid from cells and also metabolize it to eicosanoids.

Ultimately, the active participation of free radicals have been recently inscribed as an arising area in understanding the inflammatory process. Free radicals (O_2, $H2O_2$.,, OH, HOC1) can be described as chemical species, with one or more unpaired electrons in the extreme orbit. These chemical substances (produced by neutrophills, sensitized monocytes, macrophages and eosinophils) are fundamental to our biological system, for counteracting the microbes invasion into our system, in millions - but these are ruinous unless tightly controlled. There are a number of scientific reports connected to the trials of free radical scavengers (enzymes such as superoxide dismutase, catalase; iron chelators; Vit. E; plant products); such studies show promising results with the scavengers described above in concealing both acute and chronic inflammation.

Chronic inflammatory disorders are assorted on the basis of alteration in connective tissues. These include rheumatic fevers, rheumatoid arthritis, ankylosing spondylitis, polyartheritis nodosa, systemic lupus erythematosus, osteoarthritis. In rheumatic fever, the exudative changes typical of acute inflammatory condition is accompanied with proliferative changes characteristic of chronic inflammation. The prevailing feature of chronic inflammatory condition is characterized by proliferation of fibrous tissue, while the exudative changes (as observed in acute inflammation) are also evidenced and it is often perceived that chronic inflammation is preceded by acute changes.

Rheumatoid arthritis is an autoimmune disease where there is a complex interplay of genetic, immunological and local factors in the inaugural of the disease. It is a nearly common disease which affects the joints, it is a combination of chronic inflammation fibrosis and tissue degradation. Studies have unveiled that prostaglandin E_2 is associated with the alogesic response in rheumatoid arthritis. Modern studies also involve leukotrienes and PAF in tissue degeneration and fibrosis associated with rheumatoid arthritis. Studies also testify commitment of monokines including interleukin 1 and tumor necrosis factor (TNF) in synovial fibrosis and tissue damage associated with the chronic proliferative phase of inflammation. There is a spacious extent for development of suitable monokine synthesis inhibitors or receptor antagonists which in trend may be useful for treatment of this dreaded disorder.

The salicylates are one of the pioneer known drugs used in the therapy of inflammatory disorders. Hippocrates, about 2400 years ago recommended the use of willow bark for the treatment of eye diseases and ache during childbirth. In the *Papyrus Ebers* (1550BC) it is established that a treatment to dispossess rheumatic pains in the womb is to employ the dried leaves of myrtle (contain salicylates) prepared with beer, to the sacral and hypogastric regions. In China, preparations from the bark of *Populus alba* and decoctions from the young shoots of *Salix babylonica* have been included to be used since several hundred years in the therapy of rheumatic fevers, colds, hemorrhages, goitre. The drugs used in inflammatory disorders be classified as:

1. Drugs with analgesic but with insignificant anti-inflammatory actions Aniline derivative - paracetamol is the predominate member of this group now used; phenacetin is outdated.

2. Drugs with analgesic and mild to moderate anti-inflammatory actions:

   (a) Propionic acid derivatives which include ibuprofen, ketoprofen, fenoprofen, naproxen, flurbiprofen.

   (b) Anthranilic acid derivatives which comprise mefenamic acid, flufenamic acid.

   (c) Acryacetic acid derivatives which include fenclofenac, diclofenac.

3. Drugs with analgesic and marked anti-inflammatory actions:

   (a) Salicylates and derivatives which comprise aspirin, sodium salicylate, benorylate, diflunisal, aloxiprin, salsalate.

   (b) Pyrazolone derivatives which include phenylbutazone, oxyphenbutazone, azapropazone, feprazone.

   (c) Indole derivatives which include indomethacin, sulindac.

The above is not an inflexible classification since effect also depends on the dose used, but for the groups of drugs it commonly holds true.

As we frequently notice, inflammatory conditions require protracted treatment with anti-inflammatory drugs. The currently used nonsteroidal anti-inflammatory drugs have divers toxic side effects which bounds there use in long term remedial treatment.

These drugs cause several unwanted effects. The most common is an inclination to persuade gastric or intestinal ulceration that can sometimes be accompanied by a secondary anemia from resultant blood loss. These drugs diversify notably in their inclination to cause such erosions. Gastric damage by these agents can be brought about by at least two clear mechanisms. While local irritation by the drugs in the stomach allows back diffusion of acid into mucosa which can causes tissue damage.

The prevailing prostaglandins synthesized by the gastric mucosa are PGE2 and PGI2; these eicasanoids inhibits acid secretion by the stomach and encourage the secretion of cytoprotective mucus in the intestine. Such prostaglandin and their analogs can block mucosal damage including that induced by anti-inflammatory drugs. Consequently, inhibition of the synthesis of endogenous prostaglandins may render the stomach more vulnerable damage.

Inflammation: Inflammatory diseases including different types of rheumatic disorders, is a greater affair to scientists around the sphere. Today an esteemed percentage of the human population is affected by this disease. A variety of inflammatory drugs are flooding the world market today but a very few are nearly non-toxic and fit for long term use. Furthermore, discontinuation of drug remedial treatment in chronic inflammatory conditions frequently lead to recurrence of symptoms.

Gastrointestinal disorders related to the use of anti-inflammatory drugs, is an enduring dilemma of medical world even today. Modern science has seen the arrival of many new anti-inflammatory drugs, but alas! the problem still leavings.

Thus, it can be mentioned that profound research with indigenous drugs can definitely open up new vistas in inflammation remedial treatment and refined natural compounds may serve as template for synthesis of a new generation of anti-inflammatory drugs which in turn may have low toxicity and preferred therapeutic index.

Medicinal Plants with Anti-inflammatory properties

1. *Acanthus ilicifolius L.* **(Acanthaceae)**

   - *Common names:* Sanskrit: Harikusa, Beng.: Hargoza, Hindi: Harkuch (Hargoza) Kanla, Bomb.: Nivagur.

   - *Distribution:* A gregarious, sparingly branched, evergreen shrub, 0.6-1.5m in height, common in the tidal swamps of creeks and rivers along the East and West coasts; also distributed in Meghalaya and the Andamans.

   - *Parts used:* Leaves.

   - *Pharmacological activities:* Leaves are used as fomentation in neuralgia and rheumatism[1].

   - *Chemical constituents:* Analysis of fresh leaves gave the following values (dry basis): water, 78.20; carbohydrates, 20.95; lipids, 13.55; protein nitrogen, 1.87; non-protein nitrogen, 0.24; and ash, 12.2%; cobalt, 3.3; copper, 9.0; manganese, 96,7; molybdenum 16.7; and zinc, 24.7 mg/g. A new alkaloid, acanthicifolin has been isolated from the air-dried plant. The plant also contains a flavone.

2. *Alangium salvifolium (L.f.) Wang. Syn. A. /amarcW/Thw.* **(Alangiaceae)**

- *Common names:* Eng.: Sageleaved Alangium, Hindi: Dhera, Akola.

- *Distribution:* A small tree with edible fruits. Found throughout the drier parts of India, especially in forest of S.India. Parts used: Stem bark.

- *Pharmacological activities:* Anti-inflammatory activity of the bark extract was found in formaldehyde induced arthritis and Granuloma pouch oedema in animals[2].

- *Chemical constituents:* A new alkaloid – demethylcephaeline along with cephaeline, psychotrine, tubulosine and demethylpsychotrine isolated from stem bark; substance AL 60, previously reported to have hypotensive activity, shown to be mixture of psychotrine, cophaeline and demethylcephaeline; isolation and characterisation of a new sterol-stigmast-5,22,25-trien-3b(p)-ol from leaves; a mono terpenoid lactam-alangiside isolated and its structure elucidated; N-benzoyl-L-phenylaninol, mp. 169°, was isolated; structures of new D, E-cis fused neohopane derivatives - alangioliol and isoalangidiol; stereostructure and synthesis of (±) alangicine; structure and relative configuration of (±) alangimarckine determined by its partial synthesis.

3. *Allium sativum Linn.* **(Liliaceae)**

- *Common names:* Eng.: Garlic, Hindi: Lahsan, Beng.: Rasun.

- *Distribution:* A hardy perennial, 60 cm in height, native to central Asia and cultivated all over India.

- *Parts used:* Bulbs.

- *Pharmacological activities:* Garlic is an effective long term preventive treatment for all rheumatic and catarrhal conditions. It produces anti-inflammatory activity against formalin induced arthritis in albino rats. A concentrate containing the active principle, allicin and allinase proved effective in the treatment of rheumatoid arthritis[3].

- *Chemical constituents:* Isolation of biologically active compound scordinin A1 which on alkaline hydrolysis yielded a peptide, scormine and allylthiofructosiduronic acid; fine unidentified saponins found; garlic bulbs yielded a mixture of polysacchararides containing pectic acid, a D-galactone and a fructan component which contained fructose (94.4) and glucose (4.3%); a linear ineclin type structure suggested for fructan on basis of methanolysis. Garlic also contains allicin and allinase.

4. *Alpina calcarata Rose.* **(Zingiberaceae)**

   - *Common names:* Eng.: Shell ginger, Mai.: Kattuchona; Oriya: Toroni; Tarn.: Amkolingi.

   - *Distribution:* It is slender, rhizomatous herb, often cultivated in gardens in eastern and southern India for its white flowers, variegated with red and yellow in pyramidal panicles.It is frequently available in the sub-Himalayan region of Bihar, West Bengal and Assam, and is extensively cultivated all over India mostly in shady situations(rhizome).

   - *Parts used:* Leaves, flowers, herb.

   - *Pharmacological activities:* The herb is reported to possess anti-tubercular properties. The water-soluble fraction of the alcoholic extract of the air-dried plant in reported to exhibit a significant anti-inflammatory activity in albino rats similar to the beta-methasone[4].

   - *Chemical constituents:* The leaves yield an essential oil containing mostly methyl cinnamate.

5. *Anacardium occidental L.* **(Anacardiaceae)**

   - *Common names:* Eng.: Cashew nut, Beng.: Kaju Badam, Hindi: Kaju.

   - *Distribution:* A small evergreen tree, native of tropical American from Mexico to Peru and Brazil but now cultivated largely in Malabar, Kerala, Karnataka, Tamil Nadu and Andhra Pradesh and to some extent in Maharashtra, Goa, Orissa and West Bengal.

   - *Parts used:* Whole plant.

- *Pharmacological activities:* Anti-inflammatory activity of the plant extract was found in carrageenan induced edema, Cotton pellet induced granuloma, formaldehyde induced arthritis and Freund's complete adjuvant induced arthritis in animals[5].

- *Chemical constituents:* See Antidiabetic chapter.

6. *Anemone obtusiloba D. Don.* **(Ranunculaceae)**

- *Common names:* Eng.: Kumaon-Kakriya, Ratanjota; Punjab: Padar, Rattanjog.

- *Distribution:* Temperate and alpine Himalayas from Kashmir to Sikkim between altitudes of 2,100 and 4,200m, and in the Nilgiri hills, above an attitude of 1,800m.

- *Parts used:* Seed.

- *Pharmacological activities:* Oil extracted from the seed is used in rheumatism (unpublished report).

- *Chemical constituents:* The air-dried plant is reported to contain a substance similar to anemonin.

7. *Anthemis cotula Linn.* **(Asteraceae)**

- *Common names:* Eng.: Cotula, Dag Fennel, Meyweed, wild Chamo-mile.

- *Distribution:* Naturalized in vast places in Uttar Pradesh & Himachal Pradesh.

- *Parts used:* Aerial part of the plant.

- *Pharmacological activities:* The aerial part of plant provides relief in inflammation of tissues[6].

- *Chemical constituents:* The whole fresh plant yields 0.01% of reddish, bitter essential oil which is acidic in reaction. A crystalline acid (m.p. 58°) is present in both free and ester form in the volatile oil. The flowers and leaves contain alkaloids. An optically active sesquiterpene lactone isolated.

8. *Arnebia hispidissima* **(Forsk.)**

Syn. Lithospermum hispidissium Lehm. DC (Boraginaceae)

- *Distribution:* A diffuse or prostrate, xerophytic herb distributed (North West India) in upper gangetic plains, Punjab, Rajasthan and Gujrat.

- *Parts used:* Whole plant.

- *Pharmacological activities:* Plant extract showed anti-inflammatory effects in carragenin induced oedema, cotton pellet induced granuloma in animals[7].

- *Chemical constituents:* Flavonoids (Vitexin) were isolated. Roots yielded dl-alkanin (Shikalkin) as a crystalline red solid.

9. *Azadirachta indica A. Juss.*

   Syn. *Melia azadirachta* Linn. (Meliaceae)

   - *Common names:* Eng.: Margosa tree, Beng.: Nim, Hindi: Nim.

   - *Distribution:* A common tree in the plain of West Bengal and other regions in the plains of India.

   - *Parts used:* Bark.

   - *Pharmacological activities:* Sodium nimbinate isolated form plant possessed potent anti-inflammatory activity in carragenin induced oedema and formaldehyde induced arthritis in animals[8].

   - *Chemical constituents:* From the plant oil three bitter principle was isolated 1. Nimbinia Sulphur free neutral, water insoluble colorless crystalline product (m.p. 205°, yield 0.1%) 2. Nimbidin (m.p.192°, yield 0.01%) 3. Nimbidin (m.p. 90-100° yield 1.1 %) a cream colored powdered insoluble in water. A new oxophenol-nimbiol, m.p 250° in addition to known substance nimbosterol, m.p. 82° from frunk bark was isolated.

10. *Berberis asiatica Roxb. ex DC.* **(Berberidaceae)**

    - *Common names:* Beng.: Daruharitra, Garhwal: Kuigora, Sanskrit: Daruharidra.

    - *Distribution:* Is a pretty shrub 1.8 to 2.4m in height, armed with trifid spines. Commonly occurring in the Himalayas from Himachal Pradesh at 600-2,700m eastwards to Bhutan and Assam at 1,500-1,800m, and on Pareshnath hills in Bihar, Pachmarhi in Madhya Pradesh and Mount Abu in Rajasthan. It also grown in hedges.

    - *Parts used:* Stems.

- *Pharmacological activities:* The root has bitter, sharp, hot taste, as a fomentation removes inflammation and swelling[9].

- *Chemical constituents:* The alkaloids are present in this plant. Berberine and palmatine are present as chlorides. In addition, two move constituents are present in small amounts, in the roots, has been reported.

11. *Berberis petiolaris Wall, ex G.Don.* **(Berberidaceae)**

   - *Common names:* Arabic: Amberbaris, Punjab: Chachar, Urdu: Amber.

   - *Distribution:* Western Himalayas from Kashmir to Nepal up to 12,000ft. Garhwal and kumaun at 2,400m.

   - *Parts used:* Roots.

   - *Pharmacological activities:* The root has cooling effects, used in paralysis and rheumatism[10].

   - *Chemical constituents:* Berberine, berbericine and a new more polar alkaloid isolated as picrate, m.p. 160°, from roots.

12. *Bergenia ligulata Engl.*

   Syn. *B. ciliata* Sternb. (Saxifragaceae)

   - *Common names:* Sans.: Paashaanabheda, Shailagaebhaja.

   - *Distribution:* Distributed in South and Eastern Asia.

   - *Parts used:* Roots. (Rhizomes)

   - *Pharmacological activities:* Acetone extract of the rhizomes possesses potent anti-inflammatory activity but the activity decreases with increasing dosage (unpublished report).

   - *Chemical constituents:* (-) Afzelechin isolated from roots. Saxin isolated from roots was identified as bergenin. Bergenin, its C-glycoside, (3-sitosterol and (+) Catechin-3-gallate isolated from roots.

13. *Boerhaavia diffusa L*

   Syn. *B. repens* L (Nyctaginaceae)

   - *Common names:* Eng.: Horse-purslane, Hog weed, Beng.: Punarnava, Hindi: Punarnava.

- *Distribution:* A herb distributed throughout India.
- *Parts used:* Whole plant.
- *Pharmacological activities:* Plant possesses good anti-inflammatory activity (unpublished report).
- *Chemical constituents:* Hentriacontane, p-sitosterol and ursolic acid isolated from roots. A glycoprotein with a molecular weight of 16000-20000 daltons isolated from roots. Ash (11.8%), Calcium (1.2%), Potassium (2.3%), presence of alkaloids free and combined amino acids determined in aerial parts of plant.

14. *Boswellia serrata Roxb. ex Coleb.* **(Burseraceae)**

   - *Common names:* Eng.: Indian OlibanumTree, Hindi and Beng.: Salai, Luban.
   - *Distribution:* A medium to large sized, deciduous balsamiferous tree up to 18m height and 2.4m in girth commonly found in dry forests from Punjab to West Bengal, and in Peninsular India. The tree is common at the foot of western Himalayas, in Rajasthan, Gujrat, Maharashtra, Madhya Pradesh, Bihar, Orissa, Andhra Pradesh and further South in Peninsula.
   - *Parts used:* Bark.
   - *Pharmacological activities:* The detailed extract of gum exudate (oleo-gum-resin) was found to possess marked anti-inflammatory and anti-arthritic activity in animals (unpublished report).
   - *Chemical constituents:* Oleogum resin consists of three principal constituents namely turpentinic liquid, rosin like resin and gum oil resembles turpentine oil. 3a-Hydroxytirucall-8,24-dien-21 oic acid (i) its acetyl derivative (ii), 3-Ketotirucail-8,24-dien-21 Oic acid (iii) and 3(3-hydroxytirucall-8, 24-dien-21-Oic acid (iv) isolated form resin. Fresh leaves on steam distillation gave an essential oil. Non-volatile fraction (gum-rosin) of oleo-gum-resin yielded a new diterpenic alcohol.

15. *Bryophyllum pinnatum (Lam.) Kurz.*

    Syn. *B. calycinum* Salisb (Crassulaceae)

    - *Common names:* Beng.: Koppata, Hindi: Zakhm-haiyat, Guj.: Ghayamari.

    - *Distribution:* Bryophyllum pinnatum is believed to be a native of tropical Africa, naturalized throughout the tropics of the world. It is cultivated in garden and grows profusely on the hills of North-Western India, Deccan and Bengal.

    - *Parts used:* Leaves.

    - *Pharmacological activities:* Anti-inflammatory activity of the plant extract was found in carrageenan induced oedema cotton pellet granuloma, formaldehyde induced arthritis, Freund's adjuvant induced oedema, Turpentine induced arthritis in animals[11].

    - *Chemical constituents:* Quercetin-3-L-rhamnoside-L-arabinofuranoside isolated. Quercetin-diarabinoside, m.p. 190° and kaempferol-3-glucoside, waxes, flavonoid glycoside and rhenolic compound isolated. Alkanes C_{25}-C_{35}, alkanols C_{26}-C_M, a-amyrin, (3-amyrin and sitosterol isolated from non-saponifiable fraction. P-Coumaric, ferulic, syringic, caffeic and para hydroxybenzoic acids, quercetin and kaempferol detected in leaves; wax hydrocarbons (C_{26}-C_{36}), wax alcoholic (C_{25}-C_{35}) and fatty acids obtained from wax of leaves.

16. *Calophyllum innophyllum I.* **(Clusiacea)**

    - *Common names:* Eng.: Alexandrian laurel, Beng.: Sultana champa, Hindi: Surpan, sultan champa.

    - *Distribution:* An evergreen tree distributed on the sea shores of India, particularly Orissa, Karnataka, Maharashtra and the Andamans. Also cultivated as an ornamental tree.

    - *Parts used:* Seeds.

    - *Pharmacological activities:* Seeds yield a fixed oil known as Domba, applied externally in rheumatism. Seed extract showed anti-inflammatory activity in granuloma pouch, carrageenan induced oedema, cotton pellet induced granuloma, formaldehyde induced arthritis, Freund's complete adjuvant induced arthritis in mice and rats[12,13].

- *Chemical constituents:* Callophylloeide, Xanthones (Dehydrocycloguanadine, Callophyllin-B, Sacareubin, 6-deoxyjacareulin) isolated. 4-Phenyleoumarins-calophyllolide, inophyllolide and calophyllic acid from ripe seeds; cinnamic acid, inophyllic and calophyllic acids and a new 4-phenylcoumarin-ponnalide from unripe seeds; a new myricetin glucoside, myricetin and quercetin from androecium; leucocyanidin from petals; friedelin, 3 new triterpenes-canophyllal, canophyllol and canophyllic acid; (+) inophyllolide, mp.188°, its cis isomer, mp.149° and 12-hydroxy derivative of cis isomer, mp. 200°, from leaves; inophylloidic acid from bark resin; jacareubin, 6-deoxyjacareubin and 2-(3,3-dimethylallyl)-1,3,5,6-tetrahydroxyxanthone from heartwood.

17. *Cananga odorata Hook.f. & Thorns.*

Syn. Canangium odoratum Baill. (Annonaceae)

- *Common names:* Eng.: Ylang-ylang, Tamil: Karumugai, Maladi, Telugu: Apurvachampakamu, Malaya: Cananga, French: Bois de Bananen.
- *Parts used:* Flowers.
- *Pharmacological activities:* Flowers of the oil are used for application of cephalagia, ophthalmia and gout[14].
- *Chemical constituents:* The flowers yield "ilang-ilang" of perfumes "Cananga oil" consists of the early portions of the distillate. Canangine was isolated and found identical with eupolauridine.

18. *Canscora decussate Schutl.* (Gentianaceae)

- *Common names:* Beng.: Daukuni, Hindi: Sankhaphuli.
- *Distribution:* A herb available throughout India.
- *Parts used:* Whole plant.
- *Pharmacological activities:* Fresh juice of the plant is recommended in epilepsy, insanity and nervous debility. Extract of the plant showed anti-inflammatory activity in

carragenin induced oedema, cotton pellet induced granuloma, formaldehyde induced arthritis in animals[15].

- *Chemical constituents:* See Antifertility chapter.

19. *Cassia alata Linn.* (Caesalpiniaceae)

- *Common names:* Eng.: Ringworm Cassia, Beng.: Dadmardan, Dadmari, Hindi: Dadmurdan, dadkapat, Benanakhi, Vilaytie aghatea.

- *Distribution:* A large handsome shrub or a small tree, 1-5m in height introduced from the West Indies and cultivated in the gardens, and also found wild almost throughout India and in the Andaman Islands.

- *Parts used:* Plant.

- *Pharmacological activities:* The plant is reported to possess anti-inflammatory property[16].

- *Chemical constituents:* The leaves contain cassiaxanthone, kaempferol, and its glycoside, aloe-emodin, chrysophanol, rhein, physicion-l-glucoside and p-sitosterol. The roots contain quinine derivatives. Crysophenol, emodine, rhein and aloe-emodine isolated from leaves and fruits; glycoside of rhein, aloe-emodine and emodine obtained from leaves and roots.

20. *Cassia fistula Linn.* (Leguninosae)

- *Common names:* Eng.: Golden-shower, Indian Laburnum, Beng.: Amaltas, Hindi: Bandarlathi.

- *Distribution:* A deciduous, medium sized tree up to 24m in height and 1.8m in girth, cultivated almost throughout India. The tree is one of the most widespread in the forests in India, usually occurring in deciduous forests throughout the greater part of India, ascending up to an altitude of 1,220m in the sub-Himalayan tract and outer Himalayas. It is common - throughout the Gangetic valley, particularly abundant in the bhabar tracts. Central India, and South India.

- *Part used:* Root, bark.

- *Pharmacology activities:* The aqueous extract of the rootbark exhibits anti-inflammatory activity[17].

- *Chemical constituents:* The rootbark yields a mixture of three flavonoids, one of them way identified as fistucacidin. The rootbark also contains tannins, phlobaphenes, reducing sugars, and oxyanthraquinones. Fruits pulp contain rhein, glucose, sucrose, fructose, and pod contain fistulic acid and leucopeler gonidin. Fistucacidin m.p. 245° obtained from bark.

21. *Cedrus deodara (Roxb.) Loud. Syn. C. libani Barrel* **(Pinaceae)**

- *Common names:* Eng.: Himalayan cedar, Deodar. Beng.: Devadaru, Hindi: Deodar.

- *Distribution:* A tall, evergreen tree distributed in N.W. Himalayas from Kashmir to Garhwal. Forests of deodar occur in Kulu, Kashmir, Chamba, Tehri-Garhwal, Almora, Simla, Chakrata and Mussoorie hill stations.

- *Parts used:* Bark, leaf.

- *Pharmacological activities:* The bark is useful in fever and rheumatism. All parts bitter, hot, pungent, light, oleagenous, useful in belching inflammations. The leaves lessen inflammation[18].

- *Chemical constituents:* Flavonoids (Several dihydro flavonols), ascorbic acid, etheral oil (0.056%) isolated from plant. Wood yields an oleoresin and a dark colored oil. Isolation and characterization of alfa-himachalene, bp. 93°/2 mm. and beta-himachalene, bp. 121°/4 mm. from essential oil; (+) lengiborneol and two new sesquiterpene alcohols - himachalol, mp. 67° and allohimachalol, mp. 85° from essential oil; deodarin, mp. 248° from the stem bark. Centdarol isolated and characterised as 2(3, 7p-dihydroxy-himachal-3-ene; isolation and structure of isocendarol; structure determination oxidohimachalene isolated from essential oil; structure of isohimachalane, isolated from wood essential oil; structures of deodarclione and limone carboxylic acid isolated from wood.

22. *Chrysanthemum indicum L.* **(Asteraceae)**

- *Common names:* Eng.: Japanese chrysanthemum, Beng.: Chrysanthemum Hindi: Guldaudi.

- *Distribution:* Native to china and Japan, cultivated in India as ornamental.
- *Parts used:* Leaves.
- *Pharmacological activities:* Leaves prescribed for migraine (unpublished work).
- *Chemical constituents:* dl-camphor, azulene and p-3-carene, bp. 70°/ 30 mm, obtained by distillation of flowers; chrysanthenone from essential oil; isolation of a new sesquiterpene lactone-yehuja lactone-along with chamazulene from flowers.

23. *Cimicifuga foetida Linn.* (Ranunculaceae)

- *Common names:* Eng.: Bugbane, French: Acteefetide, cimicaire, German: Wanzen kraut, Punjab: Jiunti.
- *Distribution:* Temperate Himalayas, from Kashmir to Bhutan (7,000-12,000ft), E. Europe, Siberia.
- *Parts used:* Root.
- *Pharmacological activities:* The root is poisonous. In Europe the root is considered a mild emetic-purgative. In China and Indo China, it is used as antiperiodic and prescribed in rheumatic infections[19].

24. *Cocculus hirsutus (L.) Diels*

Syn. *C. villosus* DC. (Menispermaceae)

- *Common names:* Sans.: Vasnati tikta, Beng.: Huyer, Hindi: Jamti ki bel, Kharetaki.
- *Distribution:* A climbing shrub occurring throughout tropical and subtropical tracts of India from the foot of Himalayas to S. India.
- *Parts used:* Roots, stems.
- *Pharmacological activities:* Roots are useful in chronic rheumatism and venereal diseases. Extracts of stems, roots are sedative, spasmolytic. Roots are used in stomach ache children[20].
- *Chemical constituents:* D-Trilobine and DL-coclaurine from roots; P-sitosterol, ginnol and monomethyl ether of inositol, mp.226° isolated; essential oil, bp.127° and two alkaloids were also isolated but not characterised.

25. *Crotalaria leburnifolia Linn.* **(Papilionaceae)**
    - *Common names:* Hindi: Mura, Tel.: Pedda-galligista.
    - *Distribution:* West Bengal and some other places of India.
    - *Parts used:* Whole plant.
    - *Pharmacological activities:* Possessed potent anti-inflammatory activity in carrageenan induced oedema, cotton pellet induced granuloma, formaldehyde induced arthritis. It also possessed Anti-hyaluronidase activity[21].
    - *Chemical constituents:* An alkaloid-crotalaburnine, mp. 185°, a pigment-lutexin and p-sitosterol isolated from seeds; a pyrrolizidine alkaloid-anacrotine, mp.197° - isolated from seeds, shown to be a cyclic diester of senecic acid.

26. *Cryptolepis buchanani Roem. and Schult* **(Asclepiadaceae)**
    - *Common names:* Hindi: Karanta, Telugu: Adaripalatige.
    - *Distribution:* Throughout India.
    - *Pharmacological activities:* Latex of the plant mixed with hot water and is applied on knees to cure rheumatism[22].
    - *Chemical constituents:* Isolation and structure of a pyridine alkaloid-buchananine.

27. *Curcuma dotnestica Val.*

    Syn. *C. tonga* L. (Zingiberaceae)
    - *Common names:* Eng.: Turmeric, Beng.: Halud, Hindi: Haldi.
    - *Distribution:* A perennial herb cultivated mainly in Tamil Nadu, Andhra Pradesh, Maharashtra, Bihar, Kerala, Orissa and West Bengal. Parts used: Rhizomes.
    - *Pharmacological activities:* Wide medicinal uses. It is used in stomachic toxic, blood purifier, antiseptic, also applied in sprains[23,24]. Chemical constituents: See Anti-fertility chapter.

28. *Cyperus rotundus L.* **(Cyperaceae)**
    - *Common names:* Eng.: Nut grass, Beng.: Muthaghas, Hindi: Motha.

- *Distribution:* A perennial sedge distributed throughout India.

- *Parts used:* Whole plant.

- *Pharmacological activities:* Plant extract showed potent anti-inflammatory activity in carrageenan induced oedema, cotton-pellet induced granuloma and pyrexia in rats[25].

- *Chemical constituents:* p-sitosterol and an essential oil. Cyperene-1 (a tricyclic sesquiterpene) and cyperene-2 (a bicyclic sesquiterpene hydrocarbon) isolated from tubers; patchoulenone, mp.52°; a new sesquiterpene ketone-mustakone, bp.128°/1mm- from essential oil, has same skeleton as copaene; isolation, structure and absolute configuration of cyperotundone; mp.46°, from tubers, cyperolone, mp.41 °, from tubers; a new sesquiterpenoid-sugetriol triacetate, mp.132° from tubers of Japanese nut grass; 27 compounds separated from essential oil by GLC and four of these copadiene, bp. 13071 mm, epoxyguaiene, bp. 102°/ 1mm, rotundone, bp. 12871 mm. and cyperolone, bp. 12070.1mm -characterised; sesquiterpenic ketol-sugeonol; structure and absolute configuration of cyperol and isocyperoi; structure of alfa-rotunol, mp.87°, and p-rotunol, mp.118°; two nor-sesquiterpenoids - kobusone and isokobusone.

29. *Dalbergia lanceolaria Lf.* (Papilionaceae)

- *Common names:* Beng.: Chanemdia, Hindi: Bithua, Mar.: Daudous.

- *Distribution:* A tall deciduous tree available throughout India. Parts used: Whole plant.

- *Pharmacological activities:* Plant extract showed potent anti-inflammatory activity in carragenin induced oedema and Formaldehyde induced arthritis in rats[26].

- *Chemical constituents:* Lanceolarin, mp.165", from root bark, characterised as biochanin A-7-apiosyl-glucoside; psi-baptigenin isolated from flowers and leaves identified as 7-hydroxy-3',4'-methylenedioxy-soflavone.

30. *Desmodium gangeticutn DC* **(Papilionaceae)**

- *Common names:* Beng.: Salpani, Hindi: Sarivan, Sans.: Shalapanini.

- *Distribution:* A shrub distribution throughout India.

- *Parts used:* Whole plant.

- *Pharmacological activities:* Anti-inflammatory and antipyretic activity was shown in carrageenan induced oedema, cotton pellet induced granuloma, writhing response and pyrexia in rats by the plant extract[27].

- *Chemical constituents:* A new pterocarpan-gangetin-isolated an characterised as 7a, 12a-dihydro-13-methoxy-3-3-dimethyl-11-(3-methyl-2-butenyl)-3H, 7H-benzofuro [3,2C] pyrano [3,2, -g] benzopyran-10-01; detection of 5 phospholipids in seeds by TLC; twelve alkaloids of four structural types (carboxylated and decarboxylated tryptamine, beta-carbolines and p-phenylethylamines) isolated; two pterocarpanoids -gangetinin and desmodin isolated and their structures determined.

31. *Dysoxylum binectariferum Hook, f.* **(Meliaceae)**

- *Common names:* Beng.: Lassumi, Tarn.: Aganivagil, Kan.: Agilu.

- *Distribution:* Sikim, Assam, West Bengal, Western Ghats and Andaman island.

- *Parts used:* Whole plant.

- *Pharmacological activities:* Anti-inflammatory activity of the plant extract was tested in carrageenan induced oedema in animals[28].

- *Chemical constituents:* A new tetranortriterpene - disobinin – isolated from fruits and characterised.

32. *Echinops echinatus Roxb.* **(Asteraceae)**

- *Common names:* Sans.: Kantalu, Hindi: Utakanta, Mar: Kadechudoak.

- *Distribution:* A herb occurring throughout India.

- *Parts used:* Roots and other parts.

- *Pharmacological activities:* Plant extract showed anti-inflammatory activity in acute carrageenan paw oedema, formaldehyde induced arthritis and Adjuvant-induced acute and chronic arthritis in rats[29].

- *Chemical constituents:* Isolation of (3-amyrin and lupeol.

33. *Elephantopus scaber I.* **(Asteraceae)**

- *Common names:* Beng.: Gojialata, Hindi: Gobhi, Sanskrit: Gojihva.

- *Distribution:* Throughout hotter parts of India.

- *Pharmacological activities:* Plant paste without sugar is applied externally in rheumatism[30].

- *Chemical constituents:* Epifriedelinol, lupeol, stigmasterol and a mixture of triacontan-1-ol and doltriacontan-1-ol isolated. A new sesquiterpene ditactone – isodeoxy-elephantopin isolated.

34. *Flacourtia indica (Burm.f.) Merr.* **(Flacourtiaceae)**

- *Common names:* Beng.: Bincha, Hindi: Bailangra, Sanskrit: Swadukartaka.

- *Distribution:* Sub-Himalayan tract ascending up to 1200m, Indus plains, upper gangetic plains.

- *Pharmacological activities:* Seeds are made into paste and used in rheumatism[31].

35. *Garcinia mangostana L.* **(Guttiferae)**

- *Common names:* Eng.: Mangosteen, Beng.: Mangustan, Hindi: Mangustan.

- *Distribution:* Tree native to Malaysia and is now cultivated in lower slopes of Nilgiris.

- *Parts used:* Fruits.

- *Pharmacological activities:* Possess anti-inflammatory properties in Freund's complete adjuvant induced arthritis in animals[32].

- *Chemical constituents:* Three new xanthones-gartanin, 8-deoxy-gartanin and normangostin-isolated from fruits; mangostin isolated and its structure confirmed; 1,3,6,7-tetrahydroxyxanthone and its glucoside isolated from heartwood; cyanidin-3-sophoroside and cyanidin-3-glucoside from rinds.

36. *Glycyrrhiza glabra* **L. (Papilionaceae)**

   - *Common names:* Eng.: Liquorice, Beng.: Jashtimadhu, Hindi: Mulhatti.

   - *Distribution:* A perennial herb, native to the Mediterranean region and is now grown in Punjab, Jammu and Kashmir and S. India.

   - *Parts used:* Roots.

   - *Pharmacological activities:* Root extract was tested in formaldehyde induced arthritis, Freund's complete adjuvant induced arthritis, Pyrexia and cotton pellet induced granuloma in animals and its anti-inflammatory and antipyretic activity was confirmed[33].

   - *Chemical constituents:* See Antiulcer chapter.

37. *Hedychium coronarium Koenig ex Retz.* **(Zingiberaceae)**

   - *Common name:* Ginger lily.

   - *Distribution:* An ornamental rhizometous herb occurring throughout the moist parts of India.

   - *Parts used:* Rhizome.

   - *Pharmacological activities:* Essential oil, obtained from rhizome is active against gram positive bacteria and fungi. Powdered rhizomes are used in medicines as febrifuge, decoction is considered as antirheumatic and tonic[34].

   - *Chemical constituents:* Essential oil (0.1%) from rhizomes contained eucalyptol.

38. *Hibiscus vitifolius* **L. (Malvaceae)**

   - *Common names:* Beng.: Bankapas, Hindi: Bankapas.

   - *Distribution:* A bushy shrub distributed in hotter parts of India.

   - *Parts used:* Seeds.

   - *Pharmacological activity:* Seeds are reported to possess powerful anti-inflammatory activity. Activity was tested in carrageenan induced oedema, Granulama pouch, Mediator induced oedema in animals[35].

   - *Chemical constituents:* A new gossypetin glucuronide-hibifolin isolated from flowers along with gossypin and characterised.

39. *Juniperus communis Linn.* (Cupresaceae)

- *Common names:* Eng.: Juniper, Hindi: Avaraar, haubera, abhal, Beng.: Havcesha, Mar.: Hosha.

- *Distribution:* The plant widely available in Northern part of India at the altitude of more than 1350m.

- *Parts used:* Leaves.

- *Pharmacological activities:* Potent anti-inflammatory activity of leaf extract was confirmed in carrageenan induced paw oedema, granuloma pouch in rats. East induced pyrexia in rat was significantly reduced by leaf extract[36].

- *Chemical constituents:* Communic acid, m.p. 228° (0.12%) from bark of J. Communis and longifolene, Juniperol, (3-sitosterol, stigmasterol and disterpene phenol-totarol isolated from its bark. Production of essential oil and tropolone by plant tissue culture has been reported.

40. *Madhuca longifolia (L.) Macb.*

Syn. Bass/a longifolia K. (Sapotaceae)

- *Common names:* Eng.: South Indian Mahua, Beng.: Rainjani, Assam: Awnapat, Hindi: Mohua.

- *Distribution:* Cultivated in U.P., Bihar, A.P., Karnataka, Bengal and Maharashtra.

- *Parts used:* Bark.

- *Pharmacological activities:* Plant extract showed anti-inflammatory activity in carrageenan induced oedema, formaldehyde induced arthritis in rats[37].

- *Chemical constituents:* A new saponin - bassianin - isolated which on hydrolysis yielded bassic acid, glucose, arabinose, xylose and rhamnose; P-sitosterol- (3-D-glucoside, stigmasterol, n-hexacosanol and 3(3-caproxy-olean-12-en-28-ol isolated from leaves; p-carotene, n-octacosanol, sitosterol, its p-D-glucoside, stigmasterol, 3p-palmitoxyolean-12-en-28-ol, oleanolic acid, quercetin, erythrodiol and palmitic acid isolated from leaves myricetin and its 3-0-L-rhamnoside isolated from leaves; structure elucidation of saponins A and B isolated from seeds; quercetin, myricetin-3-O-L-rhamnoside and quercitrin isolated; soil bacterial hydrolysis of saponins of seed kennels yielded protobassic acid and prosapogenol; Mi-saponin A and Mi-saponin B isolated from seeds and characterised as 3-0-p-D-glucopyranosyl-28-0-[a-L-rhamnopyranosyl-(1-3)-p-D-xylopyranosyl (1-4)-oc-L-rhamnopyranosyl (1-2) a-L-arabinopyranosyl]-protobassic acid and 3-0-p-D-glucopyranosyl-28-0-[3-0-p-D-apio-D-furanosyl-4-0-(a-L-rhamnopyranosyl-(1-3)-p-D-xylopy-ranosyl)-ot-L-rhamnopyranosyl (1-2)-a-L-arabinopy-ranosyl]-protobasic acid respectively; Mi-saponin C isolated from seed kenels, characterised as 3-0-p-D-gluco-pyranosyl-28-0-[(3-0-a-L-rhamnopyranosyl-4-0-p-D-gluco-pyranosyl]-p-D-xylopy-ranosyl (1 -4)-a-L-rhamnopyranosyl (1 -2)-a-L-arabino-pyranosyl)-protobassic acid.

41. *Mammea longifolia Planch. & Triana*

Syn. *Ochrocarpus longifolius* Benth. & Hook.f. (Clusiaceae)

- *Common names:* Eng.: Alexandrian laurele, Beng.: Nagesar, Hindi: Nagkesar.
- *Distribution:* A tree cultivated in S. India.
- *Pharmacological activities:* Plant possesses potent anti-inflammatory properties (unpublished report).
- *Chemical constituents:* Squalene, cycloartenol compesterol, stigmasterol and p-sitosterol. Flowers contained vitexin and mesoinositol. Two new 4-alkylated coumarins-surangin A and B from roots.

42. *Mesua ferrea L.* (Guttiferae)

- *Common names:* Eng.: Iron wood, Beng.: Nagkeshar, Guj: Nagchampa.
- *Distribution:* A tree found in eastern Himalayas, Assam, West Bengal, W.Ghata, Travancore and the Andaman Islands.
- *Parts used:* Seeds.
- *Pharmacological activities:* Seeds yield a fatty oil used as an embrocation in rheumatism. Anti-inflammatory activity was tested in carrageenan induced oedema cotton pellet induced granuloma and Granuloma pouch in animals[38].

- *Chemical constituents:* Mammeisin isolated from seeds; a new 4-phenylcoumarin mesuagin isolated from seed oil and characterised; mammeigin and mesuol isolated from seed oil; a new biflavanone-mesuaferrone A-isolated from stamens and characterised as 8, 8'-binaringenin; structure elucidation of another biflavone-mesuaferrone B-isolated from stamens.

43. *Michelia champaca Linn.* (**Magnoliaceae**)

   - *Common names:* Beng.: Champa, Assam: Phulchopa, Bombay: Champa, French: Champac, Eng.: Golden champa, yellow champa.

   - *Distribution:* A large tree, cultivated mainly in South India, West Ghats Assam and Bengal.

   - *Parts used:* Root, root bark.

   - *Pharmacological activities:* The dried root and root bark, mixed with curdled milk is useful as an application to abscesses, clearing away or maturing the inflammation[39].

44. *Moringa oleifera Lamk.*

   Syn. *Moringa pterygosperma* Gaertn. (Moringaceae)

   - *Common names:* Eng.: Drum stick tree, Beng.: Sajina, Hindi: Sahinjna, Soanjna.

   - *Distribution:* A small tree native to India. Parts used: Seeds.

   - *Pharmacological activities:* Oil obtained from seeds is used medicinally in gout and acute rheumatism[40].

   - *Chemical constituents:* See Antifertility chapter.

45. *Myrtus communis L.* (**Myrtaceae**)

   - *Common names:* Eng.: Myrtle, Beng.: Sutrasowa, Hindi: Vilatimehendi, Murad.

   - *Distribution:* A small tree cultivated in N.W. India.

   - *Parts used:* Berries.

   - *Pharmacological activities:* Myrtle oil applied in rheumatism and considered rubefacient[41].

   - *Chemical constituents:* Isolation and structure elucidation of two acylphloroglucinols A and B; limonene (23.4), linanool (22.2), alfa-pinene (14.5), cineol (11.6), P-cymol (1.8), camphene (0.5), p-pinene (0.3%) and traces of car-3-ene found in leaf essential oil.

46. *Nyctanthes arbor-tristis* L. (Oleaceae)

- *Common names:* Eng.: Tree of Sorrow, Night flowering jasmine, Beng.: Shefali, Hindi: Harsinghar.seoli.

- *Distribution:* A large shrub or small tree grown as an ornamental.

- *Parts used:* Leaves.

- *Pharmacological activities:* Leaves used in rheumatism and fevers; decoction given in sciatica[42].

- *Chemical constituents:* Flavanol glycosides- astragalin and nicotiflorin isolated from leaves. A new iridoid - nyctanthoside - isolated and characterised; crocin-1 (p-digentiobioside ester of a-crocetin), and crocin-3 (p-monogentio-bioside ester of a-crocetin) isolated from flowers; D-mannitol isolated from flowers; detection of astragalin and nicotiflorin by chromatography; a new glycoside   naringenin-4'-0-p-D-glucopyranosyl-a-xylo-pyranoside isolated from stem along with P-sitosterol.

47. *Ocimum basilicum* L. (Lamiaceae)

- *Common names:* Eng.: Common basil, Beng.: Bantulsi, Hindi: Babui tulsi.

- *Distribution:* Indigenous to the lower hills of Punjab cultivated throughout the greater part of India.

- *Parts used:* Whole plant.

- *Pharmacological activities:* Plant considered antipyretic[43] agent.

- *Chemical constituents:* See Antiulcer chapter.

48. *Paederia scandens (Lour.) Merrill.*

Syn. *P. tomentosa* Blume (Rubiaceae)

- *Common names:* Beng.: (Prasarani) Gandal, Hindi: Ghandhali, Somaraji, Guj: Gandhana.

- *Distribution:* Found in C. and E. Himalayas extending to Calcutta.
- *Parts used:* Leaves and stems.
- *Pharmacological activities:* Plant extract showed anti-inflammatory activity stronger than that of acetylsalicylic acid and weaker than that of hydrocortisone[44].
- *Chemical constituents:* Hentriacontan, hentriacontanol, methyl mereaptan, ceryl alcohol, palmitic acid, sitosterol, stimasterol, campesterol, ursolic acid and iridoid glycosides-asperuloside, paederoside and scandoside isolated from leaves and stems.

49. *Pinus roxburghii Sarg.*

Syn. P. longifolia Roxb. (Pinaceae)

- *Common names:* Eng.: Long leaved pine, Beng.: Pine, Hindi: Chir, Salla.
- *Distribution:* Found in Eastern and Western Himalayas.
- *Parts used:* Stem.
- *Pharmacological activities:* Oil terpentine oil obtained by purification. From oil of terpentine oleoresin is used in rheumatic pains (unpublished report).
- *Chemical constituents:* Oleoresin obtained from oil of terpentine. Friedelin, ceryl alcohol and p-sitosterol isolated from bark, hexacosyl ferulate isolated and structure confirmed by synthesis.

50. *Piper longum L.* **(Piperaceae)**

- *Common names:* Eng.: Long pepper, Beng.: Pepul, Hindi: Pipar, Piplamul.
- *Distribution:* Native of India and cultivated in W.Ghats, Karnataka and Tamil Nadu, to some extent in W. Bengal.
- *Parts used:* Roots and fruits.
- *Pharmacological activities:* Roots and fruits are used as counter-irritant and analgesic for muscular pain and inflammations[45]. Chemical constituents: Two new monocyclic sesquiterpenes, b.p. 235° (15.5) and b.p.247° (11.1%) from essential oil; two new alkaloids-piperlong-

umine (piplartine), mp.124° and piper-longuminine-from roots and stem bark, characterised as N-(3, 4, 5-trimethoxycinnamoyl)-piperidin-2-one-5-ene and isobutyl-lamide of piperic acid respectively; a new sesquiterpenic hydrocarbon containing tetra substituted double bond from essential oil; sesamin isolated; isolation of N-isobutyldeca-trans-2-trans-4-dienamide, mp.69°.

51. *Pluchea indica Less.* **(Asteraceae)**

- *Common names:* Beng.: Kakronda, Manjuriukha.

- *Distribution:* A shrub found in salt marshes in Sundarbans. Distributed in new world tropical and sub-tropical regions of Asia. It contains around 50 species out of which 6 have been recorded in India.

- *Parts used:* Roots and leaves.

- *Pharmacological activities:* Roots and leaves are antipyretic, leaves infusion is used in lumbago[46].

- *Chemical constituents:* Endesmane derivatives of the enactahemone. Pluchea indica is known to contain 3-(2', 3'-diacetoxy-2'-methylbutyryl) -cuanhtemone (molecular formulae $C_{24}H_{36}O_8$), colourless prism shaped crystals of m.p. 165°C. The plant is also known to contain linaloylapiosyl glucoside (colourless viscous oil, molecular formulae $C_{21}H_{30}O_{10}$), linaloyl glucoside (colourless viscous oil, molecular formulae $C_{16}H_{28}O_6$),9-hydroxylinaloyl glucoside (colourless viscous oil, molecular formulae $C_{16}H_{28}O_7$), plucheisude A (amorphous powder and B. Plucheoside B (amorphous powder).

52. *Pluchea lanceolata C. B. Clarke.* **(Asteraceae)**

- *Common names:* Punjab: Sarmei, Hindi: Rasna, Marmandai, Sans.: Rasna.

- *Distribution:* A small shrub, found commonly in Punjab and U.P.

- *Parts used:* Whole plant.

- *Pharmacological activities:* Plant used in rheumatoid arthritis[47].

53. *Psoralea corylifolia Linn.* (Fabaceae)

- ***Common names:*** Eng.: Bakuchi, Beng.: Barachi, Hindi: Babchi.

- ***Distribution:*** A common herb, available in India. Parts used: Seeds.

- ***Pharmacological activities:*** Seeds are specially recommended for inflammatory diseases of skin[48].

- ***Chemical constituents:*** Isolation and separation of psoralone and isopsoralone from seeds; isolation and separation of psorlen and isopsoralen from seeds; a new isoflavone-neobavaisoflavone- and a new chroneno-chalcone-bavachromene isolated from seeds and fruits; bavachin, psoralidin, 4'-0-methylbavachalcone, 7-0-mehylbavachin and isobavachalene isolated from seeds; a novel monoterpene phenol-(+)bakuchiol-from seeds; its structure and absolute configuration [(S)-chirality] assigned; a new isoflavone-corylin-isolated and characterised as 7-hydroxy-6", 6"-dimethylpyrano (2", 3", 4', 3') isoflavone; partial synthesis of corylin; high yield of psoralen and angelicin found in seeds; new coumestrol-corylidin - isolation from seeds together with triacontane and p-sitosterol-p-D-glucoside; new formylated chalcone-neobava-chalcone-isolated from seeds and its synthesis; a new isoflavone-carylinal - isolated from seeds together with neobavaiso-flavone as their methyl ethers; isolation and structure elucidation of another isoflavone psoralenol from setds.

54. *Ranunculus aquatilis Linn. var. trichophyllus Hook. f.* (Ranunculaceae)

- ***Common names:*** Eng.: Water crowfoot, water Fennel.

- ***Distribution:*** Punjab Plain, W. Himalaya from India to Kumaon, Baluchisthan, Afghanistan, N. Africa and Europe.

- ***Pharmacological activities:*** The leaves are applied as blister to the wrists in rheumatism[49].

55. *Ranunculus avensis Linn.* (Ranunculaceae)

- *Common names:* Eng.: Corn Crowfoot, Crows-claws, French: Bassinet des champs, Malta: Devil's claws. Punjab: Chambul.

- *Distribution:* Western Himalayas from Kashmir to Kumaon, Mt. Abu, Afganisthan, Europes N. Africa.

- *Pharmacological activities:* In Europe the plant is used in intermittent fevers, gout[50].

56. *Ranunculus muricatus Linn.*

Syn. R. cabulicus Boiss. (Ranunculaceae)

- *Common name:* Eng: Field crow foot.

- *Distribution:* Punjab Himalayas, Punjab, Kashmir, W. Africa, Europe, temperature N. America.

- *Pharmacological activities:* In Europe the plant is used in intermittent fevers, gout[51].

57. *Ricinus communis L.* (Euphorbiaceae)

- *Common names:* Eng.: Castor-seed, Castor oil plant, Beng.: Bheranda, Hindi: Erandi.

- *Distribution:* A small tree cultivated chiefly in Andhra Pradesh, Maharashtra, Karnataka and Orissa. It is also found as wild.

- *Parts used:* Roots.

- *Pharmacological activities:* Decoction of roots is useful in lumbago[52].

- *Chemical constituents:* See Antidiabetic chapter.

58. *Sagittaria sagittifolia L.* (Alismataceae)

- *Common names:* Eng.: Old-world arrowhead, Beng.: Muya muya, Hindi: Chotakut.

- *Distribution:* A herb found throughout India.

- *Parts used:* Leaves.

- *Pharmacological activities:* The leaves are used in sore throat and inflammation of breast[53].

- *Chemical constituents:* Hentriacontanone and sitosterol isolated; a diterpene - sagitariol - isolated and characterised as labda-7,14-diene-13(5), 17-diol.

59. *Semecarpus anacardium Lf.* **(Anacardiaceae)**

- *Common names:* Eng.: Marking-nut tree, Beng.: Bhela, Hindi: Bhilawa.

- *Distribution:* A tree occurring in hotter parts of India.

- *Pharmacological activities:* Fruits used for rheumatism[54].

- *Chemical constituents:* Bhilawanol from fruits was found to be a mixture of 1,2 dihydroxy 3 (pentadecenlyl-8') benzene 1,2 dihydroxy-3-(pentaclecadienyl-8'.11')-benzene; studies on methylated bhilawanol showed that it contained more than seven components; two major components identified as dimethyl ethers of 1-pentadeca-8-enyl-2,3-dihydroxy benzene (I) and 1 -pentadeca-7,10-dienyl-1,3-dihydroxy benzene (II); defatted nuts yielded three biflavones A, B, and C; latter two compounds characterised as 3'8-binaringenin and 3',8-biliquiriligenine; reexamination of bhilawanol showed it to be comprised of two components, 1, 2-dihydroxy-3-pentadecenyl benzene (32-32%) and its corresponding diene analogu (68-70%); a new biflavan-tetrahydroro bustafalvone-and tetrahydro amentoflavone isolated from nuts; leaves yielded only amentoflavone.

60. *Sida acuta Burm.f.*

Syn. S. Carpinifolia Masters (Non-L.f) (Malvaceae)

- *Common names:* Beng.: Sweet berela, Hindi: Bariara, kharenta, Mar.: Tupharia.

- *Distribution:* A common under shrub.

- *Parts used:* Leaves and roots.

- *Pharmacological activities:* Leaves used in rheumatic affections. Roots are used as antipyretic[55].

- *Chemical constituents:* Ecdysterone isolated from the plant.

61. *Tinospora crispa (Linn.) ex. Hook. f. & Thorns.* **(Menispermaceae)**

- *Common names:* Hindi: Gulancha, Beng.: Goloncha.

- *Distribution:* A climbing shruts, found throughout the tropical parts of India known by the same regional names as Tinospora cordifolia and used medicinally.

- *Parts used:* Leaves.

- *Pharmacological activities:* In the Philippine Islands it is considered to be a panacea to be applied to all bodily afflictions. It is given in chronic rheumatism[56].

- *Chemical constituents:* Sodium, Potassium, Calcium, Iron, Aluminium, Copper and Zinc estimated in leaves; two unidentified alkaloids, one hydroxy compound, mp.95°, y-sitosterol and another sterol and essential oil, b.p.116°, isolated from leaves.

62. *Tinospora malabarica (Lam.) Miers.* (Menispermaceae)

- *Common names:* Beng.: Padma gulameha, Hindi: Gulancha, Gurch, Marati: Gulvel, Tamil: Potchindil, Oriya: Gulochi, Guduchi.

- *Distribution:* Bengal, Assam, Khasiam Orissa, Kankan, Kanara and nearly all districts of Tamil Nadu.

- *Parts used:* Leaves and stems.

- *Pharmacological activities:* In China and Tong king the fresh leaves and the stems are used in the treatment of chronic rheumatism, fumigations are recommended in piles and ulcerated wounds[57].

63. *Tylophora asthmatica W. & A.*

Syn. T. indica Merrill. (Asclepiadaceae)

- *Common names:* Oriya: Mendi, Beng.: Anantomul, Hindi: Antanul.

- *Distribution:* A climber distributed in Assam, West Bengal, Orissa and Peninsular India.

- *Parts used:* Whole plant.

- *Pharmacological activities:* Plant extract was used in different animal models like carrageenan induced oedema, cotton pellet induced granuloma and granuloma pouch and found significant anti-inflammatory activity[58].

- *Chemical constituents:* Three alkaloids A,B and C isolated; alkaloids B and C characterised as desmethyl-tylophorine and desmethyltylophori-nine respectively; crystal structure of tylophorinidine and relative stereochemistry of tylophorinine and tylophorinidine; (+) septicine and (+) isotylocrebrine also isolated from fresh leaves; dehydrotylophorine, anhydrodehydrotylophorinine and anhydrodehydrotylophorinidine isolated; sterio-chemistry of tylophorinine and tylophorinidine; absolute configuration of tylophorine; tylophorine and tylophorinine content in leaves is a function of plant growth phase and is highest during flowering period; gama-fagarine and skimmianine isolated from roots and aerial parts.

References

1. Dictionary of Economic plants of India, Council of Agricultural Research, New Delhi, p-5.

2. Prasad, D.N., Bhattacharya, S.K. and Das, P.K., Ind. J. Mod Res., (1966), 54, 582.

3. Turner, B., Acta phytother., (1964), 11, 141.

4. Chopra, ef a/, Indian J. Med. Res., (1954), 42, 385.

5. Agarwal, O.P., Agents Actions, (1982), 12, 298.

6. Krochmal, A., Eco. Bot, (1954), 8, 3.

7. Pravakar, M.C., Kuwar, I., Shenshi, M.A. and Khan, M.S.Y., Planta Med., (1981), 43, 396.

8. Pillai, N.R. and Shantha Kumari, G., Planta Med., (1980), 43, 59.

9. Atal, O.K. and Kapoor, B.M., Cultivation and utilization of Medicinal Plants, Reg. Res. Lab, C.S.I.R Jammu-Tawi, (1982), 545.

10. Ibid , P- 545.

11. Pal, S and Nag Chowdhury, A.K., Fitoterapia, ('1990), 61(6), 527.

12. Nath, R., Saxena, R.C., Palit, G., Nigam, S.K. and Bhargava, K.P., Ind. J. Pharmac., (1979), 11, 39.

13. Bhalla, IN., Saxena, R.C., Wigam, S.K., Misra, G. and Bhargava, K.P., Ind. J. Med. Res., (1980), 72, 762.

14. Kirtikar, K.R. and Basu, B.D., Indian Med. Plants (1981), Vol. I, International Book Distributors, Dehradun, 65.

15. Shankarnarayan, D., Gopalkrishnan, C. and Kameshwaran, L, Ind. J. Pharm. Sci., (1979), 41, 78.

16. Silva, and Abraham, Fitoterapia, (1981), 52, 195.

17. Nair, et al, J. Res. Indian Med. Yoga, (1977), 12(1), 77.

18. Indigenous Drugs of India (1982) 2nd edition, Academic Publisher, Calcutta, p-500.

19. Kirtikar, K.R. and Basu, B.D., Ind. Med. Plants, (1981), Vol.1, International Book Distributors, Dehraduna, 25.

20. Indigenous Drugs o! India, (1982) 2nd edition, Academic Publishers, Calcutta, p-501.

21. Singh, H. and Ghosh, M.N., Ind. J. Physiol. Pharmacol., (1968), 12, 22.

22. Atal, C.K. and Kapoor B.M., Cultivation and Utilization of Med. Plants, Reg. Res. Lab C.S.I.R Jammu-Tawi, (1982), 545.

23. Ghatak, N. and Basu, N., Ind. J. Expti, Biol., (1972), 10, 235.

24. Deodhar, S.D., Sethi, R. and Srimal, R.C., Ind. J. Med. Res., (1980), 71, 632.

25. Gupta, M.B., Nath, R, Shivastava, N, Shankar, K., Kishore, K. and Bhargava, K.P., Planta Med., (1980), 39, 157.

26. Tripathi, S.N. and Kishore, P., Ind. J. Med Res., (1967), 1, 155.

27. Ghosh, D., Anantharam, M. and Purashothaman, K.K., Ind. J. Pharmac., (1980), 12, 210.

28. Tandon, R., Jain, G,K, and Singh, S., Ind. J. Pharmac., (1982), 14, 103.

29. Singh, B., Gambhir, S.S., Panday, V.B. and Joshi, V.K., J. of. Ethnopharm., (1989), 25, 189.

30. Atal, C.K. and Kapoor, B.M., Cultivation and utilization of Med Plants, Reg. Res. Lab. C.S.I.R. Jammu-Tawi, (1982), p-545.

31. Ibid p-545.

32. Gopalkrishan, C., Shankaranarayan, D., Kameshwaran, L, and Nazimuddeen, S.R., Ind, J. ExptlBiol., (1980a), 18, 843.

33. Siddiqui, H.H., Ind. J. Pharm., (1965), 27, 80.

34. Singh, Umrao, Wadhwani, A.M., and Johri, B.M., Dictionary o! Economic Plants of India, I.C.A.R, New Delhi, (1983), p-97.

35. Parmar, N.S. and Ghosh, M.N., Ind. J. Pharmac., (1980a), 12, 201.

36. Chatterjee, I, Ghosh, C., and roychowdhuri, P., Indian Drugs, (1991), 28, 430.

37. Gupta, M.B., Bhalla, T.N., Gupta, G.B., Mitra, C. and Bhargava, K.P., Jap. J.Pharmaco.,/ (1971), 21, 377.

38. Gopalkrishnan, C., Shankaranarayan, D., Nazimuddeen, S.K., Viswanathan, S. and Kameshwaran, L., Ind. J. Pharmacol., (1980a), 12, 181.

39. Kritikar, K.R. and Basu, B.D., Indian Med. Plants, (1981), Vol. I, International Book Distributors, Dehradun, p-57.

40. Indegenous Drugs of India, (1982), 2nd edition, Academic Publishers, Calcutta, p-365.

41. The useful plants of India, (1986), Publications and Information Directorate, CSIR, New Delhi, p-390.

42. Ibid, p-400.

43. Ibid, p-404.

44. Rastogi, R.P. & Mehratra, B.N., Compedium of Indian Medicinal Plants, Vol.2, (1991), CDRI, Lucknow and PID, CSIR, New Delhi, p-503.

45. The useful plants of India, (1986), Publications and Information Directorate, CSIR, New Delhi, p-460.

46. Sen, I, Ghosh, T. K. & Nag Choudhuri, A.K., Life Sci., (1993), 52, 737.

47. The useful plants of India, (1986), Publications and Information Directorate, CSIR, New Delhi, p-500.

48. Anand, K.K., Sharma, M.L, Singh, B. and Roy Ghatak, B.J., Ind. Exptl, Biol, (1978), 16, 1216.

49. Kirtikar, K.R. and Basu, B.D., Indian Med. Plants, (1981), Vol.l, International Book Distributors, Dehradun, 14.

50. Ibid, p-16.

51. Ibid, p-17.

52. The useful plants of India, (1986), Publications and Information Directorate, CSIR, New Delhi, p-526.

53. Ibid, p-539.

54. Ibid, p-566.

55. Ibid, p-573.

56. Kirtikar, K.R. and Basu, B.D., Indian Med. Plants, (1981), Vol. l, International Book Distributors, Dehradun, 77.

57. Ibid, p-76.

58. Gopalkrishnan, C., Shankaranarayan, D., Kameshwaran, L and Natarajan, S., Ind. J. Med. Res., (1979), 69, 513.

6 *Medicinal Plants with Anti-Microbial Properties*

The science of microorganisms is a somewhat current branch of biology. About 130 years ago, Louis Pasteur (1857) fashioned his first report on lactic acid fermentation to the Scientific Society at Lille. At the close of the corresponding year he reported to the Academy of Sciences of France on the alcoholic fermentation. In this communication Pasteur hinted at the operative role of microorganisms in conversions of the substrate substances. This statement contradicted the ordinarily accepted concepts matured by Liebig. The year of 1857 can therefore be suitably considered the year of foundation of physiological microbiology, microbiology as an autonomous science.

The science of microorganisms owes its advance primarily to the study of fermentation processes, and also advances in medicine and veterinary (later agriculture and soil microbiology).

Many scientists postulated that human diseases might be treated with preparations which would execute selectively pathogenic microbes without touching man. The known physician Paracelsus (1493-1541) used arsenic to treat syphilis but was a flop. There hundred years later, Paul Ehrlich (1854 -1915), a German physician, bacteriologist, and initiatory in immunology and chemotherapy, synthesized in 1912 the compound of arsenic that killed *in,* utility agent of syphilis. He named his preparation Salvarsan and established its chemical structure.

The Soviet chemist Kraft showed (1949) that compound of arsenic cannot have the As = As bond. He proved that Salvarsan is a mixture of polymer homologues of the following structure:

Unfortunately, the structure of the Salvarsan molecule is still described by many authors in the form as it was first shown by Ehrlich.

Salvarsan remained the only chemotherapeutic preparation for a prolonged time (except quinine which was familiar to the Indians of South America from ancient times; they used it to treat malaria).

New organic preparations, e.g. sulpha drugs, were achieved in the '30s of this century. Prontosil was the first efficient sulphanilamide to combat oppressive streptococcus infections. The anti-coccal action of sulfanilamide was first discovered in experiments on animals by the German bacteriologist Domagk (1934). But soon (1935) it was shown that prontosil decomposes in the alive body to give a extremely active sulfanilamide and the toxic compound tri-aminobenzene, which has no antibacterial properties:

Sulphapyridine was synthesized in the Soviet Union in 1937. This preparation was resembling in its properties to prontosil. Other sulfa drugs, such as sulphathiazole, sulphaethidole, phthalasul-phathiazole, were promptly synthesized to substitute sulphapyridine.

The discovery of sulfa drugs and their use in medicine for treatment of infectious diseases, e.g. meningitis, sepsis, pneumonia, erysipelas, and gonorrhea, was a significant occurrence in medicine.

But different biologically active substances obtained by biosynthesis, i.e. compounds produced by microorganisms during their life cycle, presented the premium welfare for medicine.

In 1877, Pasteur and Joubert reported that aerobic bacteria could restrain the development of Bacillus anthracis. In the late 19th century, the Russian therapist Manassein (1841) and Polotebnov (1838-1908), a pioneer in the Russian dermatology, showed that Penicillium fungi can hinder in vivo the growth of microbes causing skin diseases of man.

Mecknikov (1845-1916), who was awarded the Nobel Prize (together with Ehrlich) for studies on phagocytosis, showed in 1894 that some saprophytic bacteria might be used to check pathogenic microorganisms.

In 1896, Gosio isolated a crystalline substance from the culture fluid of Penicillium brevi-compactum. This was mycophenolic acid which inhibited the growth of anthrax microbe.

Emmerich and Low (1899) noted the discovery of an antibiotic substance formed by Pseudomonas pyocyanea, which they called pyocyanase; the preparation was used as a local antiseptic.

Black and Alsberg (1910-1913) isolated penicillic acid from Penicillium fungus; it had antimicrobial properties as well.

Unfortunately, these and other findings and discoveries were not developed in suitable time, but they gave a strong motive to later studies of biologically dynamic property of metabolism of micro-organisms.

Alexander Fleming discovered in 1929 a new preparation, penicillin, which was isolated in the crystal state only in 1940. This new and very potent chemotherapeutic substance was obtained from the microorganisms, i.e. by biological synthesis.

The year of 1940, when penicillin was isolated, is the date of birth of the new branch in science, the science of antibiotics. This branch has been speedily developed during the past three decades.

The discovery of penicillin has become a great victory of modern biology, medicine and chemistry. The importance of this discovery was demonstrated very vividly during the years of the World War II. Many lives were saved by penicillin. Penicillin, and especially its derivatives, are no less important in our days.

"The high efficacy of penicillin in combative miscellaneous infections and inflammatory processes has become a powerful impetus to the search for new more efficacious antibiotic substances produced by various microorganisms (bacteria, streptomycetes), lower plants (yeast, algae, molds, high fungi), and higher plants and animals.

The persistent search was crowned by the discovery of many new microorganisms producing antibiotics. The examination of these discoveries is completely characteristic. In 1896 Gosio isolated mycophenolic acid, in 1899 Emmerich and Low described pyocyanase, in 1937 Welsh described the first antibiotic actinomycetin, in 1939 Krasilnikov and Korenyako obtained mycetin and Dubos isolated ivrothridn. In other words, in 1940, i.e. the year when crystalline penicillin was prepared, five antibiotics were already known. The number of these substances then rapidly increased in subsequent years.

The count of antibiotics is now greater than 6500 but only about 100 of them are used in medicine to treat patients with diversified inflammatory processes (pneumonia, peritonitis, furunculosis), various forms of tuberculosis, and numerous infectious diseases, which were formerly considered either remediless or troublesome to cure. Fatality rate of sepsis, meningitis, crupous pneumonia, etc. considerably decreased due to antibiotics.

Majority antibiotics are not used in medicine because of their toxicity, instability in the patient body, and for other logic.

The definition of an antibiotic by Waksman in 1951 confined them to substances produced by microorganisms, but the definition must now be stretched to encompass resembling substances prepared synthetically or present in some of the higher plants. Many a worthy number of both microbes and higher plants are acclaimed to have antibiotic properties for the treatment and remedies of microbial infections which testify the extent of further research and progress in a country like India where endemic species contribute a rich flora.

List of some plants are given below which possess antimicrobial properties.

Medicinal Plants with Anti-microbial Properties

1. *Aegle marmelos Coor.* **(Rutaceae)**
   - *Common names:* **Eng.:** Bael Tree, Hindi, Beng. & Mar.: Bel.
   - *Distribution:* A tree, attaining a height of 12m growing wild and also cultivated throughout the country, particularly in the dry regions.
   - *Parts used:* Leaves.
   - *Antimicrobial activities:* Leaf extract possessed antifungal activity[1].
   - *Chemical constituents:* See Anti-diabetic chapter.

2. *Allium sativum Linn.* **(Liliaceae)**
   - *Common names:* Eng.: Garlic, Hindi & Guj.: Lasan, Beng. & Mar: Lasum.
   - *Distribution:* Cultivated all over India.
   - *Parts used:* Bulbs.
   - *Antimicrobial activities:* Bulb extract showed antibacterial activities
   - *Chemical constituents:* See Hepatoprotective chapter.

3. *Alpinia officinarum Hance* (**Zingiberaceae**)

  - *Common names:* Hindi: Kulinjan, Beg.: Sugandha bacha.

  - *Distribution:* A native of China.

  - *Parts used:* Rhizome.

  - *Antimicrobial activities:* A flavonoid from rhizome showed strong antifungal activity against *Trichophyton rubmm, I mentagogrophyts, Epidermophyton floccosum* responsible for skin diseases. It also showed activity against a member of gram positive and gram-negative bacteria and pathogenic & non-pathogenic yeasts[3].

  - *Chemical constituents:* Galargin, Kaempferide, Kaempferol and a glucoside obtained from roots.

4. *Anaphalis contorta D. Don* (**Asteraceae**)

  - *Distribution:* Himalayas from Kashmir to Sikkim, altitude 2000-4000m and Meghalaya, alt: 1200-2000m.

  - *Parts used:* Flowers.

  - *Antimicrobial activities:* Fungicidal activity was found in oil[4]. Flower head and the hairs are employed for stopping bleeding.

  - *Chemical constituents:* A new glycoside - Tiliroside isolated from flowers and characterised as kaempferol-3-p-D (6"-0-p-coumaroyl) glucoside 1,8-cineoie and d-limonene as major components of oil.

5. *Aristolochia bracteata I.*

   Syn. *Aristolochia bacteolata* Lamk. (Aristolochiaceae)

  - *Common names:* Eng.: Bracteated birthwort, Sans.: Dhumra-patra, Hindi: Kiramar, Guj.: Kidamari, Tel.: Gadidha-gadappa.

  - *Distribution:* All over India.

  - *Parts used:* Leaves.

  - *Antimicrobial activities:* The plant contains aristolochic acid[5] which stimulate phagocytosis and give improvement in defense substances of the body in bacterial infections.

- *Chemical constituents:* Ceryl alcohol, p-sitosterol, aristolochic acid and KCI from leaves.

6. *Arnebia nobilis Reichb. F.* **(Boraginaceae)**

- *Distribution:* Grows wild in Afghanistan from where roots are imported to India.
- *Parts used:* Whole plant.
- *Antimicrobial activities:* Plant extract shows anti-microbial as well as Anticancer Activities[6].
- *Chemical constituents:* Three new napthoquinones-5, 8-dihydroxy-2-(1'-p, |3-dimethylacryloxy-4'-methylpentyl)-1,4-napthoquinone (I), 5,8-dihydroxy-2-(4'-hydroxy-4'-methylpentyl)-1-4-napthoquinone (II) and 2-(1 '-acetox 1 '-hydroxy 1 '-methyl pentyl)-5,8-dihydroxy-1,4-naptho-quinone (III) - isolated along with alkanin, 5, 8-dihydroxy-2-(1'-(3, f}-dimethylacryloxy-4'-methylpent-1'enyi)-1, 4-napthoquinone and 5, 8-dihydroxyl-2-(1'-acetoxy-4'-methylpent-3'enyl)-1, 4 napthaquinone ; hexacosanoic acid and sitosterol were isolated.

7. *Aster peduncularis Wall.* **(Asteraceae)**

- *Distribution:* Western Himalayas from Himachal Pradesh to Kumaon altitude 1200-2700m.
- *Parts used:* Leaves.
- *Antimicrobial activities:* Essential oil from leaves showed antibacterial activity[7].

8. *Aster thomsonii Clarke* **(Asteraceae)**

- *Distribution:* Western Himalayas from Kashmir to Nepal, alt. 2100-3900m.
- *Parts used:* Leaves.
- *Antimicrobial activities:* Leaves extract showed antibacterial activity[8].
- *Chemical constituents:* Essential oil.

9. *Atylosia trinervia* **DC. (Papilionaceae)**

- *Distribution:* The Nilgiris up to 2000m.
- *Parts used:* Whole plant.

- *Antimicrobial activities:* Atylosol exhibited antibacterial activity against Bacillus subtilis and Staphylococcus aureus[9].

- *Chemical constituents:* A new biphenyl derivative atylosol isolated together with lupenone, lupeol and sitosterol and its structure determined.

10. *Azadirachta indica A. Juss.*

   Syn. Melia azadirachta Linn. (Meliaceae)

   - *Common names:* Eng.: Margosatree, Beng.: Nim, Hindi: Nim.

   - *Distribution:* A common tree in the plain of West Bengal and other regions in the plains of India.

   - *Parts used:* Bark.

   - *Antimicrobial activities:* The leaf extract processes antibacterial properties[10].

   - *Chemical constituents:* See Anti-inflammatory chapter.

11. *Capparis moonii Wight* (**Capparaceae**)

   - *Common names:* Sans.: Rudanti, Mar.: Wagati.

   - *Distribution:* Throughout Western Ghats.

   - *Parts used:* Whole plant.

   - *Antimicrobial activities:* Plant extract showed little effect *in vivo* and *in vitro* on growth of Mycobacterium tuberculosis or its lesions in susceptible animals, it did not show any bacterio-static property *in vitro*[11].

   - *Chemical constituents:* Rutin, |5-sitosterol and 1-stachydrine, m.p. 232°, isolated from fruits.

12. *Carpesium abrotanoides Linn.* (**Asteraceae**)

   - *Common name:* Kashmir: Wotiangil.

   - *Parts used:* Whole plant.

   - *Antimicrobial activities:* Carpesiolin showed antibacterial and cerabrone showed antifungal activity[12].

   - *Chemical constituents:* Granilin isolated and its stereochemistry established; carpesiolin and carabrone isolated; structure of carpesiolin elucidated.

13. *Cassia fistula Linn.* (Leguminosae)

- *Common names:* Eng.: Golden-shower, Indian Laburnum, Beng.: Amaltas, Hindi: Bandarlathi.

- *Distribution:* A deciduous, medium sized tree up to 24m in height and 1.8m in girth, cultivated almost throughout India. The tree is one of the most widespread in the forests in India, usually occurring in deciduous forests throughout the greater part of India, ascending up to an altitude of 1,220m in the sub-Himalayan tract and outer Himalayas. It is common throughout the Gangetic valley, particularly abundant in the bhabar tracts. Central India, and South India.

- *Part used:* Fruit.

- *Antimicrobial activities:* An aqueous extract of fruit pulp exhibited antibacterial activities[13].

- *Chemical constituents:* See Anti-inflammatory chapter.

14. *Centaura calcitrapa Linn.* (Asteraceae)

- *Parts used:* Leaves.

- *Antimicrobial activities:* Cenicin showed hypoglycaemia activity and also antibiotic activity against Bruce/la abortus, *Staphylococcus aureus* and *Psendomonas aeruginosa*[14].

- *Chemical constituents:* Polyphenols, sterol, amino acids and triterpenes from leaves, flowers and green branches; two alkaloids, mp 198° and 118°, p-smyrin and p-sitosterol isolated from Egyptian plant; lipid and carbohydrate contents of plant also studied; a bitter germacranolide -cnicin - isolated from leaves.

15. *Coleus forskohlii Briq.* (Lamiaceae)

- *Common name:* Eng: Kaffie Potatoes.

- *Distribution:* Himalayas from Garhwal to Nepal ascending to 2500m, Parasnath Hills in Bihar and hills of Deccan Peninsula.

- *Parts used:* Leaves, roots.

- *Antimicrobial activities:* Essential oil showed antimicrobial activity[15].

- *Chemical constituents:* A new diterpenoid methylenequinone - coleon-E isolated from leaves and its structure elucidated; a new diterpenoid barbatusin isolate from leaves and its crystal structure determined; Coleon-from leaves characterised; Crystal structure of Cyclobutatusin isolated from leaves; three new lab done diterpenoids (I, II & 111) isolated from roots and their stereo structure determined; 3p-hydroxy-3-deoxybarbatusin isolated and characterised; isolation and crystal structure of coleneol; three new diterpenes coleonol-B, coleonol-C and deoxycoleonol, isolated from roots; isomeric coleonol-B and C shown to be 6p-acetoxy-8, 13-epoxy-1, 7, 90c-trihydroxylabd-14-en-11-one and deoxycoleonol characterised as 70c-acetoxy-8, 13-epoxy-1cc, 6p-dihydroxylabd-14-en-11-one; another diterpene-coleosol isolated and characterised.

16. *Euphorbia microphylla Linn.* **(Euphorbiaceae)**

- *Common names:* Beng.: Chota keruee; Santhal: Dudhiaphul.

- *Distribution:* Plains of Bengal, Eastern India gangitic plains.

- *Parts used:* Stem along with other plant parts.

- *Antimicrobial activity:* Crude plant extract showed antibacterial activity against both gram positive and gram negative bacterial at the level of 100mg/mL concentration[16].

- *Chemical constituents:* The plant contains wax ester (C_H-C_{66}), straight chain alcohol (most likely composition is $CH_3(CH_2)_{28}CH_2OH$, sterol glucoside (p-sitosterol-p-D-glucopyranoside) flavonoid-7-O-p-D-glucoside.

17. *Euphorbia thymifolia Linn.* **(Euphorbiaceae)**

- *Common names:* Sans: Laghu dudhika, Hindi: Choti-dudhi, Beng.: Shwet-keruee, Mar.: Ghakdidudhi, Tel: Reddivari manubala, Tarn.: Sittrapaladi.

- *Distribution:* Mainly Eastern and Southern Indian Plains.

- *Parts used:* Stems and leaves.

- *Anti-microbial activities*: Plant employed as a cure for ringworm. Compound A and C inhibited growth of Escherichia co//'and Bacillus subtitis but had no effect on B. cercus and Staphytococcus aureus. Compound B did not inhibit growth of any of these four organisms[17].

- *Chemical Constituents*: Compounds A, mp 187°, B and C isolated.

18. *Gossypium hirsutum L.* **(Malvaceae)**

- *Common names*: Eng.: American cotton; Ben.: Tula.

- *Distribution:* Uplands of Asia, America and Africa.

- *Parts used:* Flower buds.

- *Antimicrobial activities:* Antibiotic activity against Heliothis virescens was attributed to a condensed tannin (M.W. 4850) present in flower buds[18].

- *Chemical constituents:* Bisaboline oxide isolated from cotton buds and characterised; total phospholipids in seeds estimated as 1.6%; revision in the structure of laciniline C and isolation of its 7-methyl ether from bracts; gossypol, 6-methoxygossypol, 6, 6'-dimethoxygossypol, hemigossypol and methoxyhemi-gossypol isolated from roots; a sestertespenoid - heliocide H2- isolated and its structure determined; gossypol isolated from pigment glands. Glands in young green tissues contained hemigossypolone as predominant terpenoid aldehyde; as glands aged in green tissues sesquiterpenoid quinones replaced by several C25-terpenoids; two new sesterpenoids - heiiocide H, and heliocide H4 - isolated and their seterostructures determined; heliocide H3, an isomer heliocide H5, isolated from young cotton balls.

19. *Hibiscus syriacus I.* **(Malvaceae)**

- *Common names:* Eng.: Rose of Sharon; Beng.: Swet jaba; Hindi: Gurhul; Orriya: Gurhul; Punj.: Gurhul.

- *Distribution:* Native of China, grown in Indian gardens.

- *Parts used:* Bark.

- *Antimicrobial activities:* Canthin-6-one-and a fatty acid fraction which contained lauric, myristic and palmitic acids showed antifungal activity against *Trichophyton interdigitele*[19].

- *Chemical constituents:* Carotenoid pigments-crytoxanthin, chrysanthemaxanthin and antheraxanthin isolated from buds, leaves and flowers; Canthin-6-one [6H-indolo(3,2,1 - d, e)(1,5) napthyri-dine-6-one] and a fatty acid fraction composed of lauric, myristic and palmitic acids isolated from bark.

20. *Hunnemania fumariaefolia Swet* (Papaveraceae)

- *Common name:* Eng: Mexican Tulip poppy.

- *Distribution:* Cultivated in Indian gardens at medium and high elevation.

- *Parts used:* Roots.

- *Antimicrobial activities:* Pseudoaleoholates of chelery-thrine and sanguinarine showed enhanced antimicrobial activity over the parent alkaloids and appeared to be useful drugs[20].

- *Chemical constituents:* A new flavanol glycoside iso-hamnetin-3-p-D-gluco-pyranoside-7-a-L-arabinopyranoside (I) isolated from petals; artifactually formed pseudo-methanolats of chelerythrin (II, III) and sangunarine (IV, V) isolated from roots along with parent alkaloids.

21. *Hypericum perforation Linn.* (Hypericaceae)

- *Common names:* Eng.: St. John's Wort, Hindi: Bassant, balsana, dendhu.

- *Distribution:* Parts of Eastern India.

- *Parts used:* Whole plant.

- *Antimicrobial activities:* Hyperforin was active against gram positive bacteria[21].

- *Chemical constituents:* Isolation of pseudohypericin and its structure elucidation, hyperforin isolated and characterised; eleven saturated straight chain C_{2131} hydrocarbons detected in wax, C_{29} compound being major (83.0%) constituent.

22. *Indigofera suffruticosa Mill.* **(Papilionaceae)**
    - *Common names:* Eng.: West Indian Indigo, Hindi: Vilaiti nil, Tarn.: Shimaiyaviri, Tel.: Shimanili, Kan.: Shimenili.
    - *Distribution:* Native of tropical America and West Indies, introduced in India.
    - *Parts used:* Whole plant.
    - *Antimicrobial activities:* Louisfieserone showed antibiotic activity against gram positive and negative bacteria and inhibited sprouting and growth of seeds of dicotyledons[22].
    - *Chemical constituents:* Isolation and crystal structure of an unusual flavone - derivative-louisfieserone from Mexican plant; (3-sitosterol and (+) pinitol isolated.

23. *Jateorhiza palmate (Lam.) Miers.* **(Menispermaceae)**
    - *Common names:* Hindi: Kalamb-ki-jar, Tel.: Kalamba-vera, Tarn.: Kalambaver, Oriya: Kolombo, Marathi: Kalamb-Kachari, Colombo.
    - *Distribution:* Southern, Western and some parts of Eastern India.
    - *Parts used:* Root.
    - *Antimicrobial activities:* Root extract exhibited antifungal activities against eight fungi[23].
    - *Chemical constituents:* Bitter constituents columbin, chasmanthin, palmarin and jateorin present; constitution of palmarin determined.

24. *Juniperus communis Linn.* **(Cupresaceae)**
    - *Common names:* Eng.: Juniper, Hindi: Avaraar, haubera, abhal, Beng.: Havcesha, Mar.: Hosha.
    - *Distribution:* The plant widely available in Northern part of India at the altitude of more than 1350m.
    - *Parts used:* Leaves.
    - *Antimicrobial activities:* All Gram positive and Gram negative bacteria were found to be sensitive to a concentration of 250 ug/mL of the leaf extract[24].
    - *Chemical constituents:* See Anti-inflammatory chapter.

25. *Lycopersicon lycopersicum (L.) Karsten* **(Solanaceae)**

- *Common names:* Eng.: Tomato, Beng.: Tomato, Bilaiti Begun, Hindi: Tomator.

- *Distribution:* Cultivated as agricultural plant throughout India and abroad.

- *Parts used:* Whole plant.

- *Antimicrobial activities:* Tomatine of the plant showed antibacterial and fungicidal activities[25].

- *Chemical constituents:* Preparation of crude tomatine from drug; (3-1 -to-matine (0.81 %) identified as main alkaloid in some experimentally produced mutants of plant; tomatine, mp. 278°, isolated.

26. *Medicago saliva Linn.* **(Fabaceae)**

- *Common names:* Eng.: Alfalfa, Hindi: Lasunghas, Punjab: Lusan.

- *Distribution:* A perennial herb of temperate Europe, Asia and North Africa widely cultivated as feeder for live Hock.

- *Parts used:* Whole plant.

- *Antimicrobial activities:* Sativin showed antifungal activity against *Cladosporium cucumerinum*[26].

- *Chemical constituents:* See Antifertility chapter.

27. *Moms alba Linn.* **(Moraceae).**

- *Common names:* Eng.: White Mulberry, Hindi: Tut, Beng.: Toot.

- *Distribution:* Cultivated throughout the plain parts of India.

- *Parts used:* Leaves.

- *Antimicrobial activities:* Muberrofuran A showed antibacterial activity against *Staphylococcus aureus* and *Fusarium roseum*[27].

- *Chemical constituents:* See Antifertility chapter.

28. *Ophiorrhiza mungos L.* **(Rubiaceae)**

- *Common names:* Hindi: Sarahati, Beng.: Gandhanakuli, Mar.: Mugusavela, nagvelli, Guj.: Mungusavel, Tel.:

Chettu, Tarn.: Keerippundu, Kan.: Mungisigida, parala garuda, Sarpari, Mai.: Avilpori.

- *Distribution:* Eastern and Southern India.
- *Parts used:* Leaves.
- *Antimicrobial activities:* 10-methoxycamptothecin at a concentration of 10 and 20 mg/ml of nutrient agar overlay showed 89 and 100% inhibition respectively herpes virus plaques[28].
- *Chemical Constituents:* Camptothecin and 10-methoxy-camptothecin isolated from leaves.

29. *Oxalis corniculata Linn.* **(Oxalidaceae)**
    - *Common names:* Eng.: Indian sorrel, Hindi: Amrul sak, Beng.: Amrul sak.
    - *Distribution:* Throughout India and Nepal.
    - *Parts used:* Whole plant.
    - *Antimicrobial activities:* Alcoholic extract of leaves showed complete inhibition of growth of *Staphylococcus typhi, S. aureus, S. albus* and S. *citrus* at 6.5 mg/ml[29].

30. *Petiveria alliacea L.* **(Phytolaccaceae)**
    - *Distribution:* Native of warmer region of America, introduced into Indian gardens.
    - *Parts used:* Roots, stems.
    - *Antimicrobial activities:* An antimicrobial substance isolated from roots and stems and its structure elucidated as benzyl-2-hydroxyethyltri-sulphide(l)[30].
    - *Chemical constituents:* Benzyl-2-hydroxyethyltrisulphide (l) present in plant extract.

31. *Piper longum Linn.* **(Piperaceae)**
    - *Common names:* Eng.: long pepper, Hindi: Pipal, Beng.: Piplamor.
    - *Distribution:* Cultivated in West Bengal, Karnataka and Tamil Nadu.
    - *Parts used:* Roots, leaves and fruits.

- *Antimicrobial activities:* The oil showed antibacterial activity against gram positive and gram-negative bacteria[31].

- *Chemical constituents:* Piperlongumine, piperlonguminine piperine, sisamine, methyl 3,4, 5 trimethoxycinnamate isolated from roots.

32. *Pueraria tuberosa Roxb. ex. Willd. DC.* (Papilionaceae)

- *Parts used:* Tubers.

- *Antimicrobial activities:* From the benzene extract of the plant a new pterocarpan tuberosin was isolated. The material tuberosin showed anti-staphylococal, anti-tubercular and antifungal activities[32].

- *Chemical constituents:* (3-sitosterol, stigmasterol, daidzein, puerarin, tuberos in and a new isoflavone C-glycoside - 4', 6"-diacetyl-puerarin were isolated from roots.

33. *Quassia amara L.* (Simaroubaceae)

- *Common name:* Eng.: Surinam quassia.

- *Distribution:* Indigenous to Brazil and guiana, grown in Indian Garden.

- *Parts used:* Whole plant.

- *Antimicrobial activities:* 18-hydroxy quassin obtain from the plant showed antiamoebic properties[33].

- *Chemical constituents:* p-sitosterol, and (3-sitostenone from wood oil obtained. Isolation of quassin, isoquassin, neoquassin and a new amaroid- 18-hydroxyquassin, m.p. 233° obtain from the plant.

34. *Rosa indica L.* (Rosaceae)

- *Common names:* Eng.: Rose china, Beng: Golap, Hindi: Gulab.

- *Distribution:* Cultivated as garden plant throughout India and other countries.

- *Parts used:* Flowers.

- *Antimicrobial activities:* Gallic acid at 3% concentration showed fungicide property against *Alternaria, Fusarium* and *Aspergillus* species[34].

- *Chemical constituents:* Fatty acids C_{18}(10.7), C_{20}(81.6) and C_{22} (11.7%) present seed oil; gallic acid isolated from flowers.

35. *Salvia officinalis L.* (Lamiaceae)

- *Common names:* Eng.: Sage, Garden sage, Hindi: Salvia sefakuss.

- *Distribution:* Cultivated as garden plants.

- *Parts used:* Leaves.

- *Antimicrobial activities:* Picnosalvin, a bitter substance isolated from the leaves, has a bacteriostatic effect on several organisms[35].

- *Chemical constituents:* Genkwanin, 6-methoxygenk-wanin, lutedin, 6-methoxyluteolin and its 7-methyl ether and hispidulin from leaves; royleanone, its 7-a-hydroxy and acetoxyderivatives as well as 6,7-dehydroroyleanone isolated from roots; salvin and its monomethyl ether isolated from flowers and their structures elucidated; essential oil contained salvin, a-pinene, p-pinene, camphor, myrcone, cineole and a-thujone; total ketone content of essential oil was 62.05% o which thujone constituted 61.63%; C_{16} (Saturated) and C_{182} (unsaturated) acids as man fatty acids found in seed oil along with p-sitosterol (91.3% of total sterol fraction); a new flavone-5-metho-xysolvigenin, mp.166° isolated from leaves.

36. *Selinum filicifolia* (Edgew.) Clarke (Apiaceae)

- *Common names:* Simla: Khes havo, Kash.: Bhootakeshi.

- *Distribution:* Himalayas from Kashmir to Nepal, alt. 1800-4300m.

- *Parts used:* Roots.

- *Antimicrobial activities:* Oil from root part showed antibacterial activity[36].

- *Chemical constituents:* Heraclenin, bergapten and imperatorin isolated from roots; heraclenol and 8-geranyloxypsoralen from roots; isoimperstorin (0.07,0.07), osthol (0.07,0.02), oxypeuce-danin (0.4,1.2) and imperatorin (0.036, 0.007%) isolated from inflorescence and roots respectively; detection of limonene, elemol, terpineol, geraniol and eudesmol in root oil by GC.

37. *Sophora tomentosa I.* **(Papilionaceae/fabaceae)**

- *Common names:* Eng.: Seacoast laburnum, silver bush, Burm.: Thimbawmagyi.

- *Parts used:* Aerial portion of the plant.

- *Antimicrobial activities:* Sophoraisoflavanone A exhibited antifungal activity[37].

- *Chemical constituents:* Anagyrine, N-acetylcystisine, baptifoline and oxymatrine isolated from aerial parts; a new 3-hydroxyflavanone-sophoronol isolated from roots and its structure determined; a new diprenylated isoflavanone isosophoranone along with isosophoronol isolated and characterised; two new fiavonoids – Sophoraisoflavanone A, m.p. 178° and sophora - flavonone-B, m.p. 193° along with isobavachin and 1-octadecyl laffeate, m.p. 108° isolated from aerial parts; two new benzifuran derivatives-l, m.p. 235 and II m.p. 179° along with 1 - maackiain, stigmasterol, medicagol, formononetin and 2', 4', 4-trihyxychalcone (liquiritigenin isolated from aerial parts; structure of I & II determined as 2-(2', 4'-dihydroxyphenyl)-5, 6-methylenedio-xybenzofuran and 2-(2'-hdroxy-4'-methoxyphenyl)-5, 6-methylenedioxy-benzo-furan respectively.

38. *Withania somnifera Dunal* **(Solanaceae)**

- *Common names:* Eng.: Ashvaganda, Hindi: Asgand, Beng.: Ashvaganda.

- *Distribution:* This is an erect shrub found throughout the drier parts of India, in waste places and on bunds; also cultivated to a limited extent for the medicinal roots.

- *Parts used:* Roots and tuber roots.

- *Antimicrobial activities: In vitro* and *in vivo* antibacterial activity against 13 organisms investigated; A_1, A_2, A_3 and to lesser extent A_4 and A_5, were effective against aerobic bacilli. None of them were active against gram negative bacteria and anaerobic bacilli[38]; an unsaturated bactone, mp 159°, was active in a concentration of 10g/mL against acid fast bacilli and pathogenic turgid but was inactive against gram negative organisms[39].

- *Chemical constituents:* See Antifertility chapter.

39. *Xanthium strumarium Linn.* (Compositae)

- *Common names:* Eng.: Burweed, Hindi: Gokhru, Chhota-gokhuru, banokra, Beng.: Chota-dhatura, Guj.: Gadariun, Kan.: Marulleummatti.

- *Distribution:* Annual herbs, found throughout the warmer parts of India, generally as weeds.

- *Parts used:* Seeds.

- *Antimicrobial activities:* Xanthumin from seeds showed antibacterial activity[40].

- *Chemical constituents:* See Antifertility chapter.

References

1. Rastogi, R.P. & Mehrotra, B.N., *Compendium of Indian Medicinal Plants,* (1991), Vol-2, Central Drug Research Institute, Lucknow and Publications & Information Directorate, New Delhi, CSIR, p-17.

2. Vaselin, P., *DeutApoth. Ztg.,* (1966), 106(51), 1861.

3. Rastogi, R.P. & Mehrotra, B.N., *Compendium of Indian Medicinal Plants,* (1991),Vol-2, Central Drug Research Institute, Lucknow and Publications & Information Directorate, New Delhi, CSIR, p-34.

4. Ibid, p-43.

5. Chopra, R.N., Nayar, S.L & Chopra, I.C., *Glossary Indian Med. Plant,* (1956), Publications & Information Directorate, CSIR, New Delhi, p-24.

6. Shukla, Y.N., Tandon, J.S., Bhakuni, D.S. and Dhar, M.M., *Phytochemistry,* (1971), 10, 1909.

7. Rastogi, R.P. & Mehrotra, B.N., *Compendium of Indian Medicinal Plants,* (1991), Vol-2, Central Drug Research Institute, Lucknow and Publications & Information Directorate, New Delhi, CSIR, p-82.

8. Ibid, p-82.

9. Tripathi, V.D., Agarwal, S.K. and Rastogi, R.P., *Phytochemistry,* (1978), 17, 2001.

10. Chopra, R.N., Nayar, S.L., and Chopra, I.C., *Supplementary to Glossary of Indian Medicinal Plants,* (1986), Publications & Information Directorate, CSIR, New Delhi, p-10.

11. Rastogi, R.P. & Mehrotra, B.N., *Compendium of Indian Medicinal Plants,* (1990),Vol-1, Central Drug Research Institute, Lucknow and Publications & Information Directorate, New Delhi, CSIR, p-76.

12. Masao, M. and Sonoe, 0., *Phytochemistry,* (1977), 16, 782.

13. Khaleque, A., Haroon, S.N., *Sci. Res. (Dacca, Pak),* (1970), 7(203), 63.

14. Karawya, M.S., Hilal, S.H., Hifnawy, M.S., EI-Hawary, S.S., *Egypf. J. Pharm. Sci,,* (1975), 16(4), 445.

15. Pizsolitto, A.C., Pozetti, G.L., Mancini, B., Loschagin, E., Mancini, M.A.D., *Rev. Fac.*

16. Chatterjee, T.K. and Pathak, M., Medical Sci. Res., (1991), 19, 785.

17. Rastogi, R.P, & Mehrotra, B.N., Compendium of Indian Medicinal Plants, (1990), Vol-1, Central Drug Research Institute, Lucknow and Publications & Information Directorate, New Delhi, CSIR, p-184.

18. Chan, E.G., Waiss, A.C. Jr., Lukefahr, M., J. Insect. Physiol., (1978), 24(2), 113.

19. Yokota, M., Zenda, H., Kosuge, T., Yamamoto, I, Yakugaku Zasshi, (1978), 98(11), 1508.

20. Mitscher, LA., Park, Y.H., Clark, D., Clark III, G.W., Hammwafahr, P.O., Wu, W.N.and Beal, J.L, Uyodia, (1978), 41,145.

21. Bystrov, N.S., Chernov, B.K., Dobrynin, V.N. and Koloaov, M.N., Tetrahedron Letters, (1975), 32, 2791.

22. Dominguez, X.A., Martinez, C., Calero, A., Dominguez, X.A. Jr., Hinojosa, M. and Zamudio, A., Tetrahedron Letters, (1978), 5, 429.

23. Horn, I., Steffen, K., Pharm. Ztg., (1968), 113(26), 945.

24. Chatterjee, T.K., Ghosh, C.M. and Achary, P.M.R., Indian Journal of Microbiology, (1993), 33(4), 275.

25. Truhaut, R., Shuster, G. and Tarrade, A.M., Ann. Pharm. Fr., (1967), 25(9-10), 621.

26. Rastogi, R.P. & Mehrotra, B.N., Compendium of tute, Lucknow and Publications & Information Directorate, New Delhi, CSIR, p-450.

27. Ibid, p-471.

28. Tafur, S., Nelson, J.D., Delong, D.C. and Suoboda, G.H., Uoydia, (1976), 39, 261.

29. Rastogi, R.P. & Mehrotra, B.N., Compendium of Indian Medicinal Plants, (1991), Vol-2, Centra] Drug Research Institute, Lucknow and Publications & Information Directorate, New Delhi, CSIR, p-503.

30. Ibid, p-523.

31. Rastogi, R.P. & Mehrotra, B.N., Compendium of Indian Medicinal Plants, (1991),Vol-1, Central Drug Research Institute, Lucknow and Publications & Information Directorate, New Delhi, CSIR, p-316.

32. Meier, B. and Sticher, 0., "Internation Congress lor research in Medicinal Plants (Lec-ture)", Munich B-10 Sep'1976.

33. Atai, C.K. and Kapur, B.M., Cultivation and Utilization of Medicinal Plants, (1982), RRL Council of Scientific and indentrial Research, p-42.

34. Tripathi, S.C. and Dixit, S.N., Experientia, 1977, 33, 207.

35. Chopra, R.N., Nayar, S.L., and Chopra, I.C., Supplementary to Glossary of IndianMedicinal Plants, (1986), Publication & Information Directorate, CSIR, New Delhi, p-89.

36. Rastogi, R.P. & Mehrotra, B.N., Compendium of Indian Medicinal Plants, (1991),Vol-2, Central Drug Research Institute, Lucknow and Publications & Information Directorate, New Delhi, CSIR, p-621.

37. Ibid, p-639.

38. Ibid, Vol.1 p-436.

39. Ibid, p-436.

40. Ibid, Vol. 2, p-711.

7 *Medicinal Plants with Anti-Ulcer Properties*

Pharmacology of the Digestive System

The Salivary Glands

Saliva contains an amylase (ptyalin) which passes with the food into the stomach where it begins the digestion of starch. Saliva serves a number of other advantageous functions: by keeping the mouth and lips moist, it aids vocalization and by moistening and lubricating the food and facilitates swallowing. Stopping of salivary discharge causes the feeling of thirst which signals a descend in the body's water makeup.

In the common subject, the entry of a bolus of food at the foremost part of the esophagus initiates a peristaltic wave which carries it towards the cardiac sphincter. Concurrent reflex relaxation of the cardiac sphincter allows the peristaltic wave to carry the bolus into the stomach. Here, churning movements and peristaltic waves assure that the food circulates and becomes completely mixed up with the gastric secretions, pepsin, hydrochloric acid (HCl) and mucus.

The constituents of gastric juice, essential for assimilation are pepsin (a proteolytic enzyme) and hydrochloric acid which simultaneously commence the digestion of protein. Salivary amylase furthermore operates in the stomach till hydrochloric acid penetrates the food mass and arrests amylase action. Transformation of protein and starch continues, and that of other substances commences, in the duodenum, which receives the pancreatic secretions. In the remainder of the small intestine, success entericus is secreted.

Hydrochloric acid is created by the oxyntic (or parietal) cells of the stomach. These cells also discharge Castle's intrinsic factor, the substance essential for the absorption of vitamin B12. Hydrogen ions, borrowed from water, are secreted by the gastric glands in exchange for a density slope using dynamism obtained from a sequence of oxidative reaction. The hydroxyl ions conglomerate with carbon dioxide supporting the power of carbonic anhydrase and the attributable to bicarbonate ions pass into the blood, following ion exchange with chloride ions, which escort the hydrogen ions into the glandular lumen. Accordingly, this detachment of the hydrogen and hydroxyl ions, results in the origination of hydrochloric acid in the stomach and of bicarbonate in the blood. It may furthermore be mentioned in this reference that more powerful the secretion of acid the more alkaline will be the blood exit the stomach, which is due to the 'alkaline tide' in the blood which accompanies gastric digestion.

Secretion of gastrin, which controls the creation of pepsinogen and HCl, is stimulated by the attendance of food inside the lumen and is inhibited by the occupancy of increase levels of HCl in the gastric antrum. On that account, the secretory action of the stomach in turn depends on the amount of food inside the lumen.

Peristaltic waves move the food via the pylorus, which intermittently relaxes synchronously with the stomach, thereby consenting the chyme to enter the duodenum. Co-ordination of gastric and duodenal movement ensures the one-way outpouring of chyme from the stomach via the pylorus.

At this state, two different hormones, secretin and cholecystokinin pancreozymin (CCKPZ) are secreted by the upper small intestine. Secretin inhibits gastric secretion and stimulates the pancreas to bring about an abundant watery fluid with an elevated bicarbonate content, which passes into the duodenum and is essential for neutralization of the remainder gastric HCl and inactivation of pepsin, consequently protecting the duodenal mucosa from injury by gastric acids.

CCKPZ lowers the muscle pitch of the cardiac, stimulates the secretion of pancreatic fluid rich in digestive enzymes, causing the gall bladder to shrink. As an outcome, a mixture of bile and pancreatic juice enters the duodenum and the course of digestion continues in an alkaline medium.

The Digestive System

The process of digestion causes breakdown of food material by chemical action and to convert them into more simple forms. These simpler forms can be absorbed into the blood and utilized by the various tissues of the body according to their requirements.

The process of digestion takes place in the alimentary canal. It is aided by certain accessory organs; the salivary glands, liver and pancreas. The digestive process can be described in four stages:

(a) Ingestion,

(b) Digestion,

(c) Absorption,

(d) Excretion.

Anatomy of Gastrointestinal (G.I.) Tract

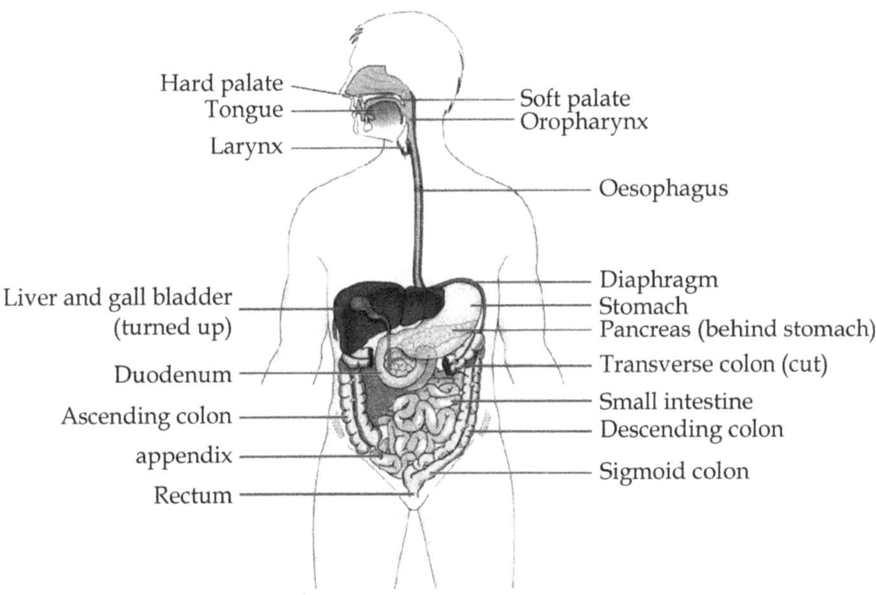

Fig. 7.1 Anatomy of Gastrointestinal tract.

The human digestive tract is comprised of the following parts:

• Mouth

• Pharynx

• Esophagus

- Stomach
- Small Intestine
    - duodenum
    - jejunum
    - ileum
- Large Intestine
- Rectum
- Anus

Mouth

The mouth is the upper portion of the alimentary canal.

The buccal cavity is found between the inner walls of the cheeks and the gums which contain the teeth. The salivary glands which open into the buccal cavity are:

(a) Parotid

(b) Submandibular

(c) Sublingual

Saliva has a pH 6.7.

Pharynx

The pharynx is a musculo membranous tube whose constricted part ends in the esophagus.

Esophagus

The esophagus is a muscular tube about 10 inches (25 cm.) long. It extends from the pharynx and transports the bolus of food to the stomach by a series of peristaltic movements.

Stomach

The stomach is a dilated portion of the alimentary canal. Shape of the normal stomach is generally like the letter 'J'. The capacity of the average stomach is about 1.12 to 1.70 litres.

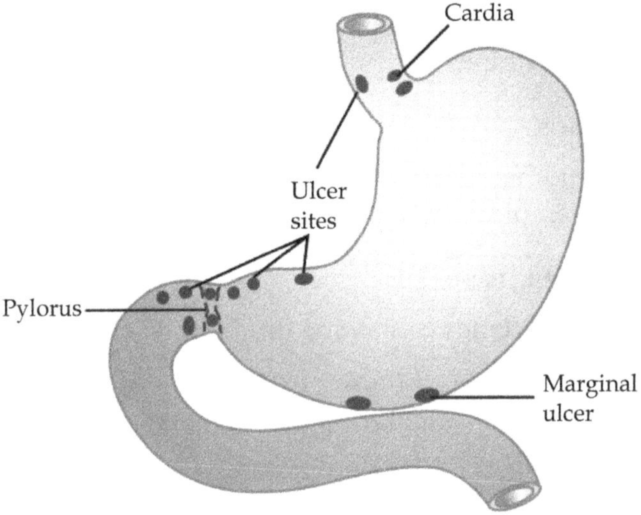

Fig. 7.2 Peptic ulcer in stomach and duodenum.

The stomach consists of the following parts:

(a) The opening at the upper end known as the cardiac orifice, where the esophagus meets the stomach.

(b) The Fundus, the upper part which in general contains a bubble of air.

(c) The body, constituting the main part of the stomach.

(d) The antrum forms the lower part of the ']' and leads to the pyloric sphincter which separates the stomach from the duodenum.

The stomach-wall consists of four coats:

(a) An outer peritoneal coat, which is a serous coat membrane and forms a part of the peritoneum.

(b) A muscular coat having three layers:

    (i) Longitudinal fibres.

    (ii) Circular fibres.

    (iii) Oblique fibres.

(c) A submucous coat containing blood vessels and lymphatics.

(d) A mucous coat which is lined by columnar epithelium and containing numerous lymphatic. All the cells secrete mucus.

The inner surface is covered by tiny ducts of the gastric glands. The epithelium of the secreting part of the gland differs in various parts of the stomach.

Cardiac Glands

This gland is located near the esophageal end. These are tubular glands, either simple or branched, and secrete an alkaline mucus.

Glands of the Fundus

These are tubular glands containing different types of cells:

Peptic cells	—	Produce pepsin
Oxyntic cells	—	Produce hydrochloric acid (HCl)
Mucus neck cells	—	Produce mucin

Pyloric Glands

The glands in the pyloric canal are also tubular in character. They produce mainly alkaline mucus.

The secretion from the body and the fundus glands is rich in acid and enzymes, whereas the secretion of the pylorus is alkaline, rich in mucus and poor in enzymes.

Small Intestine

The small intestine is the portion of the alimentary tract extending from the pyloric and of the stomach and continues till the large intestine (the caecum). It is about six meters long and consists of three parts:

(a) The Duodenum

(b) The Jejunum

(c) The Ileum

The Duodenum — The first ten inches of the small intestine is shaped like a horse shoe, the curve encircling the head of the pancreas. The bile ducts and the pancreatic duct open into the ampulla of Vater (ampulla Vateri).

The Jejunum occupies the upper two fifths of the remaining small intestine.

The Ileum occupies the rest of the small intestine.

The wall of the small intestine, like the stomach wall, has also four coats, viz.:

1. Serous coat (part of the peritoneum)
2. Muscular coat
3. Submucous coat
4. Mucous Membrane (inner membrane)

As in the stomach, the mucous membrane is arranged in folds. These folds increase the surface area from which secretion and absorption can take place. The surface of the mucous membrane is slightly roughened by minute projections called VILLI. Each villus contains capillaries into which the end products of food are absorbed and a central lymphatic vessel (lacteal) where fats are absorbed.

The mucous membrane of the small intestine contains glands which secrete the intestinal juice (SUCCUS ENTERICUS).

Large Intestine

The large intestine extends from the end of the ileum to the anus.

Diseases of the Stomach and Duodenum

Peptic Ulcer

In the western hemisphere, peptic ulcer is one of the commonest diseases of the alimentary tract. It affects particularly the working years of a patient's life and its social implications are therefore considerable and this disease is a perennial problem encountered by the clinicians around the world.

Etiology

The term 'peptic ulcer' refers to an ulcer found in the lower end of the esophagus, the stomach, the duodenum, in the small intestine after surgical anastomosis to the stomach, or rarely at the junction of a Meckel's diverticulum with the small intestine. Although the immediate cause of peptic ulceration is digestion of mucosa by acid and pepsin of the gastric juice, the sequence of events that leads to the development of the ulcer are unknown. Digestion by acid-pepsin cannot be the only factor involved, since ulcers do not develop in some normal people who secrete acid and pepsin in substantial amounts. The problem is aptly stated in the question. 'Why does the_ stomach not digest itself?' The answer lies on the fact that normal stomach is capable of resisting digestion by its own secretions, so that the problem of ulcer etiology may be written.

Acid Plus Pepsin versus Mucosal Resistance

Theoretically, peptic ulceration may be caused due to either increase in gastric secretion or if the withstanding of the mucosa is reduced. It is favorable to think about the factors believed to be involved in the progress of chronic peptic ulcers according to for what reason they may reverse either side of the balance.

1. *Hypersecretion of gastric juice:* There is strong documentation to verify that ulcers happen only in the occupancy of acid and pepsin. Peptic ulceration has at no time been found in patients with pernicious anemia, and it is greatly ambiguous if a benign chronic ulcer always happens in alliance with achlorhydeia. On the other hand, oppressive obstinate peptic ulcer occurs in patients influenced with the Zollinger ellison syndrome, which is characterized by severely augmented gastric secretion. Further, patients with duodenal ulcer discharge about twice as much acid as compared to healthy individuals, and duodenal ulcer heals when gastric hypersecretion is reduced by vagotomy. Nevertheless, gastric hypersecretion does not appear in all patients with duodenal ulcer. Consequently, factors affecting mucosal resistance need be considered in patients with gastric ulceration.

2. *Renew of gastric mucosa:* Alkaline mucus is the first line of fence for the gastric mucosa, and it may act plainly as a protecting obstacle. Furthermore, the external layer of the gastric mucosa renews itself in every two or three days and of that kind lesser injury in the mucosa are quickly healed under normal state of affairs. Change in the rate of cell recurrence in the upper alimentary mucosa may explanation for the advancement of ulcers from acute to chronic grade.

3. *Change due to inflammation:* Gastritis, which may be both comprehensive and oppressive, ordinarily occurs in patients with gastric ulcer and because there is no certain indication, it seems probable that the gastritis in reality precedes the progress of the ulcer; if so, the inflammatory alteration may well prearrange the

progress of ulceration by altering the hindering of the mucosa from assimilation by the gastric discharge.

4. ***Reflux of bile:*** Regress of bile and other secretions into the stomach occurs more repeatedly in patients accompanied by gastric ulcers than in usual mankind and in patients with duodenal ulcers, this may he attributed to an irregularity of pyloric sphincter. Irrespective of the device, the elevated density of bile salts in the stomach intervene with the perfection of the gastric mucosa, consequently predisposing to the progress of ulceration.

5. ***Supply of blood of mucosa:*** One of the distinguished theories of ulcer development is that the withstanding of the mucosa to assimilation is reduced as an outcome of handicapped blood stock; such detriment could happen either as a consequence of venous or arterial thrombosis, or due to 'shunting' of blood within the mucosa. Despite it is implausible that this is the basis of peptic ulceration in common but the same may notice for the comprehensive ulceration that occurs in the old.

   Disassociated from these native implements, multiform general or inherent conditions are known to be allied with the evolvement of peptic ulcer.

6. ***Family history:*** There is no hesitancy that peptic ulcer tends to happen in families, and the inclination tends to stream authentic to type, so that the children of parents with duodenal ulcer acquire duodenal ulcer, and similarly for gastric ulcer. A convincing family history is repeatedly detected in patients who acquire ulcer in childhood or puberty.

   There is an alliance among duodenal ulcer and blood group 'O'.

7. ***Sex group:*** There are prominent differences couple in the frequency and behavior of peptic ulcer. Duodenal ulcer occurs 5 to 10 times more frequently in men than in women, and puncture occurs 20 times more frequently in men. Despite these effects may be due to differences in the life pattern of men and women, there arc basr assuming that the female sex hormones in some manner guard against peptic ulcer. Women seem to be specially shielded fronting ulceration meanwhile pregnancy, when agile ulcers are practically unfamiliar; ulcer symptoms which postpone at the time of pregnancy ordinarily happen again promptly after that. The occurrence of ulcer symptoms and

ulcer complications expand distinctly in women at about the menopause. The sex variance in the frequency and behavior of gastric ulcer is ample less than for duodenal ulcer.

8. *Factors related with environment:* There are marked variations in the incidence of gastric and duodenal ulcer between different countries, and even between different parts of the same country e.g., the proportion of duodenal ulcer to gastric ulcer is very much higher in Scotland than it is in London. There are also differences in the incidence of ulcer as between social classes so that duodenal ulcers tend to be evenly distributed throughout the entire population, while gastric ulcer occurs more commonly amongst poor people, especially in Britain. South Indian people are more prone to peptic ulcer than North Indian people.

9. *Anxiety:* There is a certain alliance between the outgrowth of acute ulcers in the stomach or duodenum and physical or mental shock or surgical operations; correspondingly there is minute hesitancy that acute anxiety is a consequential consideration in precipitating ulcer recurrences and occasionally ulcer complications such as hemorrhage or perforation. Despite these properties are probably mediated via the central nervous system. How stress or anxiety temper the incident or behavior of peptic ulcer is not conceived.

10. *Seasonal variations:* There are mighty seasonal factors which can be shown to power the occurrence of ulcer symptoms and fatality rates; in Britain, ulcer lethality is at its bottommost in August and September and begins to upsurge in October, with a longer exacerbation of ulcer symptoms in the Spring. The basis of these seasonal variations is unascertained.

11. *Other factors:* The frequency of peptic ulceration appears to be elevated in patients with chronic lung disease, chronic liver diseases and hyperparathyroidism; likewise, anti-inflammatory drugs such like the salicylates, phenylbutazone and indomethacin have all been analogous with an increased occurrence of peptic ulcer, distinctively of gastric ulcer. Corticosteroids are also postulated to basis peptic ulcer.

In the early eighties, Robin Warren and Barry Marshall in the Royal Perth hospital, Western Australia, isolated a spiral Gram negative bacteria from a patient's stomach which was named initially *Campylobacter pyloridis* and now has been referred to as *Helicobacter pylori*. In 1993, Graham and Go, described the impact of the association of this fascinating microbe with peptic ulcer disease. Infection with *Helicobacter pylori* has been fixed as an important cause of chronic gastritis. There is much indication to advocate the blameworthy role of the organism in the growth of peptic ulcer disease. It has been even involved in the course of gastric carcinogenesis.

An estimated 50% in the adult population in developed countries, and about 90% in the developing countries may be contaminated with *H. pylori.*

H. pylori infection tends to clump in families and people living in crowded or closed environments, suggesting a person-to-person transmission of the organism.

In the light of the preceding, *H. pylori* infection can be regarded as and significant and prevalent health problem, meriting serious attention and interference by the medical profession. Most methods to detect *H. pylori* are directly or indirectly based on urease produced by the organism. The non-invasive tests include serologic and urea breathe tests. Invasive tests are based on obtaining biopsy or gastric juice for urease study and microscopy to determine *H. pylori* infection.

Combinations of three drugs incorporating proton pump inhibitor (Omeperazole), Nitronidazole (Tinidazole) and antibiotic (Amoxycillin) have been shown to be best reported thus far.

Pathology

Ulcers occurring in the stomach and duodenum may be acute or chronic, the difference being that a chronic ulcer penetrates the muscularis mucosae, whereas an acute ulcer or an erosion does not. Chronic ulcers occur with exceptional regularity in certain sites: in the stomach on the lesser curvature just above the angulus or less frequently at or near the pylorus, while duodenal ulcers occur within 1 cm of the pylorus on the anterior or posterior wall. Acute lesions are frequently multiple and are less regularly distributed. Benign ulcers occur only occasionally on the greater curvature or on the anterior wall of the stomach.

Clinical Features

While there is good basis for believing that gastric and duodenal ulcers are different diseases with different etiology and natural history, it is appropriate to describe the general features of 'peptic ulcer' as inclusive of both, nothing differences where they occur.

Peptic ulcer may manifest in different ways. The commonest presentation is of chronic, episodic dyspepsia extending over months or years. However, the ulcer may come to notice as an acute episode with bleeding or perforation, with little or no previous history. Occasionally the patient presents with the symptoms of gastric outlet obstruction, having had insignificant dyspepsia previously.

Pain: This is the characteristic symptom of peptic ulcer, and it has three distinguished features- sharp localization to the epigastrium, relationship to food, and periodicity. Ulcer pain is commonly referred to the epigastrium, in the midline or to the right; wherever it occurs, it is usually distinctly localized so that the patient can point to the site. This feature of ulcer pain is so noticeable as to be called 'the pointing sign'. Occasionally ulcer pain is not distinctly localized; it may be referred diffusely in the epigastrium, the lower chest or to the back in the interscapular region in the fifth to eighth thoracic segments. Pain referred to the interscapular area, especially if it is a new feature, suggests the possibility that the ulcer has penetrated posteriorly, involving structures such as the pancreas. The description of the pain is not especially useful, although patients commonly describe it as gnawing or burning. Pain varies greatly in severity, and it is sometimes helpful to ask the patient to qualify the symptom as 'pain' or as 'discomfort' as a measure of its intensity.

Most patients recognize a relationship of the pain to food, although the relationship varies between patients, and in the same patient from time to time. Duodenal ulcer-pain tends to appear between meal times, so that the patient may describe it as 'hunger' pain, which is characteristically relieved by food. A distinguished feature of duodenal ulcer is pain awakening the patient from sleep between 2 and 4 a.m. The pain of gastric ulcer occurs less regularly; it often occurs within an hour of eating, is less often relieved by food, and it rarely occurs at night. Besides the characteristic relief obtained after eating, ulcer pain is almost always relieved by antacids, by vomiting and by bed rest in hospital.

Ulcer pain is characteristically episodic occurring regularly each day for days or weeks at a time, then disappearing, to reappear weeks or months later. Between attacks, the patient feels quite well, and may eat and drink with impunity. Bouts of pain may at first persist only a day or so at a time and occur only once or twice a year. As the natural history evolves, however, episodes begin to last longer and occur more frequently, so that in extreme cases remissions of pain may be short lived and pain or discomfort becomes more or less incessant. The cause for these relapses is difficult to substantiate. Seasonal factors may be operative, sometimes cognitive stress may be blamed, sometimes dietary imprudence, and sometimes alcoholic excess. Most commonly, no explanation can be found for the relapse.

Pain is sometimes absent or so insignificant as to be dismissed by the patient. Such individuals may complain of other symptoms such as a feeling of 'distension' in the epigastrium or a poorly defined sense of discomfiture after eating. Other complaints include episodic nausea and sometimes anorexia, as well as heartburn or water brash. Nausea, anorexia, vomiting and weight loss occur more frequently in gastric ulcer than in duodenal ulcer. Vomiting in ulcer patients almost always relieves pain and when it is continuous may result in weight loss. This helps to distinguish it from vomiting of psychological cause, in which weight is usually maintained. Persistent vomiting in an ulcer subject usually indicates some degree of gastric outflow obstruction, whether due to spasm or organic constriction of the gastric outlet. In such patients, vomiting is usually abundant, so that the patient is 'surprised' at the volume; the patient often recognizes food eaten twelve or more hours earlier, and he is aware of the unpleasant smell of the vomitus. Although there is no constant change in bowel rhythm during an ulcer relapse, some patients are conscious of constipation or diarrhea when dyspepsia reappears.

Physical signs: The only physical sign that may be present is 'the pointing sign' by which the patient perfectly indicates the site of pain; when accompanied by localized tenderness the sign is virtually diagnostic of an ulcer. However, tenderness may be completely absent. In patients with gastric outlet obstruction, the stomach may be visibly distended, a succession splash may be present, and gastric peristalsis may be seen.

Diagnosis

The diagnosis of peptic ulcer can usually be made from the characteristic history, but it requires corroboration by barium meal examination or endoscopy. In some patients the peptic ulcer may present with bleeding, perforation or even pyloric stenosis with few or no prior symptoms. The patient with troublesome dyspepsia, in whom barium meal analysis is negative, presents difficulties. Some of these patients will be found to have an ulcer at endoscopy and surely some may be found to have an early carcinoma. Some clinical judgment must be applied in order to distinguish between dyspepsia of psychological origin and that due to organic lesions which have not been detected radiologically. In general, the history in the former is more diffuse, the symptoms very seldom as clear cut, the pain poorly localized, and there are no sharply defined tender areas. Categorical evidence of a psychological abnormality can usually be obtained. It is a good rule that patients who develop dyspepsia for the first time in middle age should be investigated endoscopically if the X-ray is negative. Probably all patients with gastric ulcer should be examined endoscopically since the lesion can be inspected more closely and biopsies taken to rule out a carcinoma. This procedure is also suggested if the physician has any doubt about the nature of the disorder.

Gastric secretion test: Although this test is of restricted diagnostic value, a high acid output tends to support the diagnosis of duodenal ulcer and sustains a decision to operate; a low acid output is more consistent with a gastric than a duodenal ulcer.

Occult Blood: The faces should be tested for the presence or absence of occult blood in all patients with gastrointestinal symptoms. The test may be carried out of a smear of the stool obtained on rectal examination.

Treatment

There are three objectives in the control of peptic ulcer, namely, the alleviation of symptoms, the healing of the ulcer and the prevention of its recurrence, while there are effective methods for relieving symptoms and from accentuating ulcer healing, at present we have no means of preventing ulcer recurrence nor of altering the natural tendency of ulcer symptoms to remit and relapse. A major problem in interpreting the effectiveness of any specific treatment is the fact that ulcer symptoms do not necessarily reflect ulcer activity. Relief of symptoms can take place in a few days, whereas healing may take weeks. Thus, the relief of symptoms, which is naturally the main consideration of the patient, does not necessarily mean that the ulcer has healed; some ulcers may persist for many months without any further recurrence of pain, and without any change in size. The more chronic the ulcer, the less chance there is of obtaining healing, because the tissues are contorted by fibrosis. It seems a reasonable aim, therefore, to try to produce ulcer healing in the early stages, in the hope of preventing irrevocable changes. Unfortunately, this ideal is difficult to attain for financial reasons, since the patient is frequently unable to take sufficient time off-work, and in any case admission to hospital cannot usually be offered to all patients with an active ulcer but has to be preserved for patients with complications such as stenosis, bleeding or intractable pain.

Rest: The single most effective procedure for the relief of ulcer pain and the promotion of healing is bed-rest. This may be undertaken at home under the care of the family doctor or more effectively in hospital; undoubtedly rest in hospital confers additional benefit, possibly because of the freedom from domestic and business worries. Whatever be the reason, pain usually disappears after a few days of bed-rest in hospital.

Diet: It is usually said that an appropriate diet for ulcer patients should be mechanically and chemically non-irritating and should consist of small frequent meals. However, there is little experimental evidence to support this recommendation. It has been shown, for example, that hourly feedings of milk bring about more acid secretion in the stomach than does the ordinary routine of four meals a day, and there is no testimony that the rate of ulcer healing can be accelerated by the traditional bland ulcer diet. Indeed, persistence with such diets may "be harmful since they may lead to suboptimal intake of vitamin C. Nevertheless, when symptoms are extreme, the patient often appreciates frequent feeds and is helped by dietetic advice.

Tobacco smoking: There is good evidence to show that stoppage of making accelerates the healing of gastric ulcers, and it is likely that this also applies to duodenal ulcers. Thus, tobacco smoking should be prohibited and totally rejected.

Drugs

Antacids: Gives symptomatic relief. Recent studies show that they promote healing and lessen recurrences. Mainly there are two types of antacids.

(i) *Absorbable antacids:* Sodium bicarbonate and calcium bicarbonate for short term periodic relief. Repeated use may cause alkalosis or milk alkalosis syndrome. Since symptoms of this complication are not unique (nausea, headache, weakness), the disorder may progress unrecognized causing kidney damage. These antacids should not be used by patients who have vomited, who are dehydrated, or who have hypertension or renal function loss. There is evidence that calcium salts increase acid secretion by local action on the gastric mucosa.

(ii) *Non-absorbable antacids:*

    (a) Aluminium hydroxide is almost safe and very frequently used. Nevertheless, there is minor risk of phosphate depletion. Symptoms include anorexia, weakness and malaise. If the loss is very uncompromising, then long term use may result in osteomalacia.

    (b) Magnesium salts may give rise to diarrhea. Some compounds consist of both magnesium and aluminium hydroxide or aluminium hydroxide and magnesium trisilicate. Magnesium preparation should be given with caution to patients with renal damage.

    (c) *Anticholinergics:* Are given primarily to delay emptying of the stomach and thus longing antacid holding. Normally used preparations are glycopyrrolate 1 mg, propantheline 7 to 15 mg or isopropamide 5 mg generally given orally in form of tablets.

    Anticholinergics can cause dry mouth and blurred vision. Difficulty in urinating, enlarged prostate, indication of acute narrow angle glaucoma are some of the common contraindications for anticholinergics.

    (d) Histamine H_2 receptor blocking agents: Most commonly used therapeutic agent. They act as a competitive inhibitor of histamine at H_2 receptors. In the stomach it blocks gastric acid secretion stimulated by histamine, gastrin (a gastric hormone), parasympathetic activity and food and diminishes both basal and nocturnal gastric acid secretion. Pepsin, secretion, gastric juice volume and intrinsic factor secretion are also reduced. In the gall bladder, H_2 blockers potentiate chokcystokinin induced contraction.

The first compound which was in prevalent use was Cimetidine. Fewer compounds like Ranitidine and Famotidine are also now in use. Roxatidine is the latest drug in these class.

With Cimetidine, the symptoms are commonly relieved within the 1st week, recuperation may take 2 to 8 weeks. The dose for Cimetidine is 800 mg. q.i.d. (with meals and at bed time).

Though cimetidine is generally well tolerated, a moderate increase in serum creatinine and serum transaminases often occurs with apparent clinical significance. Diarrhea, rash, drug fever and myalgias have been reported and mental confusion with excitement may develop in elderly patients with renal impairment. Other rare side-effects comprise illness in patients with extensive burns, sinus bradycardia, hypotension after rapid I.V. injection and hyperglycemia.

(e) *Sucralfate:* It is a sucrose and aluminium containing disaccharide. It is reported to combine with proteins and proteolytic enzymes (e.g. pepsin) and to form in the base of the ulcer a protective coating that assists healing.

(f) Omeprazole (proton-pump-inhibitor): Blocks gastric acid secretion by inhibiting H^+, K^+ - ATP- ase in parietal cell membrane. This is used in the therapy of peptic ulcer. Omeprazole produces nausea, diarrhea, abdominal pain paraesthesia, dizziness. Toxicological studies suggested that the drug forms carcinoid rumors in gastric mucosa in animals. The new drug in this classification is lansoprazole.

(g) Tri Potassium Di-citro Bismuth.

(h) Radiation therapy and surgery: For specific cases of duodenal ulcer.

Disturbances in the gastrointestinal function, are accountable for various illnesses and discomfort in human beings. Over the past few decades, there have been a rise in research activity, directed towards development of effective and safer antiulcer drugs both synthetically and from natural resources. In the 1960's, research with the roots and rhizomes of liquorice (Glycerrhiza glabra) showed that the plant showed great promise in treatment of peptic ulcer. Doll et al (1962), reported their findings on clinical trial of triterpenoid liquorice compounds as antiulcer agents. Since then, a significant amount of investigation has been done on Glycyrrhizin, thus leading to the development of carbenoxolone sodium. Similar studies with other indigenous plants have led to the identification of various Indian herbs with significant antiulcer activity.

Medicinal Plants with Anti-ulcer Properties

1. *Adhatoda vasica Nees.* **(Acanthaceae)**
   - *Common names:* Hindi: Arusha, Beng.: Basak or Vasaka.
   - *Distribution:* It is sub-herbaceous bush, found throughout the year in plains and sub-Himalayan tracts in India, ascending up to 1200 meters flowers during February-March and also at the end of rainy seasons.
   - *Parts used:* Leaves.
   - *Pharmacological activities:* Produced anti-ulcer activity in the form ofherbal or herbo-mineral preparations[1].
   - *Chemical constituents:* See Anti-diabetic chapter.

2. *Aloe barbadensis Mill.*

   Syn. **A. vera** Tourn. Ox. Linn. (Liliaceae)
   - *Common names:* Eng.: Curacao Aloe, Barbadose Aloe, Hindi: Ghee-Kunvar, Beng.: Ghrita-Kumari.
   - *Distribution:* It is xerophilic, arborescent or herbaceous, the fleshy and strongly cuticularised leaves usually pricky at the margin and arranged in dense rosettes. It is naturalized in India. It is planted in many Indian gardens and available all over India.
   - *Parts used:* Leaves.

- *Pharmacological activities:* Oral administration of the plant extract significantly reduced both the number of ethanol induced gastric lesions as well as lesion index in experimental rats[2]. It produced anti-ulcer activity in experimental rats[3].

- *Chemical constituents:* Leaf latex contains aloin, isobarbaloin, emodin, aloe-emodin, 3-barbaloin.

3. *Alpinia galanga Willd.* (Zingiberaceae)

- *Common names:* Eng.: The greater Galangal, Hindi: Kulanjan, Beng.: Kulanjan.

- *Distribution:* Found in South India and Bengal.

- *Parts used:* Rhizomes.

- *Pharmacological activities:* Ethanolic extract exhibited gastric anti-secretary anti-ulcer and cytoptotective activities in rats[4].

- *Chemical constituents:* See Anti-diabetic chapter.

4. *Althaea rosea Cav.* (Malvaceae)

- *Common names:* Eng.: Holly-Hock, Hindi: Gulkhera.

- *Distribution:* A herb, often grown in gardens for showy flowers, which yield a red dye.

- *Parts used:* Stem.

- *Pharmacological activities:* The damages of mucus membrane of rat stomach, caused by aspirin, atophan considerably decreased by the polysaccharides, obtained from stem[5].

- *Chemical constituents:* 3-Glucoside of kaempferol, quercetin, cyanidin, kaempferol, quercetin, a flavanol glycoside-herbacin and 3-rutinoside were isolated from the plant.

5. *Antirrhinum majus Linn.* (Scrophulariaceae)

- *Common name:* Eng.: Snapdragon.

- *Distribution:* Cultivated as garden plant.

- *Parts used:* Leaves.

- *Pharmacological activities:* Luteolin showed marked anti-ulcer action when given orally to guinea pigs at 10 mg/kg/day during 5 days of histamine treatment 8 to rats for 12 days preceding pyloric ligation under same conditions apigenin was much less effective[6].

- *Chemical constituents:* Alkaloid-4-methyl- 2,6-maphthyridine, three other tertiary alkaloids, sixteen amino acids such of which eleven were identified as alanine, aspartic acid, cysteine, glutamic acids, glutamine, glycine, lysine, serine, threonine tyrosine and valine were isolated from aerial parts and cyanidin-3-glucoside and cyanidine-3-rutinosde from flowers.

6. *Asparagus racemosus Wild.* **(Liliaceae)**

- *Common names:* Hindi: Sata war, Beng.: Satamuli.
- *Distribution:* Found throughout tropical and subtropical parts of India, up to 4000ft in the Himalayas.
- *Parts used:* Roots.
- **Pharmacological activities:** Produced anti-ulcer activity in the form of herbal or herbomineral preparation[1]. Oral administration of powder of dry roots prevented the formation of duodenal ulcer in rats[7]. Root exhibited ulcer healing effect in patients probably via strengthening the mucosal resistance or cytoprotection. It did not produce any antacid activity[8].
- **Chemical constituents:** Leaves contain quercetin-3-gucuronide, of m.p. 204°.

7. *Azadirachta indica* A. Juss.

Syn. *Melia azadirachta* Linn. (Meliaceae)

- *Common names:* Eng.: Margosa Tree, Hindi: Neem, Beng.: Neem.
- *Distribution:* A large tree with rough bark. Native to India, grown all over India, Grows wild in the dry forests of the Decan.
- *Parts used:* Leaves, Fruits and Seeds.
- *Pharmacological activities:* Aqueous extract leaves, exerted anti-ulcer effect in rats on oral administration[9]. Aqueous extract of leaves produced anti-ulcer activity in rats exposed to cold restraint stress or given ethanol orally[10]. A significant anti-ulcer effect was found in

nimbidin, one of the constituents of oil of the seed[11]. Some active ingredients isolated from the lipid parts of fruits, exhibited anti-ulcer activity in stress induced ulcers in male rats[12].

- *Chemical constituents:* See Anti-inflammatory chapter.

8. *Benincasa hispida* **(Thunb.) Cogn.**

Syn. B. cerifera Savi (Cucurbitaceae)

- *Common names:* Eng.: White squash or Ash Gourd, Hindi: Petha, Beng: Chalkumra.
- *Distribution:* A large climber and annual plant. Cultivated throughout India, fruits used as vegetable. Flowers are large yellow.
- *Parts used:* Fruits.
- *Pharmacological activities:* Fruits produced anti-ulcer activity in shay rats[13].
- *Chemical constituents:* See Anti-diabetic chapter.

9. *Boerhaavia diffusa Linn.* **(Nyctaginaceae)**

- *Common names:* Eng.: Spreading, Hog-weed, Hindi: Sant, Beng.: Rakta-punarnava.
- *Distribution:* A perennial creeping weed, with pinkish flower, found at almost all parts of India.
- *Parts used:* Aerial parts.
- *Pharmacological activities:* It showed protection against stress induced ulcer in albino rats/mice[14].
- *Chemical constituents:* See Anti-inflammatory chapter.

10. *Brassica oleracea Linn. Var. Capitata Linn.* **(Brassicaceae)**

- *Common names:* Eng.: Cabbage, Hindi: Band-Gobi, - Beng.: Bandhakapi.
- *Distribution:* Cabbage is a Commonly used vegetable like cauliflower and available throughout India.
- *Parts used:* Leaves.
- *Pharmacological activities:* Leaf powder did not affect the ulcer index significantly, but its aqueous extract reduced the index[15].
- *Chemical constituents:* See Anti-diabetic chapter.

11. *Catha edulis Forsk.* **(Celastraceae)**

    - *Common name:* Eng.: African tea.

    - *Distribution:* An evergreen shrub, native to South Africa, introduced into India at Mysore and Bombay. Leaves and buds have stimulating effect.

    - *Parts used:* Aerial parts.

    - *Pharmacological activities:* Extract produced anti-ulcer activity and a non-specific neuro-muscular blocking effect[16].

    - *Chemical constituents:* Leaves and young shoots contain d-norisoephedrine and amino acids, beside this, an alkaloid, l-ephedrine and cathine (d-norpseudo-ephedrine) were isolated.

12. *Centella asiatica* **(*Linn.*) Urban.**

    Syn. *Hydrocotyle asiatica* Linn. (Apiaceae)

    - *Common names:* Eng.: Indian pennywort, Hindi: Brahma-mandiki; Beng.: Thol-khuri.

    - *Distribution:* A herb, found throughout India.

    - *Parts used:* leaves.

    - *Pharmacological activity:* Plant extract inhibited significantly gastric ulceration induced by cold and restraint stress in rats[17].

    - *Chemical constituents:* Thankunic acid, m.p. 314°, triterpene glycoside-thankuniside mp. 239°, asiatic acid as methyl ester, brahmic acid, m.p. 293°, isobrahmic acid, m.p. 263°, brahmoside, m.p. 242° and brahminoside, m.p. 223°, isothankuniside, m.p. 250°, isothamkunic acid, m.p. 288°, madecassoside, m.p. 220° and madecassic acid, m.p. 265°. A new triterpene acid-isolated and characterized as 2a, 3(3, 6(3-trihydroxynes-12-en-oic acid; polyacetylenes and nine other acetylenes isolated from subterranean parts.

13. *Cephalandra indica N Wight & Arn.* **(Cucurbitaceae)**

    Syn. *Coccinia indica* W & A

    - *Common names:* Eng.: Ivy Gourd, Hindi: Kanduri, Beng.: Telakucha.

- *Distribution:* Found throughout India, wild and cultivated.
- *Parts used:* Leaves.
- *Pharmacological activities:* Aqueous, alcoholic extract and a crystalline compound of the leaf produced anti-ulcer effect in white albino rats[18].
- *Chemical constituents:* See Anti-diabetic chapter.

14. *Cinnamomum cassia Bliue.* (Lauraceae)

- *Common name:* Eng.: Casia lignea.
- *Distribution:* An evergreen tree with aromatic bark. Bark is used as stomachic and carminative.
- *Parts used:* Bark.
- *Pharmacological activities:* Cassioside and cassiol, two components y obtained from bark produced anti-ulcer activity[19].
- *Chemical constituents:* Bark yields volatile oil known as "Oil of cassia" contain high percentage of cinnamic aldehyde.

15. *Cocos nucifera Linn.* (Arecaceae)

- *Common names:* Eng.: Coconut, Hindi: Nariyal, Beng.: Narikel, dab.
- *Distribution:* The tree is cultivated mostly in hot and humid parts of India, particularly near sea, for its great commercial value.
- *Parts used:* Seed.
- *Pharmacological activities:* Produced anti-ulcer activity in the form of herbal or herbomineral preparations[1].
- *Chemical constituents:* Coconut contains protamine, albumine, composed of glutamic acids, alanine, serine, cystine, leucine, isoleucine, valine, aspartic acid and other amino acids, globulin. Detection of phenol, P-cresol, caproic acid and p-hydroxybenzoic acid by TLC in shell fibres; in addition, tar from shells contained crotonaldehyde, furfural and acetic acid.

16. *Curcuma zedoaria Rose.* (Zingiberaceae)

- *Common names:* Eng.: Zedoary, Hindi & Beng.: Kachura.

- *Distribution:* A stem less herbs, root stock is tuberous. Rhizomes are considered as stimulant carminative and stomachic. The herb found in some parts of India.

- *Parts used:* Rhizome.

- *Pharmacological activities:* A significant inhibition in ulcer formation was produced on oral and subcutaneous administration of the extract in restrained and water immersed mice[20].

- *Chemical constituents:* Rhizome contains zedoarone, curcolone, curcumenol, a furanodiene, m.p. 44 °and beside these sesquterpenoid-zederone, pyrocurzerenone m.p. 76° and curcumol, m.p. 141°. Isolation of main component of essential oil-curzerenone-and its structure elucidation; absolute structure of zederone established; another sesquiterpene- dehydrocurdione isolated and characterized; synthesis of pyrocurzerenone; curzerenone, pyrocurzerenone and new furanosesquiterpenoids-furanodienone (I), isofuranodienone (II) and epicurzere-none-isolated and their absolute configurations established.

17. *Eclipta alba (Linn.) Hassk.* **(Asteraceae)**

- *Common names:* Hindi: Bhangra, babri, Beng.: Kesuti, keshukti.

- *Distribution:* Herbs - found throughout India, particularly moist ground. It is used for darkening hair.

- *Parts used:* Aerial parts.

- *Pharmacological activities:* Produced anti-ulcer activity in the form of herbal or herbomineral preparations[1].

- *Chemical constituents:* It contains desmethyl wedelo-lactone-7-0-glucoside, sixteen polyacetylenic thiophenes and nicotine.

18. *Emblica officinalis Gaertn.* **(Euphorbiaceae)**

- *Common names:* Eng.: Emblic Myrobalan, Hindi: Amla, amlika, Beng.: Dhatri, Amlaki.

- *Distribution:* A small or medium sized tree, found throughout tropical part of India, ascending to 1300m, cultivated in gardens and home yards.

- *Parts used:* Fruits.
- *Pharmacological activities:* Produced anti-ulcer activity in the form of herbal or herbomineral preparations[1].
- *Chemical constituents:* In addition, with vitamin C fruits contain corilagin, ellagic acid, and Trigalloyl glucose.

19. *Ficus racemosa Linn.*

Syn. *F. glomerata* Roxb. (Moraceae)

- *Common names:* Eng.: Cluster fig, Country fig, Hindi: Coular, Beng.: Jagyadumar.
- *Distribution:* A large deciduous tree distributed throughout India particularly in evergreen forests, moist localities. It is cultivated in village for sauce and edible fruits.
- *Parts used:* Bark.
- *Pharmacological activities:* Anti-ulcer and anti-secretary activities wereproduced in experimental rats by the aqueous extract of the dried bark[21].
- *Chemical constituents:* Leaf contains glycoside and bark contains tannin.

20. *Glycyrrhiza glabra Linn.* **(Papilionaceae)**

- *Common names:* Eng.: Liquorice, Hindi: Mulhatti, Beng.: Jashtimadhu.
- *Distribution:* A perennial native to the Mediterranean region and is now grown herb, cultivated in South India, Punjab and Kashmir.
- *Parts used:* Rhizome.
- *Pharmacological activities:* Anti-ulcer effect was observed in it[22]. Produced anti-ulcer activity in the form of herbal or herbomineral preparations[1]. Liquorice may be applied for symptomatic relief from the pain of peptic ulcer[23]. Anti-ulcer activities along with other pharmacological properties of liquorice were described[24].
- *Chemical constituents:* The chief constituent of liquorice is glycyrrhizin, which is present in the drug in the form of potassium and calcium salts of glycyrrhizic acid. It also

contains glucose (3.8%), sucrose (2.4-6.5%), bitter principles, resins, asperagine (2-4%) and fat (0.8%). A flavonone thamnoglucoside, mp. 232°, isolated from roots; used as smooth muscle relaxant in pharmaceutical composition; twenty-seven flavonoids present in roots of these six isolated and three identified as 4',7-dihydroxyfavanone (liquiritigenin); its 4'-(3-D-glucoside (liquiritin) and 2,4', -trihydroxychalcone (isoliquiritigenin); other three are new flavonoids, -L-1, mp. 164°, L-5, mp. 150°, L-7, mp.142°, aglycones (90%) obtained by hydrolysis of flavonoid L-1, separated into liquiritigenin, mp. 207° and isoliquiritigenin, mp. 198°, two new chalcone glucosides characterised as trans-isoliquiritigenin-4'-p-D-glucopyranoside (isoliquiritin), mp.230°, liquititigenin, liquiritin and isoloquiritigenin detected by PC; 7-hydroxy-4-methoxyisoflavone (formonetin) from roots; a new flavonoid glycoside-liquraside, mp.150° - characterised as trans- isoliquiritigenin-4-0-(-0-p-D-glucopyranosyl-2-p-D-apiofuranoside); ten flavonoids identified in plant by PC and saponaretin (isovitexin) characterised; isolation and structure of new flavone glycoside-thamnoliquiritin. A new triterpenoid-loquoric acid-isolated from roots, its structure elucidated; isolation of two triterpenoid acids-11 -deoxoglycyrrhetic acid and liquiritic acid, mp. 298°, characterised as C-20 epimer of glycyrrhetic acid; structure of isoglabrolide, mp. 318°; new lactones-glabrolide, mp. 360°, deoxoglabrolide, mp. 274°and isoglabrolide-obtained from acid hydrolysate of crude glucosides, glycyrrhizic acid isolated from rhizomes and roots; isolation of glycyrrhetol, mp. 304° and 21a-hydroxy-isoglabrolide and their structures elucidated; synthesis of glycyrrhizic acid derivatives; 18cc-hydroxyglycyrohetic acid isolated from acid fraction of plant extract; 24-hydroxy-11-deoxyglycyrrhetic and 24-hydroxycyrrhetic acids isolated as their Me esters; structures of 24-hydroxyliquiritic and liquiridiolic acids determined; preparation of Me glabrate from Methyl glycyrrhetate.

21. ***Leucas aspera Spreng.* (Lamiaceae)**
    - *Common names:* Hindi & Beng.: Chota halkusa.
    - *Distribution:* A woolly herb, found throughout the plain part of India.
    - *Parts used:* Whole plant.
    - *Pharmacological activities:* Anti-ulcer activity was observed[25].
    - *Chemical constituents:* Two alkaloids m.p. 139° and m.p. 183° galac-tose, ursolic acid, [3-sitosterol, oleanolic acid and two strols m.p. 135° and 130°, a-sitosterol, (3-sitosterol and a compound A, mp. 61 ° isolated from aerial parts.

22. ***Mikania cordata (Burm.) B.L. Robinson***

    Syn. *M. scandeno* Hook. f. non Willd (Compositae)
    - *Common name:* Beng.: Taralata.
    - *Distribution:* A herbaceous climber, found at South India. Assam and West Bengal.
    - *Parts used:* Leaves.
    - *Pharmacological activities:* Potent antiulcer properties were found in rats by the plant extract[26].
    - *Chemical constituents:* Mikanolide m.p. 230° from leaves and stems, falvone-mikanin, (3,5-dihydroxy-6,7,4'-trimethoxyfalvone), fumaric acid and epifriedelinol from roots, leaves and stems, and fridelin, and stigmasterol from roots were isolated. Six new sesquiterpene dilactones-mikanolide, dihydromikanolide, deoxy-mikanolide, scandenolide, dihydroscandenolide and miscandenin isolated from aerial parts, crystal structure of mikanolide, three new labdenin acid derivatives, two kaurenic acid derivatives and four new germacranolides isolated and their structures determined.

23. ***Musa paradisiaca Linn.***

    Syn. *M. sapientum Linn.* (Musaceae)
    - *Common names:* Eng.: Edible Banana Plantain, Hindi: Kela, Beng.: Kala.

- *Distribution:* It is native in India and cultivated for its fruits.

- *Parts used:* Fruit.

- *Pharmacological activities:* Anti-ulcerogenic activity was produced in rats by the powder of plantain banana of unripe fruits on oral administration[27]. Two steryl acyl glucoside, active against peptic and duodenal ulcers, were isolated from the fruits[28]. Produced anti-ulcer effect in the form of herbal or herbomineral preparations[1].

- *Chemical constituents:* The fruits are rich source of carbohydrates, mineral and vitamins (specially B-complex) 14a-methyl-9(3, 19-cyclo-5a-ergost-24(28)-en-3p-ol isolated from plant.

24. *Ocimam basilicum Linn.* (Lamiaceae)

- *Common names:* Eng.: Common basil, Hindi: Gulal tulsi, Beng.: Bantulsi.

- *Distribution:* Indigenous to the lower hills of Punjab, cultivated throughout the greater part of India.

- *Parts used:* Aerial parts.

- *Pharmacological activities:* Its powder, aqueous extract and ethanolic extract reduced the ulcer index[14].

- *Chemical constituents:* It's volatile oil contains Ocimene, methyl chavicol, sambulene, methyl cinnamate, linalool, borneol, safrole and cineole. Sesquiterpene hydrocarbon-1-epibycyclosesqui-phellandrene, methyl charriol (90%) and linalool were also isolated.

25. *Panax ginseng Mey. C.A.*

Syn. *Aralia quinqueplia* Nees (Araliaceae)

- *Common names:* Eng.: Chinese ginseng, Asiatic ginseng.

- *Distribution:* This plant does not occur in India, but P. pseudo ginseng Wall, and few of its varieties are available at different parts of the Himalayas. The root of P. ginseng is a very important and valuable drug in Chinese system of medicine.

- *Parts used:* Leaves.

- *Pharmacological activities:* A polysaccharide obtained from leaves, produced anti-ulcer activity (29).

- *Chemical constituents:* Root contains panaxadiol, m.p. 250°, a polysaccharide, two triterpene sapogenins, oleanolic acid, b-sitosterol, three other glucosides and saponin-ginsenoside Rg-as deca-acetate. Beside these the herb also contains flavonoids kaempferol and trifolin, panaxosides A and B, steroidal hormones, pantothenic acid, niacin and an alkaloid. Panaxosides B and C isolated from roots found to be trisaccharides, carbohydrate moiety of former contained glucose units whereas that of latter contained glucose and rhamnose two of these units were linked panaxatriol isolated; ginsenoside-Rg1 isolated from roots and its structure established; ginsenosides Rb1, Rb2 and Re, mp. 197°, 200° and 199° respectively, on hydrolysis yielded 20(S)-protopanaxadiol, partial hydrolysis of these saponins yielded prosapogenin which was identified as 3-0-(2(3-D-glucopyranosyl-p-D-glucopyranosyl (20S)-protopanaxadiol; anti-inflammatory glucosides panax saponins A and C isolated, partial structure of former proposed; preparation of a cardiotonic substance which contains eight triterpenoid saponins; ginsenosides RO, mp. 239 (chikusetsusaponin V), Rb1, Rb2, Re and Rd, mp. 206° isolated from roots and their structures established; ginsenosides Re, Rf isolated along with panaxadiol, panaxatriol, daucosterol, mannitol, sucrose and glucose; ginsenosides Rd, Re, Rg1, isolated from flowers and buds; new saponins ginsenosides F1, F2 and F3 isolated from leaves and their structures established; crude saponins isolated from aerial parts (leaves, 12.8, stems, 1.6 and flowers, 6.9%); crystal structure of panaxoside A; new saponins ginsenoside Rh1 and M7cd isolated from roots and flower buds respectively and characterised as 6-0-(3-D-gluco pyranoside of 20(S)- protopanaxatriol and 20-0-(3-D-glucopyranoside of dammar 25-ene-3(3-6a, 12b, 20(S), 24S-pentaol respectively; ginsenosides Rb1, Rb2, and Re isolated from leaves and flower buds; ginsenoside F3 from flower buds; ginsenosides Rb2, Re, Rd, Re and Rg1 isolated from fruits; in addition to above, ginsenosides Ra and Rg2 isolated from roots.

26. *Plantags asiatica Linn.* **(Plantaginaceae)**

- *Common name:* Kan.: Sirapotta gida.
- *Distribution:* Herbs - commonly found at hilly parts of India, on vast places.
- *Parts used:* Leaves.
- *Pharmacological activities:* A water-soluble substance, planta glucide, isolated from leaves, exhibited anti-ulcer property[30].
- *Chemical constituents:* Planta glucide.

27. *Pluchea indica Less.* **(Asteraceae)**

- *Common name:* Beng.: Munjhu rukha, kakronda.
- *Distribution:* Shrubs, found in salt marshes in Sundarbans (W.B) distributed in new world tropical and sub-tropical regions of Asia. It contains around 50 species out of which 6 have been recorded.
- *Parts used:* Roots.
- *Pharmacological activities:* Root extract exhibited significant antiulcer activity in rats[31].
- *Chemical constituents:* See Anti-inflammatory chapter.

28. *Solanum nigrum Linn.* **(Solanaceae)**

- *Common names:* Eng.: Black night shade, Hindi: Makoi, Beng.: Kakmachi.
- *Distribution:* A shrubs, found throughout India, berries are globose and green, but turns yellow on maturity, flowers are white. A good source of solarodine.
- *Parts used:* Aerial parts.
- *Pharmacological activities:* Powder and methanolic extract significantly lowered the ulcer index[14].
- *Chemical constituents:* Solasodine like compounds in leaves and berries, tigogenin in berries, glucoalkaloids in immature berries, and solasonine and solamargine in leaves were detected.

29. ***Strychnos nux-vomica Linn.* (Loganiaceae)**
    - *Common names:* Eng.: Nux-vomica, snake-wood, Hindi: Kajra, kuchla, Beng.: Kuchila.
    - *Distribution:* A tree found almost throughout the tropical parts of India. Dried and ripe seeds are used as drug Nux-vomica used tonic, stimulant etc.
    - *Parts used:* Seed.
    - *Pharmacological activities:* Oral administration of the powder produced anti-ulcer activity in shay rats[32]. Strychnine exhibited anti-ulcer effect in shy rats[33].
    - *Chemical constituents:* Two major alkaloids of seeds are strychnine and brucine, leaves contain strychnine, brucine, methoxystrychnine and vomicine, fruits contain loganin, m.p. 222° a glycoside.

30. ***Terminalia chebula Retz. C.B. Clarke in part* (Combretaceae)**
    - *Common names:* Eng.: Chebulic myrobalan, Hindi: Harra, Beng.: Haritaki.
    - *Distribution:* A large tree, found throughout India in deciduous forests. Forests are of variable size, and rich in tannin.
    - *Parts used:* Fruits.
    - *Pharmacological activities:* Powder of dry fruits, on oral administration, prevented the formation of duodenal ulcer and reduced the ulcer index in rats, in experimentally induced acute gastric ulcerations[6].
    - *Chemical constituents:* Fruits contain terchebin a tannin compound and a glycoside of anthraquinone derivatives, and flowers contain chebulin, m.p. 249°. Palmitic, stearic, oleic, linoleic, arachidic and behenic acids isolated from fruit kernels.

31. ***Trichosanthes dioic Roxb.* (Cucurbitaceae)**
    - *Common names:* Eng.: Pointed gourd, Hindi: Parwal, Beng.: Potol.
    - *Distribution:* An annual creeping herbs, cultivated throughout the plains of N. India, extending to Assam and Bengal.

- *Parts used:* Leaves.

- *Pharmacological activities:* Produced anti-ulcer effect in the form of herbal or herbomineral preparations[1].

- *Chemical constituents:* Roots contain an amorphous saponin, hentriacontane, or phytosteril a nitrogenous bitter principle, glycosidic in nature and resembling colocynth, small amount of essential oil, little fixed oil, and traces of tannins.

32. *Trigonella foenum-graecutn Linn.* **(Fabaceae)**

- *Common names:* Eng.: Fenngreek, Hindi: Methi, Beng.: Methi.

- *Distribution:* Cultivated in many parts of India.

- *Parts used:* Seeds.

- *Pharmacological activities:* Anti-ulcer activity was evaluated in rats[34].

- *Chemical constituents:* Two flavonoid glycosides, quercetin and luteolin, and two steroidal saponins from seeds identified by PC.

33. *Zingiber officinale Rose.* **(Zingiberaceae)**

- *Common names:* Eng.: Ginger, Hindi: Adrak, Beng.: Ada.

- *Distribution:* The plant is a herbaceous perennial, producing leafy shoots which attain a height of about 1-3ft. Ginger is cultivated in many places. Cochin ginger takes the highest rank among Indian gingers but the districts of Rungpur, Midnapore and Hooghly in Bengal, Surat and Jhama in Bombay and Kumaon in Uttar Pradesh are also noted for production of good ginger.

- *Parts used:* Rhizomes.

- *Pharmacological activities:* On oral administration of acetone extract of the rhizome, zingiberone, the main terpenoid of acetone extract and gingerol, the pungent principle of the rhizome significantly prevented gastric lesions in HCI/ethanol induced gastric lesion in rats[35]. Beta sesquiphellandrene, beta-bisabolene and 6-shogaol, some active principles of Taiwan zinger produced anti-ulcer activity in HCI/ethanol induced gastric lesions in rats[36].

- *Chemical constituents:* Detection of heptone, octane, isovaleraldehyde, nonanol, ethyl pirene, camphene, p-pinene, sabinene, myrecene, limonene, p-phellandrene and 1,8-cineole in essential oil by GLC; presence of gingediol, methylgingedio and their diacetates by GC-MS; new sesquiterpenes-sequitherjene, cis-sesquisabinese hydrate and zingiberenol [2 methyl-6(trans-4'-methyl-4' hydroxycyclohex-2'-enyl)-hept-2-ene] isolated and their structures determined; car-3-ene a-terpinone, a-terpuneol, nerol, 1,8-cineole, zingiberene, nerol geranial, gexaniol and geranyl acetate identified in essential oil from rhizomes.

References

1. Singh, K.P. & Singh, R.H., *J. Res. Ayurv. Siddha*, 1985, 6(2), 132.

2. Avalos, A. A., Diaz, M.Q., Larionova, M. & Nieto, A.E., *Revista Cubana de Farmacia*, 1989, 23(3), 278.

3. Narendran, S., Saraswathi & Varadharaja, V., Seminars & Symposiam Proceedings in Med & Ammat. Plants Abstr., 1985, 7(1), 103, No.0606.

4. AI-Yahya, M.A., Rafatuilah, S., Mossa, J.S., Ageel, A.M., Al-Said, M.S. & Tariq, M., Phytotherapy Research, 1990, 4(3), 112.

5. Barnaulov, O.D., Manicheva, O.A., Trukhaleva, N.A., Kozhina, I.S., Fokina, N. E. & Salikhov, C.A., Rastit Resur., 1985, 21(3), 329.

6. Rastogi, R.P. & Mehrotra, B.N., Compendium of Indian Medicinal Plants, (1991), Vol.2, Central Drug Research Institute, Lucknow and Publications & Information Directorate, New Delhi, CSIR, p-58.

7. Dahanukar, S.A., Date, S.G. & Karandikar, S.M., Indian Drugs, 1983, 20(11), 442.

8. Singh, K.P., & Singh, R.H., J. Res. Ayurv. Siddha, 1986, 7(3-4), 91.

9. Proc. 24th Indian Pharmacol. Soc. Conference, Ahmedabad, Gujrat, India, Dec.29-31, 1991, 40.

10. Garg, G.P., Nigam, S.K. & Ogle, C.W., Plants Medica, 1993, 59(3), 215.

11. Pillai, N.R. & Santhakumari, G., Planta Medica, 1984, 50(2), 143.

12. Moursi, S.A.H. & AI-Khatib, I.M., Jpn., J. Pharmacol., 1984, 36(4), 527.

13. Jangannavar, S.L., Amruthraj, G. & Seethalakshmi, R., Seminars & Symposiam Proceedings in Med. & Aromat. Plants Abstr., 1986, 8(2), 181, No, 1157.

14. Proc. 24th Indian Pharmacol. Soc. Conference, Ahmedabad, Gujrat, India, Dec.29-31, 1991, 3.

15. Akhtar, M.S. & Munir, M., J. Ethnopharmacol., 1989, 27(1-2), 163.

16. Tariq, M., Ageel, A.M., Parmar, N.S. & AI-Meshal, I.A., Fitoterapia, 1984, 55(4), 195.

17. Chatterjee, T.K., Chakraborty, A. & Pathak, M., Indian J. of Expt, Bio., 1992, 30(10), 889.

18. Jeganathan, N.S., Manavalan, Ft., Kamaraj, G., Ravi, M., Venugopal, D. & Dharani, R., Proceedings of 42 Indian Pharmaceutical Congress, Manipal, GP03: p.90, 28-30th Dec. 1990.

19. Shiraga, Y., Fukaya, C., Yokoyama, K., Tanaka, S., Fukui, H., Tabata, M. & Okano, K., J. Pharm. Scs., 1987, 76(11), 5214.

20. Watanabe, K., Shibata, M., Yano, S., Cai, Y, Shibuya, H. & Kitagawa, I., Yakugaku Zasshi, 1986, 106(12), 1137.

21. Patel, S.M. & Vasavada, S.A., Bull. Med. Ethnobot. Res., 1985, 6(1), 17.

22. Saraswathi, P., Seninars & Symposiam Proceedings in Med. & Aromat, Plants Abstr., 1986, 8(2), 182, 1180.

23. Trease, G.E. & Evans, W.C., Pharmacognosy (11th Edition), Baillience Tindall, London, 490.

24. Lutomski, J., Nieman, C.-& Fenwick, G.K., Herba Polonica, 1991, 37(3-4), 163.

25. Reddy, M.K., Ramachandran, S. & Kameswaran, L., Seminars & Symposiam Proceedings in Med & Aromat. Plants Abstr., 1986, 8(2), 181, No.1164.

26. Pal, S., Bhattacharya, S. & Nag Chowdhuri, A.K., Phytotherapy Research, 1988, 2(4), 100.

27. Goel, R.K., Chakraborty, A. & Sanyal, A.K., Planta Med., 1985, No.2, 85.

28. Ghosal, S. & Saini, K.S., J. Chem. Res.(s), 1984, No.4,110.

29. Sun, X.B., Matsumoto, T. & Yamada, H., Planta Medica, 1992, 58(5), 432.

30. Voitenko, G.N., Lipkan, G.N., Maksyutina, N.P. & Lebedev-Kosov, V.I., Rastit. Resur., 1983, 19(1), 103.

31. Pal, S. & Nagchowdhuri, A.K., Phylotherapy Research, 1989, 3(4), 156.

32. Panda, P.K. & Panda, D.P., Indian Drugs, 1993, 30(2), 53.

33. Ibid, 30(9), 458.

34. AI-Meshal, I.A., Parmar, N.S. & Tariq, M., Seminars & Symposiam Proceedings in Med. & Aromat, Plants Abstr., 1985, 7(3), 283, No.1831.

35. Yamahara, J., Mochizuki, M., Rong, H.Q., Matsuda, H. & Fujimura, H., J.Ethnopharmacol., 1988, 2392(3), 299.

36. Yamahara, J., Hatakeyama, S., Taniguchi, K., Kawamura, M. & Yoshikawa, M., Yakugaku Zassh'1, 1992, 112(9), 645.

8 *Herb-Drug Interactions*

Herbs are plant derived materials which are used for medicinal purpose. Herb-drug interactions are interactions that occur between herbal medicines and conventional drugs. These types of interactions may be more common than drug-drug interactions because herbal medicines often contain multiple pharmacologically active ingredients, while conventional drugs typically contain only one. Some such interactions are clinically significant, although most herbal remedies are not associated with drug interactions causing serious consequences. Most herb-drug interactions are moderate in severity. The most commonly implicated conventional drugs in herb-drug interactions are warfarin, insulin, aspirin, digoxin, and ticlopidine, due to their narrow therapeutic indices. The most commonly implicated herbs involved in such interactions are those containing St. John's Wort, magnesium, calcium, iron, or ginkgo. The possibility of drug interactions, direct toxicities, and contamination with active pharmaceutical agents are among the safety concerns about dietary and herbal supplements. Although there is a widespread public perception that herbs and botanical products in dietary supplements are safe, research has demonstrated that these products carry the same dangers as other pharmacologically active compounds. Interactions may occur between prescription drugs, over-the-counter drugs, dietary supplements, and even small molecules in food — making it a daunting challenge to identify all interactions that are of clinical concern.

Concerns about herb-drug interactions are often not based on rigorous research. Most herb-drug interactions identified in current sources are hypothetical, inferred from animal studies, cellular assays, or based on other indirect means; however, attention to this issue is needed for drugs with a narrow therapeutic index, such as cancer chemotherapeutic agents, warfarin, and digoxin.

To date, well-designed clinical studies evaluating herbal supplement-drug interactions are limited and sometimes inconclusive. This issue of the 'Digest' provides information about several herbs and their potential interactions with other agents.

The mechanisms underlying most herb-drug interactions are not fully understood. Interactions between herbal medicines and anticancer drugs typically involve enzymes that metabolize cytochrome P450. For example, St. John's Wort has been shown to induce CYP3A4 and P-glycoprotein in vitro and in vivo.

Table 1 Herb-Drug interactions

Herbs	Drugs	Interaction
Scutellaria Balcalensis	Losartan	May increase drug levels
	Rosuvastatin	May decrease drug levels
Berberis vulgaris	Drugs that displace the protein binding of bilirubin, e.g. phenylbutazone	May potentiate effect on drug on displacing bilirubin
Vaccinlum myrtillus	Warfarin	Potentiation of bleeding
Cimicifuga racemosa	Statin drugs e.g. atorvastatin	May potentiate increase in liver enzymes, specifically ALT.
Fucus vesiculosus	Hyperthyroid medication, e.g. carbimazole	May decrease effectiveness of drug due to natural iodine content
	Thyroid replacement therapies, e.g. thyroxine	May add to effect of drug.
Lycopus vlrginicus, Lycopus europaeus	Radioactive iodine	May interfere, with administration of diagnostic procedures using radioactive isotopes
	Thyroid hormones	Should not be administered concurrently with preparations containing thyroid hormone.[11]
Uncaria tomentosa	HIV protease inhibitors	May increase drug level.
Capsicum spp.	Theophylline	May increase absorption.
Apiumg raveolens	Thyroxine	May reduce serum levels of thyroxine.
Coleus forskohill	Antiplatelet Medication	May potentiate effects of drug
	Hypotensive medication	May potential effects of drug
	Prescribed medication	May potentiate effects of drug
	Prescribed medication	May potentiate effects of drug
Vaccinium macrocarpon	Midazolam	May increase drug levels
	Warfarin	May alter INR (most frequently increase)

Table 1 Contd...

Herbs	Drugs	Interaction
Salvia miltiorrhiza	Midazolam	May decrease drug levels.
	Warfarin	May potentiate effect of drug.
Harpagophytum procumbens	Warfarin	May increase bleeding tendency
Echinacea angustifolia	HIV protease e.g. darunavir	May decrease drug levels.
	Immunosuppressant medication	May decrease effectiveness of drug
	Midazolam	Decreases drug levels when drug administered intravenously
Denothera blennis	Phenothiazines	May decrease effectiveness of drug.
Allium sativum	Antiplatelet and anticoagulant drugs e.g. aspirin warfarin	Aspirin: May increase bleeding time.
	Warfarin	May potentiate effect of drug. Large doses could increase bleeding tendency.
	HIV protease inhibitors, e.g. saquinavir	Decreases drug level.
Zingiber officinale	Antacids	May decrease effectiveness of drug
	Antiplatelet and anticoagulant drugs e.g. phenprocoumon, warfarin	Phenprpcoumon: May increase action of drug.
	Warfarin	Increased risk of spontaneous bleeding.
	Nifedipine	May produce a synergistic antiplatelet effect
Ginkgo biloba	Anticonvulsant medication, e.g. carbamazepine sodium valproate.	May decrease effectiveness of drugs.
	Antiplatelet and anticoagulant drugs e.g. aspirin, clopidogrel, ticlopidine, warfarin	Prolongation of bleeding and /or increased bleeding tendency
	Antipsychotic medication e.g. haloperidol, olanzapine, clozapine	May potentiate the efficiency of drug in patients with schizophrenia
	Benzodiazepines, e.g. diazepam, midazolam	May alter drug level
	HIV non-nucleoside transcriptase inhibitors e.g. efavirenz	May decrease drug levels

Table 1 *Contd...*

Herbs	Drugs	Interaction
	Hypoglycaemic drugs e.g. glipizide, metformin, pioglitazone, tolbutamide	Glipizide: May cause hypoglycaemia.
		Metformin: May enhance action of drug.
		Pioglitazone: May decrease effectiveness of drug
		Tolbutamide: May decrease effectiveness of drug
	Nifedipine	May increase drug levels or side effects.
	Omeprazole	May decrease drug levels.
	Talinolol	May increase drug levels
Hydrastis Canadensis	Drugs which displace the protein binding of bilirubin e.g. phenylbutazone	May potentiate effect of drug on displacing bilirubin
	Midazolam	May increase drug level
Camallia sinensis	Boronic acid-based protease inhibitors e.g. bortezomib	May decrease efficacy of drug.
	Folate	May decrease absorption
	Statin drugs e.g. simvastatin	May increase plasma level and side effect of drug.
	Warfarin	May inhibit effect of drug : decreased INR
Crataegus laevigata (c.owyacantha)	Digoxin	May increase effectiveness of drug
	Hypotensive drugs including betablockers	May increase effectiveness of drug
(Trigonella foenumgraecum) Gymmema sylvestre, Galega officinalis) Plantago ovata, p. psylllium, P. Indica)	Hypoglycemic drugs, including Insulin	May potentiate hypoglycaemic activity of drug
Piper methystioum	CNS depressants, e.g. alcohol barbiturates benzodiazepines	Potentiation of drug effects
	L-Dopa and other Parkinson's disease treatments	Possible dopamine antagonist effects
Panax ginseng	Antihypertensive medications including nifedipine	Genera: May decrease effectiveness of drug
		Nifedipine: May increase drug levels
	Antiplatelet and anticoagulant drugs	General: May potentiate effects of drug.
		Warfarin: May decrease effectiveness of drug

Table 1 *Contd...*

Herbs	Drugs	Interaction
	CNS stimulants	May potentiate effects of drug
	Hypoglycaemic drugs, including insulin	May potentiate hypogly-caemic activity of drug
	MAO inhibitors e.g. phenelzine	Headache and tremor, mania
Laxative: *Aloe Barbadensis, Aloe ferox, Cassia spp, Rhamnus purshlana, Rumex crispus*	Antiarrhythmic agents	May affect activity if potassium deficiency resulting from long term laxative abuse is present
	Cardiac glycosides	May potentiate activity if potassium deficiency resulting from long-term laxative abuse is present
	Potassium depleting agents e.g. thiazide diuretics, corticosteroids, licorice not (glycyrrhiza glabra)	May increase potassium depletion
Glycyrrhiza glabra	Antihypertensive medications other than diuretics	General: May decrease effectiveness of drug.
		ACE-inhibitor: May mask the development of Pseudoaldosteronism
	Cilostazol	May cause hypokalaemia, which can potentiate the toxicity of the drug.
	Digoxin	May cause hypokalaemia which can potentiate the toxicity of the drug.
	Diuretics	Spironolactone (potassium-sparing diuretic): reduced side effects of drug.
		Thiazide and loop (potassium depleting) diuretics: The combined effect of licorice and the drug could result in excessive potassium loss.
	Immuno-supressives, e.g. sirolimus	May decrease drug clearance.
	Midadazolam	May decrease drug level
	Omeprazole	May decrease drug level
	Potassium depleting drugs other than thiazide and loop diuretics e.g., corticosteroids stimulant laxatives	The combined effect of licorice and the drug could result in excessive potassium loss
	Prednisolone	May potentiate the action or increase levels of drug

Table 1 *Contd...*

Herbs	Drugs	Interaction
Athaea officinalis	Prescribed medication	May slow or reduce absorption of drugs
Fillpendula ulmaria	Warfarin	May potentiate effects of drug
Phellodendron amurense	Drugs that displace the protein binding of bilirubin e.g. phenylbutazone	May potentiate effect of drug on displacing bilirubin
Capsicum annuum, Matricaria recutita, Camellia sinensis, Tillacordata, Rosmarinus officinalis, Silyblurn marianum, Verbena officinalis	Iron	Inhibition of non-haem iron absorption
Plantago ovate, Plantago indica	Carbamazepine	Decreases plasma drug level
	Digoxin	May decrease absorption of drug
	Iron	Inhibition of non-haem iron absorption
	Lithium	May decrease absorption of drug
	Prescribed medication	May slow or reduce absorption of drugs
	Thyroxine	May decrease efficacy of drug
Schisandra chinensis	Immuno supressives e.g. tacrolimus	May increase drug levels
	Midazolam	May increase drug levels
	Prescribed medication	May accelerate clearance from the body
	Talinolol	May increase drug levels possible effect on inhibiting p-gp
Eleutherococcus senticosun	Digoxin	May increase plasma drug levels
Ulmus rubra	Prescribed medication	May slow or reduce absorption of drugs
Hypericum perforatum	Amitriptyline	Decrease drug levels
	Anticonvulsants e.g. carbamazepine me-phenytoin, phenobarbitone, phenytoin	May decrease drug levels via CYP induction
	Antihistamine e.g. fexofenadine	Decreases drug levels
	Antiplatelet and anticoagulant drugs e.g. clopidogrel, phenprocoumon, warfarin	Clopldogrel: May potentiate effects of drugs
		Phyenprocoumon: decreases plasma drug levels.
		Warfarin: decreases drug levels and INR

Table 1 *Contd...*

Herbs	Drugs	Interaction
	Benzodiazepines, e.g. alprazolam midazolam quazepam	Decreases drug levels and is probably dependent upon the hyperforin content
	Calcium channel antagonists e.g. nifedipine verapamil	Decreases drug levels
	Cancer chemotherapeutic drugs e.g. irinotecan imatinib	Decreases drug levels
	Digoxin	Decreases drug levels
	Finasteride	May decrease drug levels
	HIV non-nucleoside transcriptase inhibitors e.g. indinavir	Decreases drug levels
	Hypoglycaemic drugs e.g. gliclazlide, tolbutamide	Gliclazide: May reduce efficacy of drug by increased clearance
		Tolbutamide: May affect blood glucose
	Immuno supressives e.g. cyclosporine, tacrollmus	Decreases drug levels
	Labradine	May decrease drug levels
	Methadone	Decrease drug levels possibly inducing withdrawal symptoms.
	Methylphenidate	May decrease efficacy
	Omeprazole	May decrease drug levels
	Oral contraceptives	May increase metabolism of drug
	Oxycodone	Decrease drug levels
	SSRls, e.g. paroxetine, trazodone, sertraline and other serotonergic agents e.g. nefazodoneveniafaxina	Potentiation effects possible with regard to serotonin levels
	Statin drugs	May decrease effect and / or drug levels
	Talinolol	May decrease drug levels
	Theophylline	May decrease drug levels
	Voriconazole	Decreases drug levels
	Zolpidem	May decrease drug levels (but with wide inter subject variability)
Silybum marianum	Hypoglycaemic drugs, including insulin	May improve insulin sensitivity
	Immuno suppressives e.g. sirolimus	May decrease drug clearance
	Metronidazole	May decrease absorption rate of drug

Table 1 *Contd...*

Herbs	Drugs	Interaction
	Omidazole	May increase drug levels
	Talinolol	May increase drug levels
Agrimonia eupatoria, Arctostaphylos uvaursh, Geranium maculatum, Vitis vinifera, Camellia sinensis, Crataegus app, Melissa officinalls, Filpendula ulmaria, Menthax piperita, Pelargonium sidoides, Pinusmas sonlana, Rubus idaeus, Salvia fruticosa, Hypericum perforatum, Salix spp.	Minerals especially iron	Iron: May reduce absorption of non-haem iron from food Zinc: May reduce absorption for food. Clinical studies with healthy volunteers: results conflicting for effect on zinc (unrefined tea, black tea consumed at or immediately after food.
Curcuma longa	Tainolol	May decrease drug levels
Valeriana eduilis, Valeriana officinalis	CNS depressants or alcohol	May potentiate effects of drug
Salix aiba, Salix daphnoides, Salix purpurea, Salix fragilis	Warfarin	May potentiate effect of drug.

Different herbs (in fruit juice forms)-Drugs interactions

JUICE	DRUG	MOA	ADR
Apple juice (AJ)	Flexofenadine Cyclosporine Aliskiren	AJ inhibits OAPT (Organic Anion Transport Polypeptide) and decreases the absorption of drug.	Diminished therapeutic efficacy.
Orange juice	Flexifebadine Aliskiren beta blockers (atenolol, Celeprolol, talindolol) Or fluoroquinolones (cipro-floxacin, Levofloxacine)	Decreases the absorption of drugs by inhibiting the OAPT (Organic Anion Transporting Polypeptide).	Reduction of therapeutic efficacy.
Pomelo orange	Felodipine, Cyclosporine or Tacrolimus	Pomelo orange inhibits the CYP3A4 mediated metabolism	Increased risk of adverse effects.
Seville orange	Dextrometharphen, Felodipine	Furanocoumarins of Seville orange juice inhibits CTP3A4 and decrease the metabolism.	Excessive adverse effects.

9 Different Analysis Techniques to Identify the Phytochemicals of Herbs

Chemical constituents of herbs are called phytochemicals. The natural product organic chemistry and plant biochemistry are closely related to Phytochemistry. Phytochemistry deals with chemical structure, biosynthesis, metabolism and their natural distribution and their biological functions.

The purpose of writing such a chapter is to provide an opening to the available methods for the analysis of plant substances. Most importantly, students or researchers can develop their own techniques for solving their problems by taking knowledge of different instrumental analytical methods which have been used. To do the phytochemistry, it requires some chemical laboratory works which should be simple and uncomplicated. However, the common sense and the thinking ability of a laboratory worker are the first principles in the laboratory. The various practical experiments are provided here for seeking the knowledge and experience.

The major problem in phytochemical research is the huge number of distinct structures produced by plants. It is very difficult to match with the collation of existing data for each class of compounds. The new chemical structure has been discovered and described at a rate of one in a day for the pharmacological interest in novel alkaloids. Owing to the huge number of plant compounds, a short introduction has been given in each chapter of the book, indicating the structural and chemical variation with their representative formulae within each class of compounds. References and tables of recent known compounds are provided. wherever possible, the RF values, color reactions and spectral features of most of the common plant components.

The phytochemical study has been improved enormously by the development of fast and accurate screening method for a particular plant component. The chromatographic, spectral techniques and other preliminary detection methods for the particular class of compounds have been emphasized in this chapter. The term 'plant' is used to refer as a whole plant kingdom.

In general, the analytical methods applied in higher plant for the identification of alkaloids, amino acids, quinine and terpenoids can be used directly to the microbial systems. The isolation of contaminating substances such as tannin and chlorophyll is simple. Although these impurities are usually absent in the sample.

There is a number of pigments including depsidones and depsides, are analyzed by microbial methods or based on color reactions, chromatographies and other special techniques. Detail information on lichen pigments is given by Culberson (1969).

There are so many books available on the method of plant analysis. Among them, the first is entitled 'Methods in Plant Biochemistry' with P.M. Dey and J.B. Harborne as series editors. It has appeared in a 10 volumes (1989-1997). The second one is Modern Methods of Plant Analysis of a series edited by H.F. Linskens and J.F. Jacson, published in 1985 and volume of 20. There are some journals which are linked directly to plant analysis. These are the Journals of Phytochemical analysis, Chromatography, Analytical biochemistry and Chromatographic Science.

Method of Extraction and Isolation

The Plant Materials

Generally after the collection of plant materials, they should be immersed in boiling alcohol within minutes. If the plant materials are not in hand, freshly picked tissue should be stored dry in a plastic bag. It remains in good condition for several days. So, plant materials can be freshly supplied by the collectors from farther away. Before the extraction, the plant materials should be dried under controlled conditions to avoid various chemical changes. The drying should be followed up as soon as possible without applying high temperature in a good air condition. If ideally dried, plant materials can be stored for the phytochemical analysis for a longer period of time. Owing to this reason,the herbarium plant tissue is the best technique for the analysis of flavonoids, alkaloids, quinine and the terpenoids. Flavonoids and alkaloids in herbarium form are significantly stable time. According to Phillipson view, a leaf sample of *strychnos nuxvomica* collected in 1675, has been containing 1-2% by weight of alkaloid. One example of herbarium plant material is the essential oil from Mentha leaf, made before 1800 (Haley and Bell, 1967). Some of phytochemicals are the best extracted under controlled conditions rather than herbarium processing. For example, the yield of condensed tannin from willow leaves is much more in vacuum-dried process in comparison to air-dried process. Whereas, the phenolic glycosides in plants are easily extracted through simple air-drying. (Orians 1995).

The contamination is an important concern in phytochemical analysis. Plant materials should not be contaminated with other plant materials during the analysis. The plant tissue must be free from the viral, bacterial and fungal infections. The contaminations may occur when lower plant materials are mixed up with the sample plant tissues. It is essential to remove all tissues from the sample compound when the fungi growing parasitically on trees are collected. Contamination may occur in such a way where two closely similar grass species grow side by side in the same field. Such plant materials may incorrectlybe collected by the collector without any realization.

In phytochemical analysis, the botanical identification of the plant must be done by the authentic authority. During the investigation, if any, mistakes over the plant identity happened in the past that are essential to note down the plant material whenever new substances from plant or even known components from the new plant sources. There should not have a question about the identity of the plant. So, it should be authenticated by the taxonomic expert. Now a days, it is common practice in phytochemical research to deposit a voucher document of a plant, examined in a recognized herbarium center. This voucher specimen of the plant can be made as future reference as required.

Extraction

Extraction of plant materials primarily depends on the texture and water content of the compounds and on the type of substances which are being extracted. To prevent enzymatic oxidation/ hydrolysis, the plant tissues should be killed before extraction process. Boiled alcohol isgood for all purpose solvent for achieving this end. In case of exhaustive extraction, the plant materials should be macerated in a blender and then filtered. The success of the extraction of a component of a green plant tissue depends on the extent of chlorophyll which is moved to the solvent. Due to repeated extraction, when the tissue debris is free from the green color, it can be assumed that all the low molecular weight compounds have been isolated.

To get organic components of the dried plant tissue like dried roots, leaf, seed have to pack in a Soxhlet apparatus with a range of solvent, starting from ether, petroleum and chloroform and then taking alcohol and ethyl acetate. Starting solvent is used to separate lipids and terpenoids and other mentioned solvents for the extraction of more polar compounds. This process is mostly applied in the extraction when working on a gram scale.

The extracted material is clarified and then concentrated in vacuum. It can be carried out in a rotary evaporator to concentrate the bulk solution to a small volume without bumping at a temperature of 30-40°C. There are some shortcut extraction processes which are usually taken in the practice. For example, water soluble compounds are isolated from the leaf tissue by following concentration; the lipids should be removed by repeated washing with petroleum at the early stage. During evaporation of an ethanolic extract in a rotary evaporator, the lipids and almost all chlorophyll are deposited on the inner wall of the flask. By using skill, the aqueous concentration can be populated off from the flask just to the right point at which the collected materials are almost free from lipids of impurities. On standing, the concentrated extract may be deposited as crystal. This crystal product can be collected by filtration and tested for their homogeneity by using chromatography in different solvents.

A single crystal product can be purified by recrystallization and soon afterward materials are available for the phytochemical analysisbut it is difficult to separate from each other when the mixtures of substances will be present in the crystal mix. In this case, it is necessary to redissolve the substances in a suitable solvent and separate them by using chromatography. In most cases, many compounds may also remain in the mother liquor and they are subjected to isolation through the following chromatographic fractionation. The standard precaution should be taken to prevent material loss. So, the concentrated plant extracts should be kept in the refrigerator for complete phytochemical analysis. Before it, a little amount of toluene should be added to the product to inhibit the fungal growth.

One standard separation method might be followed on the alkaloid containing plant material based on the varying polarity of the solvents. The amount and type of components separated into different fractions, will vary from plant to plant.

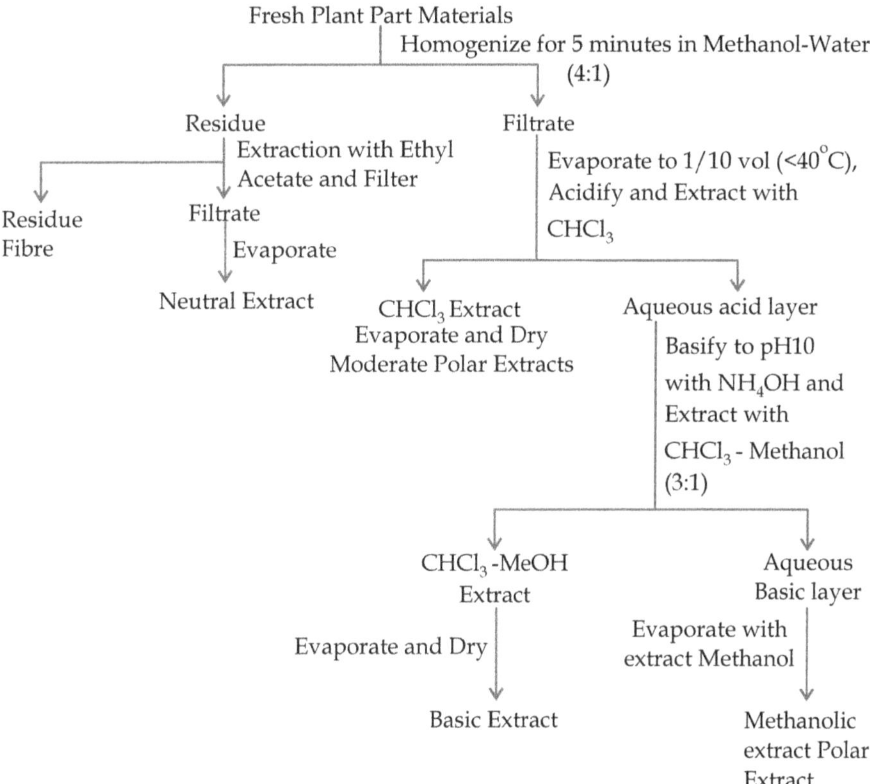

Fig. 9.1 A general procedure for extracting fresh plant tissues and fractionation into different classes according to polarity.

Method of Separation

The separation and purification of plant materials are mostly done by using one or more chromatographic techniques. Paper chromatography (PC), Thin Layer Chromatography (TLC), Gas, Liquid Chromatography (GLC) and High Performance Liquid Chromatography (HPLC) are mainly applied in components separation technique. The selection of chromatography technique depends on the solubility properties and the volatility of the plant compounds to be isolated. Paper Chromatography is mainly useful to water soluble constituents such as carbohydrates, amino acids, nucleic acid bases, organic acids and phenolic compounds. Thin Layer Chromatography is generally applied to the separation of lipids soluble components like lipids, steroids, carotenoids, simple quinine and chlorophyll also. Whereas, Gas Liquid Chromatography is suitable for the separation of compounds which are mainly volatile compounds, fatty acids, mono and sesquiterpenes, hydrocarbons and sulphur compound. There are some compounds which are not separated by GLC due to their low volatility. These plant constituents are converted to ester or trimethylsilyl ether, so that they are completely suitable for the GLC separation. By contrast, the less volatile compounds can be separated by the HPLC technique. In the HPLC technique, both column efficiency and high speed are applied to the analysis of plant materials. Most often a combination of PC and TLC, TLC and HPLC or TLC and GLC are the best choice for separating a particular class of plant component.

There is another technique widely used in phytochemical analysis that is electrophoresis. Initially, this technique was only applicable to the charged compounds such as amino acids, some alkaloids, amines, organic acids and proteins. Some neutral compounds like sugar, phenol are analyzed by electrophoresis but firstly neutral compounds should be converted to a metal complex using electric fields.

Sargent introduces some information on electrophoresis technique in 1969. One such technique: Capillary electrophoresis is carried out in a small bore fused tubes about one meter long. High voltage (30kV) and UV detection is followed during the analysis the plant sample can be applied at the anode end but the concentration should be high. This electrophoresis technique is a suitable analytical technique for the plant secondary metabolites like plant polyphenols (Tomas –Barberan, 1995).

Occasionally, some other separation techniques are also used in the phytochemical research. The simplest liquid-liquid extraction, automatic extraction of Craig counter current distribution apparatus and droplet counter-current chromatography (DCCC) has been developed when techniques fail. Droplet counter current chromatography technique is mainly adopted for the separation of water soluble phytochemicals (Hostettmann et al., 1986). Another separation technique like filtration through Sephadex gels, affinity chromatography and differential ultracentrifugation are mostly taken to the isolation of plant proteins and nucleic acids.

The main separation techniques that are usually applied in the phytochemical research have been discussed here. Chromatography is a process of separation of a mixture into individual components using a stationary phase and a mobile phase. Based on the type of stationary phase and mobile phase, chromatography can be classified into different types. They are gas solid chromatography, gas liquid chromatography, solid liquid chromatography and liquid chromatography. The principle of separation of plant compound can be either absorption or partition. Based on the principle of separation, chromatography can be called as adsorption chromato-graphy (Gas Solid Chromatography, Thin Layer Chromatography, Column Chromatography and High performance liquid chromato-graphy) or partition chromatography (Paper Chromatography).

Paper Chromatography (PC)

Paper chromatography is the technique in which the analysis of unknown substances is carried out by flowing suitable solvent on the specified filter paper. There are two types of paper chromatography. One of them works on adsorption property in which silica or alumina acts as stationary phase and solvent as the mobile phase. This technique is known as Paper adsorption Chromatography. Other one acts on the principle of partition in which moisture or water present in the pore of cellulose fibers in the filter paper functioned as stationary phase and mobile phase are used as solvent. In PC, the principal separation of phytochemicals is generally follows the partition rather than adsorption property. In partition, the phytochemicals are partitioned between a largely water –immiscible alcoholic solvents (like n-butanol) and water. The classic solvent mixture is n-butanol-acetic acid-water (4:1:5, top layer) which is still widely applied as a general solvent for the separation of plant constituents. In general, pure water is a versatile chromatography solvent to be used for the separation of purines, pyrimidines, phenolic compounds and plant glycosides.

These are commercially available with different types of filter paper which are used in paper chromatography. The choice of filter paper depends upon the techniques, thickness, flow rate and purity of plant constituents. The polarity of cellulose paper can be reduced by incorporating silicic acid or alumina into the papers which are suitable for the separation of lipids. The paper can be modified by soaking them in paraffin or silicone oil in order to carry out 'reverse phase' chromatography.

Whatman filter paper with a different grade is used in PCs. These papers differ in their sizes, shapes, porosity and thickness.

The phytochemicals are usually detected as colored or the UV-fluorescent spots in the paper chromatography. Usually phytochemicals react with the chromogenic reagent used either as a spray or as a dipping to develop the color. For the large sheet, the dipping technique is followed to be an easier one in comparison to spray technique. During the qualitative analysis of plant products through chromatography, Retardation Factor (Rf value) is very important. The Rf value of phytochemical is calculated for identifying the spots. It can be defined as the ratio of distance travelled by the solute to the distance travelled by the solvent front.

$$\text{Rf value} = [\text{Distance travelled by solute} / \text{Distance travelled by solvent front}]$$

The Rf value always appears as a fraction and may lay within the range 0.01 to 0.99. Ideally, Rf values are from 0.3 to 0.8. The Rf value is specific and constant for every plant compound in a particular stationary phase and mobile phase. When Rf value of a sample and reference compound is same, sample compound is identified by its standard. If it differs, the compound may be different from its reference standard.

The great advantage of the PC is that the separation is carried out on sheets or filter paper which act as both mediums for the isolation and the supporting material. Reproducibility of Rf value is an important parameter for a new plant compound.

Thin Layer Chromatography (TLC)

The principle of separation of thin layer chromatography is adsorption. One or more phytochemical constituents are spotted on the thin layer of adsorbent (Stationary phase) coated on a chromatography plate. The mobile phase (Eluent) solvent flows through the stationary phase due to capillary action (against the gravitational force). The components move according to their affinity towards the adsorbents. Plant components having higher affinity towards the stationary phase travels faster. So, the separation of components on the thin layer chromatography plate depends on the affinity of components towards the stationary phase.

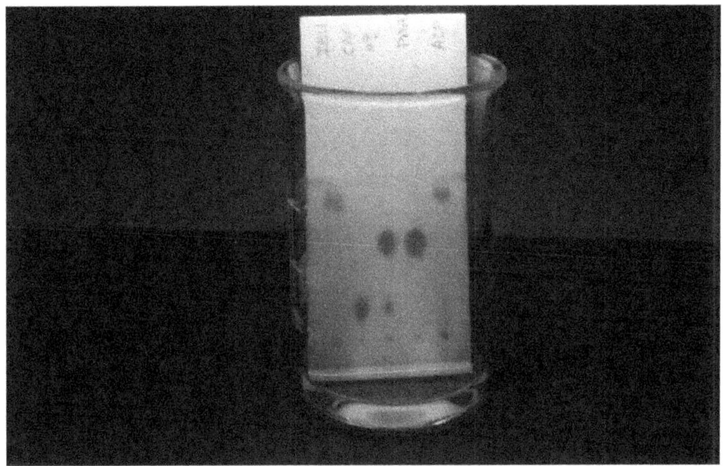

Fig. 9.2 Thin layer chromatographic technique.

TLC is more preferable in comparison to PC because of versatility, speed and sensitivity. Versatility of TLC is due to the different types of adsorbent may be spread onto a glass plate or other supporting materials employed for chromatography. Silica gel is the most widely used adsorbent in TLC. The adsorbent layer may be made up of aluminum oxide, celite, calcium hydroxide, Sephadex, poly vinyl pyrrolidone, cellulose and a mixture of two or more of the above materials. Speed of TLC is high due to the compactness of adsorbent on the TLC plate. It is advantageous for the liability compounds. The sensitivity is high because separation of fewer amounts of plant materials can be achieved. The advantage of TLC is the labor of spreading glass plate with adsorbents. The glass plate should have been cleaned carefully with acetone to remove grease. The slurry of silica gel in water should be vigorously shaken at a time interval before spreading on the plate. Due to variation in particle size of adsorbents, calcium sulfate hemihydrates (15%) may be added to help bind the adsorbent on the glass plate. The slurry or the mixture of stationary phase and water is prepared according to the required ratio. After the preparation of the slurry, the TLC plates can be prepared by following any of the techniques. Generally used techniques are pouring, dipping, spreading and spraying. Among these techniques, spreading is the best technique where the TLC spreader is used. The thickness of the stationary phase is adjusted by using a knob in the spreader. The thickness of the adsorbent layer is 0.25mm and 2mm when it is used for analytical and preparative purpose respectively. After spreading adsorbents, the plate should be allowed for setting (air dried). This is done to avoid the cracks in the surface of the stationary phases. After setting, the plates are activated by heating in an oven for 30 minutes at 100-110°C. Activation of the plates is the process where the moisture and the other adsorbed substances are removed from the surface of the adsorbent. In some cases, properties of adsorbents are modified by adding an inorganic salt (silver nitrate for argentation TLC) and it is carried out when the plates are being spread. The moisture content of silica gel can be controlled by using coated plate in the laboratory which is a crucial factor during the separation of some plant components.

Application of sample on the TLC plate is an important matter. To get a good spot, the concentration of the sample or the standard solution should be less. 2-5μL of 1% solution is spotted using a capillary tube or a micropipette. The spots should be kept at least 2cm above the base of the TLC plate. It is also kept in mind that the spotting area should not be immersed in the mobile phase in the development chamber.

Nowadays, pre-coated plates are mostly used in commercial purpose. They provide more uniform and reproducible results. The plates are available with different adsorbents, coated on a glass, aluminium sheets or plastic. These plates may be with or without a fluorescent indicator, when plates are observed in UV light of 254nm wavelength. Recently, TLC plate is coated with fine micro particles of silica that is used in the column for HPLC. It is popularly known as High Performance Thin Layer Chromatography (HPTLC). This chromatography is more efficient and effective in the rapid separation of plant components than the conventional chromatography.

The mobile phase used in TLC depends on the different factors. Some of the factors are nature of substances to be separated, nature of stationary phase used and the mode of chromatography that is normal phase or reverse phase chromatography. The solvent used in chromatography is a pure solvent or the mixture of solvents. Solvents are used in TLC according to their higher polarity. The solvent composition is carried out by trial and error method with considering the solubility, the polarity of the compounds. The Rf values of plant components in TLC are less reproducible than the paper chromatography. So, one or more reference compound as markers is included to standardize the condition for an accurate measurement of Rf value. During the development of the TLC plate, a developing tank or chamber of different sizes is used. The new development tank has a hump in the middle of the chamber which reduces the solvent. The development chamber should be lined inside a filter paper with the mobile phase. So, the atmosphere inside the chamber is saturated with the mobile phase. If the saturation of the atmosphere inside the chamber is not done, edge effect occurs where the solvent front in the middle of the TLC plate goes faster than on the edge. As a result, the spots on the TLC plate are distorted and not regular.

The detection of compounds on the TLC plate is carried out by visualizing the color spotsbut for the detecting colorless spots, any of the following techniques are employed. These are nonspecific and specific methods. In non specific method, Iodine chamber method, Sulphuric acid spray reagent, UV chamber for fluorescent compounds and Flourescent stationary phase are included. In the Iodine chamber method, brown or amber color spots on the TLC plate are observed when the plates are kept in the chamber with little iodine crystal at the bottom. Sulphuric acid reagent is a mixture of 70-80% of sulphuric acid with little potassium dichromate/ potassium permanganate or few mL of nitric acid. Here nitric acid is used as an oxidizing agent. This reagent is sprayed on the TLC plate and then heated in an oven. Black spots are noticed due to charring of compounds. If the compounds are observed under the UV chamber at 254nm (Short Wave length) or at 365nm (Long wavelength), bright fluorescent spots are seen under the black background. When the TLC plates are kept under the UV chamber, the dark spots are observed on the fluorescent stationary (Silica gel GF) background.

Specific visualizing agents are used to identify the compounds. Ferric chloride for phenolic or tannin, Ninhydrin in acetone for amino acids, Dragendroff'sreagent for alkaloids, 3,5 Dinitro benzoic acid for cardiac glycosides and 2,4 Dinitophenyl hydrazine for aldehydes and ketones are used in specific method. Densitometer is used to measure the density of the spots.

Gas Liquid Chromatography

Gas chromatography is mainly gas solid chromatography and Gas liquid Chromatography. In both types of chromatography, gas is used as the mobile phase and either solid or liquid is used as the stationary phase. The principle of separation of a compound in GLC is partitioned. Gas is used as mobile phase and liquid which are coated on to a solid support is used as the stationary phase. The mixture of compounds is to be separated firstly, converted to vapor state and then mixed with the mobile phase. The plant constituent having high solubility in the stationary phase moves slower and elute later. No compound has the same partition co-effieicent for a fixed combination of stationary phase, mobile phase. The compound can be separated according to their partition co-efficient. Partition co-efficient can be defined as the ratio of the solubility of a substance distributed between two immiscible liquids at a constant temperature and pressure. The equipment or apparatus used in GLC is more sophisticated, expensive in comparison to a PC or TLC. GLC consists of four main apparatus. These are column, heater, flow of gas and a detection device. The column is a long narrow tube usually made up glass or stainless steel in the form of coil to conserve space. It is packed with a stationary phase on an inert material. The column can be classified according to their nature and use. Depending on its use, the column may be analytical or preparative type. On the basis of nature of column, it may be packed column or capillary column and coated open tubular column. The heater is provided to heat the column at a constant rate from 50 to 350°C. Pre-heater is used in GLC to convert the sample into its vapor state and mix them with the mobile phase (Carrier gas). Carriers gas is generally inert in nature like nitrogen or argon. They are stored under high pressure. The regulator is used to deliver the gas with uniform pressure and flow rate. The separation of compounds depends on the rate of passing of vapor through the column. Detectors are the important device for the Gas Liquid

Chromatography. It is considered as the heart of the apparatus. The requirement of an ideal detector isapplying to a wide range of samples, high sensitivity, rapid response,linearity and simple and easy to maintain. A detector device is required to measure the compounds as they are left in the column. The detector device is connected to the potentiometer recorder, which produces the results of the separation in the form of a series of peaks with different intensity. Different type of detectors commonly used in GLC is Thermal Conductivity Detector (TCD), Flame Ionization Detector (FID), Argon Ionization Detector (AID) and Electron Capture Detector (ECD). The result of GLC can be expressed in terms of retention of volume, which is the volume of gas required to elute a component or sample from the column.

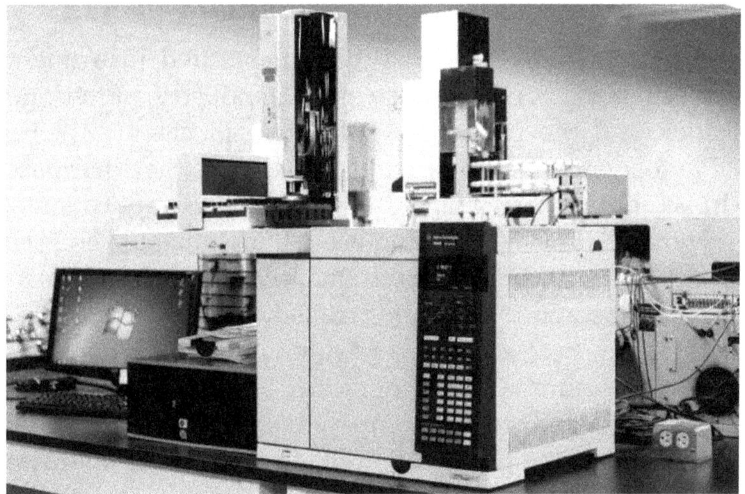

Fig. 9.3 Gas Liquid Chromatography (GLC) equipment.

Highly variable things in GLC are the nature of the stationary phase and the operative temperature. Variability of GPC's properties mainly depends on the polarity and volatility of plant compound to be separated. Some plant compounds are not isolated in the original state. So these classes of compounds are firstly converted to a derivative and then subjected to separation through the Gas Liquid Chromatography. Quantitative and Qualitative analysis of plant products can be carried out by GLC by measuring the area under the peaks on the GLC trace which are related to the concentration of different components in the mixture. There are two formulas which are used to measure the area.

1. Area= peak height X Peak width at half the height= 94% of the peak area
2. Peak area is equivalent to that of a triangle produced by drawing tangents through the points of inflection.

The peak area can be measured automatically by using an electronic integrator. The different apparatus of GLC can be arranged in such a way that the separated compounds can be further analyzed through mass spectroscopy or combined GC-MS apparatus. These techniques are employed for the analysis of phytochemicals (Simpson 1970).

There are so many books and reviews on GLC, related to phytochemical analysis.

High Performance Liquid Chromatography (HPLC)

HPLC is being widely used highly sophisticated instrument. It is used in chemical and petrochemical industry, Environmental Application and the Forensic Application, Biochemical separation Food, Phytochemical analysis and broadly in the Pharmaceutical field. In actual fact, nowadays, there is no such application area of analysis where HPLC is not being used. It is a versatile and sensitive technique which can provide both quantitative and qualitative data in a single operation. It is also called as high pressure liquid chromatography because high pressure is applied when compared to the classical column chromatography. The apparatus for HPLC is highly sensitive and costly compared to GLCbecause of all the connection within the HPLC is jointed with screw to withstand the high pressure and also a suitable pumping system is attached. The mobile phase used in HPLC is mainly a miscible solvent mixture which may either remain isocratic or may be changed continuously in its required proportion from a chamber. The column is packed with very small spherical particles of silica coated or bonded with the stationary phase. Smaller spherical particles are important because they offer more surface area over the conventional larger particles. These particles are highly sensitive to poisonous impurities. So, before injecting the plant extracts, it is essential to purify and filter the sample mixture. HPLC differs from GLC that it's a stationary phase bonded to a porous polymer which is kept in a narrow-bore stainless steel column. The liquid solvent mixture is forced through the column under the controlled pressure. The principle of separation in HPLC is adsorption. When mixtures of phytochemicals are introduced into the HPLC column, they travel according to their relative affinities towards the stationary phase. The plant component has more affinity towards the stationary phase, travel slower. The compounds are eluted off the column by means of a detector. The whole operation in HPLC can be controlled through a microprocessor. The temperature of the operation can be re-arranged in HPLC whereas it is remained fixed in GLC. HPLC is mainly used for the separation of the compounds which are mostly non-volatile in nature. These are higher terpenoids, phenols, alkaloids, lipids and all types of sugar. HPLC is the best application in the area where the phytochemicals can be detected in the ultraviolet or visible region of the spectra. HPLC is the latest technique to be used in the analysis of phytochemicals.

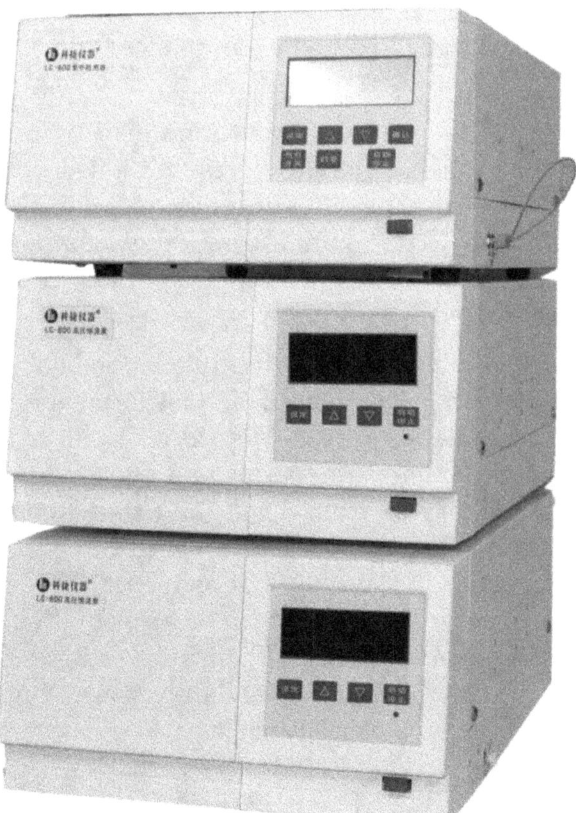

Fig. 9.4 High Performance Liquid Chromatography (HPLC) equipment.

Methods of Identification

After the separation and purification of plant compounds, it has been identified to know the class of the compound and then has been found out the particular component which is present in isolated parts. The single spot is essential for the testing of homogeneity of the compound in TLC or by otherChromatography. The compound should be clear in response to color test or its solubility or its RF value and its UV spectral characteristics. To complete the identification, Physicochemical properties of plant compound are compared with the data collected from the literature or authentic materials. These properties include melting points, boiling points, optical rotation and RF value under standard conditions.

The identification of plant compounds can also be obtainedthrough the spectral characteristics like Ultraviolets (UV), Infrared (IR), Nuclear magnetic resonance and Mass spectral measurements.

The known sample can usually be identified by using authentic materials or the available literature data. For a new compound, it is followed to confirm the identification through the chemical degradation or by the synthesizing the compounds in the laboratory. The identification of new compounds can also be done by X-ray crystallography technique.

Spectroscopy can be defined as the interaction between molecules or atoms or ions of a compound and electromagnetic radiation. Electromagnetic radiation may be absorbed or emitted whereas the energy of the molecule moves from one energy state to another state. This change may be from the ground state to an excited state or an excited state to ground state. In the ground state, molecules reserve the energy as the sum of rotational energy, vibration energy and electronic energy. This energy can be measured with the help of spectroscopy. The EMR is a different form like visible radiation, UV radiation, IR radiation, Microwave, Radiowaves, X-ray or Cosmic ray. They are different in their wavelength, frequency and energy.

Ultraviolet and Visible Spectroscopy

Any colored substance to the naked eye will absorb radiation in the region of 400nm-800 nm but for colorless compounds, the range is

200nm-400nm. The colored substances absorb light of different wavelength in a different manner and finally were getting an absorption curve (Absorbance Vs Wavelength) in a unique pattern. In the absorption curve of plant substance, the wavelength at which the maximum absorbance of radiation is happing that is called Lamda Max. It is not usually affected by the concentration of a substance and mostly useful in identifying the plant substance. The absorption spectra of plant materials can be determined by using a dilute solution (10-50µg/mL) against a blank solvent.

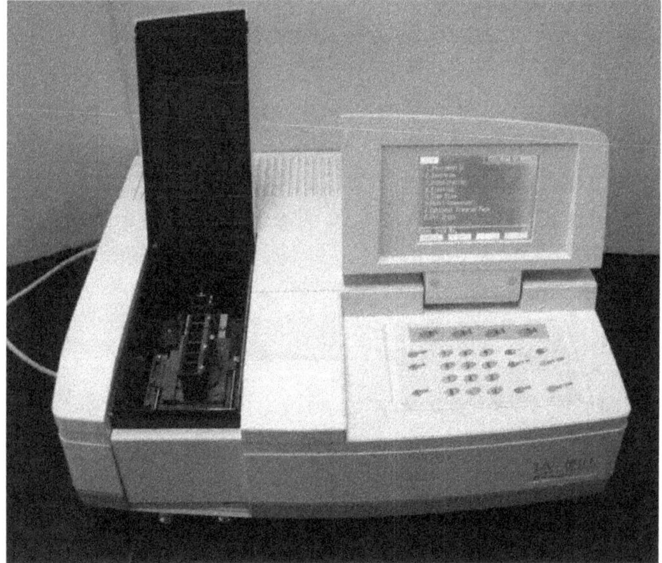

Fig. 9.5 Ultraviolet and Visible Spectroscopy equipment.

The cuvette cell (Sample cell) is used to hold the sample solution. The geometry and materials used in preparing the sample cell depend on the instruments and the sample solution to be handled. The material in a sample cell should not absorb the radiation to be applied in the sample solution. The sample cell volume of 0.5mL to 10 mL and path length of the sample 1cm to 10cm is available. Polystyrene cell is used foraqueous but not in organic solution. Quartz cell is used in the UV region. The solvent used in UV spectroscopy is 95% ethanol. The plant compounds are soluble in ethanol. Commercial ethanol should not be used because it contains residual benzene, which absorbs radiation in the short wavelength whereas chloroform and pyridine are generally not taken since they absorb radiation in the region of 200-600nm.

For the crystalline products, the intensity of wavelength maxima is expressed as logs, where formula is:A/C1 (A=absorbance, C= concentration in g moles/liter, 1= cell path length in cm). Either the molecular weight or concentration is not known, the absorbance value should be considered and Lamda Max may be taken as the most intense peak.

During the spectral study, plant compound should be highly purified otherwise it shows a characteristic properties. Until the absorption properties become constant, the plant materials should be repeatedly purified. The spectral measurement for the identification purpose can be greatly affected by either different pH values or the presence of particular inorganic salts in neutral solution. For example, if alkali is added into an alcoholic solution of a phenolic compound, the Lamda Max extends to longer wavelength (Bathocromic shift or Red shift) with increase in absorbance but alkali is added to the neutral solution of aromatic carboxylic acids. The shift leads a shorter wavelength that is known as hypothermic shifts or blue shift.

Infrared (IR) Spectroscopy

The name of IR spectroscopy is vibrational spectroscopy. It deals with the study of absorption infrared radiation which results in vibrational transitions. IR spectra are mainly applied to the plant substances to determine functional groups in the structure. It is already established that atoms or groups of atoms in a molecule are connected by bonds. These bonds are analogous to the springs. They are not rigid in nature. Due to the continuous motion of molecules, the bonds are vibrated with some frequency. This is known as the natural frequency of vibration. Absorption of IR radiation takes place and exposes a peak when the applied infrared frequency comes to equal with the natural frequency of vibration of bonds in molecules. Due to absorption of different frequency, individual bonds or functional groups show the characteristic peak. IR spectra may be observed in solution in chloroform or carbon tetrachloride (1-5%) as a ponder with specific oil or in solid state, mixed with potassium bromide.

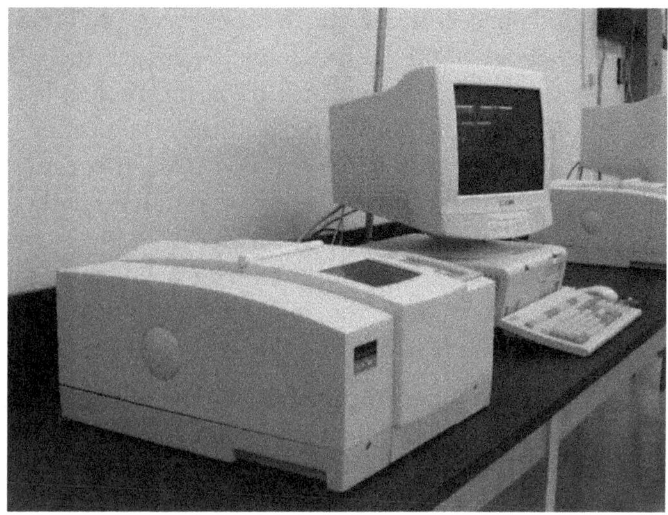

Fig. 9.6 Infrared (IR) Spectroscopy equipment.

List of characteristics and frequency of some important natural products:

S. No.	Common Functional Group	Position of Characteristic Band (cm^{-1})
1	Alkanes [C-H Stretching] and [C-H Bending]	2950-2860 and 1460-1380
2.	Alkenes [C-H Stretching] and [C=C Stretching]	3050-3010 and 1680-1650
3.	Aromatic [C-H Stretching], [C-H Bending] and [C=C Stretching]	3050, 700-860 and 1600-1500
4.	Alcohols [C-O Stretching] and [O-H Bending]	1400-1250 and 1000-1150
5.	Phenol [C-O Stretching] and [O-H Bending]	1800-1660, 1300-1400 and 1200
6.	Alkynes [C=C Stretching]	2300-2150
7.	Aldehyde [C=O Stretching]	1820-1680
8.	Ketones [C=OStretching]	1760-1705
9.	Ester [C=O Stretching]	1750-1700
10.	Lactones	2220
11.	Carboxylic Acids	2280
12.	Amine [N-H Stretching]	3600-3200
13.	Sulfide [S-H Stretching]	2610-2500
14.	Finger point region	1300-400

The range of measurement in IR spectra is 400-667 cm^{-1}. IR spectrum region above 1200-cm indicates the peaks due to vibration of individual bonds or functional groups in the molecules, whereas below 1200-cm shows the bonds/peaks due to vibration of whole molecules. The IR spectrum below 1200-cm is the region that is known as 'Fingerprint' region. The most reliable method for the identification of functional groups in molecules is the measurement of the IR spectrum. IR spectroscopy can be used as fingerprint in phytochemical studies where the natural sample compounds are compared with a synthetic sample in this IR spectrum region.

Two natural samples are closely similar in chemical structure but they can be identified with the help of IR spectra. On the basis of IR absorption spectra, IR spectroscopy can also contribute to elucidate the chemical structure of a new plant compound.

Mass Spectroscopy

Biochemical research on natural products has been eased by the application of mass spectroscopy. It provides the information about the molecular weight of a compound which is microgram in quantity.

The molecular weight of a compound can be determined in several ways. One such method is mass spectroscopy. Not only for molecular weight but also it is useful for structure elucidation. Mass spectroscopy is also known as a positive ion or line spectra. It is applied electron bombardment to convert a neutral molecule to a positive charge tangent. So, the molecule becomes a positively charged particle. The sample should be vapor to form and is allowed through the sample unit. The positively charged ions are separated from the molecules according to their mass. The equation is (*m/e* is proportionate to *r*). Where e= charge of ion, m= mass and r= radius of ion particles.

UV and IR spectroscopy are generally operated by the phytochemist, whereas the mass spectra and NMR spectroscopies are handled by the trained personnel because these instruments are more expensive and sophisticated. The plant compounds which are in volatile in nature are first converted to trimethyl silyl ether, methyl ester or other derivatives, then vaporized in the MS instruments. MS associated with GLC is applied to identify the structural complex compounds which may be present in a particular plant extract.

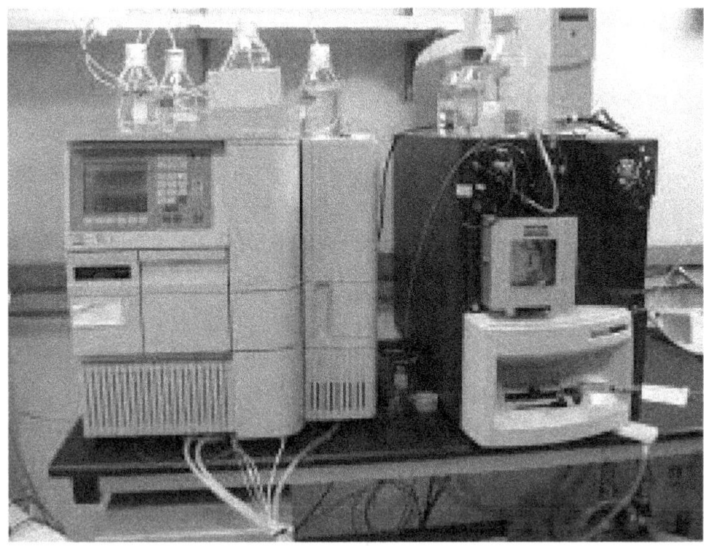

Fig. 9.7 Mass Spectroscopy equipment.

The new technique is developed to continue the emerging of spectral analysis in mass spectroscopy with Fast Atom Bombardment (FAB). By using only MS, it is difficult to detect different type of glycoside (O-glycosidic sugar) of sugar in the analysis of plant glycosidesbut it is now easy to identify the original glycoside sugar by applying HAB –MS.

Nuclear Magnetic Resonance Spectroscopy (NMR)

NMR spectroscopy is the study of spin changes at the level of nucleus of an atom due to absorption of radiofrequency energy in the presence of a magnetic field. The nucleus of atoms having an odd mass number gives NMR spectra like 1H, 13C, 35Cl etc.because they have the asymmetrical charge distribution. They have a spin quantum number like1/2, 3/2, 5/2. 1H has ½ and (2I+1) orientation. On the other hand 12C, 16O, 14N etc. do not give NMR spectra because of symmetrical charge distribution and their spin quantum number is an integral value.

Where, I= spin quantum number of atoms. The numerical value of I related to the mass number and atomic number of isotopes. By the help of an external magnetic field, the proton or nucleus with odd mass number spin on its own axis and a magnetic moment is created and result with a frequency called as processional frequency.

This state is known as the ground state. So, when the applied frequency is equal to the processional frequency, the absorption of energy happens and an NMR is recorded. Due to the absorption of energy, the protons or nucleus moves from ground state to excited state and results in changing in spin orientation. If the application of radio frequency is removed, the proton or nucleus comes down from the excited state to ground state. It should be noticed that with increasing the strength of the magnetic field, does not influence the transition from the ground state to excited state but increase the processional frequency of the proton or nucleus. Without application of an external magnetic field, it is noted that there is only one average spin of the proton. So, the radio frequency cannot be absorbed.

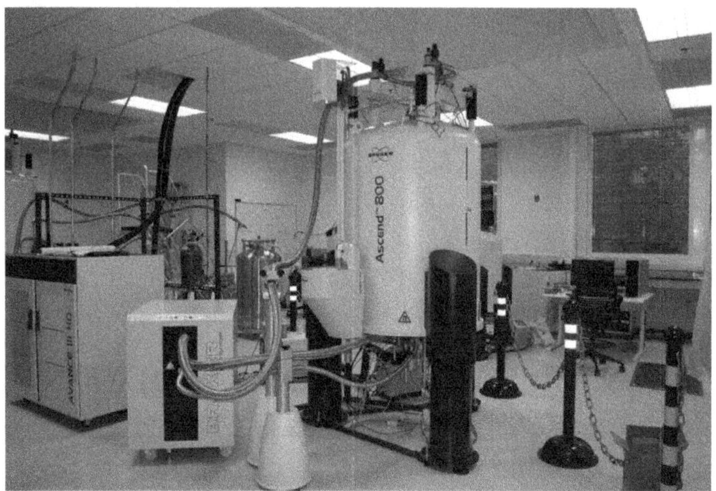

Fig. 9.8 Nuclear Magnetic Resonance Spectroscopy (NMR) equipment.

The nucleus is surrounded by the electrons. So, proton can be present within or outside the circulating magnetic field developed by the circulating electrons present in different types of bonds like double bonds, triple bond, aromatic bond etc. When a proton is present inside the magnetic field created by circulating electrons or close to an electro positive atom. The more external magnetic field is required to cause excitation. Such proton is known as shielded protons. Such effect is called as shielded effects. Whereas proton is present outside the circulating magnetic field or proton is close to an electronegative atom, the less external magnetic field is sufficient for excitation. Such proton is called unshielded proton and the effect is known as deshielded effects.

Due to differences in magnetic field 'H' atoms in a molecule, proton has a different processional frequency and different applied radio frequencies are required for excitation. Finally, the different peaks or signals for different types of proteins are gotten. In practice, the sample substance is mixed in an inert solvent and placed between the pole of a powerful magnet. The protons in a molecule undergo the different chemical shifts according to their shielding or the deshielding effects. The chemical shift is the difference between the absorption position of a sample and a reference compound. Here mostly used reference compound is tetramethylsilane (TMS) which is a mainly an inert compound. Chemical shift can be measured in delta value. It can be expressed in ppm and value range from 0 to 10 delta for the most compounds. The solvent used in NMR spectra should be inert and without protons like carbon tetrachloride, deuteron chloroform ($CDCl_3$) and deuterium oxide (D_2O). Proton NMR may be quite complex. Due to the attachment of protons to adjacent carbon atoms. The signal appears as triplets or doublets instead of a single peak. The weak magnetic moment is generated by 12C compare to a proton. In this case, the signal is much weaker. The solvent used in 13C NMR is same but 13C resonance is much greater about 0-200ppm whereas range from 0-10 ppm. The combination of C NMR and proton NMR spectroscopy is a very useful technique for the elucidation of the structure of new terpenoids, alkaloids, flavonoids and also useful in the analysis of glycosides. Both NMR spectral measurements are successfully used in the structure and analysis of protein as well as others macromolecules.

A plant compound can be identified on the basis of chromatographic and spectral technique by comparing with a standard compound. Chromatography comparison should be based on co-chromatography of the unknown substance with a standard compound by three distinct chromatography properties. There is the retention time by GLC and HPLC and RF on TLC or by RF on PC and TLC and relative mobility on electrophoresis. Practically, spectral measurement of UV, IR, MS and proton NMR should be compared to each others.

Analysis of Results

Ideally, phytochemical analysis of herb is an established discipline in all branches of plant science. The application of this subject in the biological sphere has been allowed in the last two decades. The subjects like phytogeography, ecology, paleobotany and phytochemical analysis method have become so important for solving different analytical problems. The application of mentioned phytochemical methods in agriculture, nutrition and food industry as well as pharmaceutical research have been increasing undoubtedly. The applications of phytochemical screening techniques are discussed in the following major branches of plant science.

Plant Physiology

The phytochemical analysis technique contributes an important role to plant physiology in determining chemical structure, biosynthesis and mode of action of natural growth hormones. Auxins, cytokinins, obsessions, gibberellins are natural growth hormones. Gibberellin groups of hormones with known structure have similar growth properties. The precise technique is to detect and distinct the gibberellin, is combined GC-MS.

Plant Pathology

The chemical characteristics and identification of phytotoxins and phytoalexins are primarily done by a pathologist using phytochemical analysis technique. Phytotoxins are the microbial synthetic products produced in higher plants due to invade of bacteria or fungi. Whereas phytoalexins are the metabolic products of higher plants, produced in response to microbial attack. The familiar phytotoxins are lycomerasmin and fusaric acids, amino acid derivatives, glycopeptides, naphthoquinone sesquiterpenoids. Some precautions have to be made during isolation and identification of phytotoxins. Some secondary metabolites are considered to be pre-infective substance which imparts an essential function in resistant to plant. The pharmaceutically active plant secondary metabolite may be obtained by applying the cell or tissue culture. For the identification of these plant metabolites, phytochemical analysis technique is used. Production of the requisite structure of secondary metabolite can be done in tissue culture by taking bacterial/fungal cell extract. Sometimes, the radio immune assay technique may be considered in the analysis of alkaloid as secondary metabolites which may be produced in cell culture.

Plant Genetics

The phytochemical analysis mainly applies to high plant genetics in identifying anthocyanins, flavor and carotenoid pigments in different color genotypes of plants. It has been found that plant genetic material has probable pathway of pigment synthesis. Chemical attribution in inherited plant has been successfully solved out by using phytochemical analysis technique. It has recently been used as identification tools for hybrid plants and also in a structure elucidation way as well as in the analysis of genetic varieties within plant populations.

Plant Ecology

There are two research areas in plant ecology, plant–animal and plant-plant interaction. Secondary plant constituents are important in plant ecology. Recently, plant–animal and plant–plant interaction is highly important research area. The secondary plant constituents known to be involved in plant–animalsinteraction are mainly alkaloids, cardiac glycosides, muster oil glycosides, cyanogens, steroids and volatile terpens. Here the plant compound may act as feeding attractants or repellents have some hormonal effects on insects or provides the insects with a defense mechanism against predation. On the other hand, plant –plant interaction where the plants exude from its roots or leaves are used to prevent the growth of other plant species. Generally, plant compounds are either volatile terpenes or simple phenolic acids.

Plant Tissue Culture

Phytochemical analysis plays a major role in plant tissue culture for the analysis and identification of secondary metabolic products. The amount of secondary metabolic products depends on applied plant hormones, the presence of light and factors.

Plant Systematic

At present, on the hybrid discipline between chemistry and taxonomy is rapidly developing that is biochemical systemic or chemotaxonomy. Practically, it deals with the chemical survey of restricted plants and the application of data are utilized in plant classification. The class of compounds comes into the matter are flavonoids, alkaloids, and protein amino acids, terpene and sulfur compounds. These compounds are potentially useful in getting new information for taxonomic purpose. At the highest level of classification, chemical analysis of amino acid sequence of plant proteins has been accounted for systemic problems.

Medicinal Plant Research

The plant kingdom is a huge source of biochemically active molecule and macromolecules but a few numbers of plants with medicinal activity have been passed. Nowadays, major medicine is available for the treatment, comes from plant origin. So, the researchers are highly devoted to phytochemical investigation which is associated with enthnobotanical information. Isolated plant constituents are first for a particular activity and then the active fractions are screened for different type of biological activity by using phytochemical analysis technique. A number of bioassay is now available to the phytochemist to analyze the phytochemicals.

References

1. Bajaj, Y.P.S. (ed.) (1996) *Medicinal and Aromatic Plants,* Volume 9, Springer, Berlin.

2. Buckingham, J. (ed.) (1994) *Dictionary of Natural Products,* Chapman and Hall, London.

3. Dey, P.M. and Harborne, J.B. (eds) (1989-1997) *Methods in Plant Biochemistry,* in 10 volumes, Academic Press, London.

4. Harborne, J.B. (1993) *Introduction to Ecological Biochemistry,* 4th edn, Academic Press, London.

5. Harwood, L.M. and Claridge, T.D.W. (1996) *Introduction to Organic Spectroscopy,*University Press, Oxford.

6. Heftmann, F. (1992) *Chromatography: Fundamentals and Applications of Chromato-graphic and Electrophoretic Techniques,* 5th edn., Elsevier, Amsterdam.

7. Wagner, H. and Bladt, S. (1996) *Plant Drug Analysis,* 2nd edn, Springer, Berlin.

8. Grayer, R. and Harborne, J.B. (1994) *Phytochemistry, 37,19.*

9. Harbome, J.B. (1969) *Phytochemistry 8,* 419.

10. Hostettmann, K. (ed.) (1991) *Methods in Plant Biochemistry*, Vol. 6, *Assays for Bioactivity*, Academic Press, London.

11. Orians, C.M. (1995) /. *Chem Ecol*, 21, 1235.

12. Stafford, A.M. and Pazole, C.J. (1997) in *Phytochemical Diversity - A Source of New Industrial Products* (ed. by S. Wrigley, M. Hayes, R.

13. Thomas and E. Chrystal), Royal Society of Chemistry, Letchworth, Herts. Tomas-Barberan, F.A. (1995) *Phytochemical Analysis* 6,177.

14. Sankar, R. S. (2010) *Text book of Pharmaceutical Analysis*, 4th edn, RX Publications, Tirunelveli-627006, India.

15. Sharma, Y.R. (2013) Elementary Organic Spectroscopy, Principles and Chemical Applications, fifth revised edn, S. Chand and Company PVT. LTD., New Delhi-110055, India.

Appendix

A) The Foods that prevent Cancer
- Eat plenty of fruits and vegetables
- Sip green tea throughout your day
- Eat more tomatoes
- Use olive oil
- Snack on grapes
- Use garlic and onions abundantly
- Eat fish

B) Foods to fight cancer

12 foods to fight cancer:

One of the easiest things for a person touched by cancer to address is their diet. And here are 12 foods from it that can each play a role in fighting one or more steps in the multi-step cancer process. Remember that ´good nourishment´ is a crucial weapon in the fight against cancer and any illness. Good cancer nutrition can be vital in increasing your personal odds of survival. Remember too that bioactive natural compounds are likely to do you a lot more good than synthetic pills! Many such compounds have strong and proven benefits.

So here are a few additions to your cancer diet, as a part of your own Integrated Cancer Treatment Programme.

1. **Oily-Fish**

   Fish oil will provide long chain omega-3, a powerful anti-inflammatory in the body that minimizes COX-2 and its abilities to drive localised negative hormones called eicosanoids which cause inflammation - driving cancer and metastases. Omega-3 has been shown to re-lengthen telomeres, which shorten when you have cancer putting the DNA structure at risk and reducing longevity. Fish oils also contain vitamin A, an important vitamin in the fight against cancer (herring, mackerel and salmon are top of the list). Fish oils have been linked to reduced levels of prostate, breast and colon cancer. Research shows they help prevent cachexia when having chemotherapy. You'll also get a little vitamin D is short-chain from them, another proven cancer-fighter. Omega 3 from fish is an important ingredient in your cancer diet. Please note that the omega 3 from flaxseed, equally important but has different benefits (for example, it helps oxygenate the tissues and provides essential fibre).

2. **Carotenoids-Carrots, peppers and greens**

   Along with apricots, red and yellow peppers, greens like kale and spinach and sweet potatoes, carrots provide anti-cancer carotenoids like beta-carotene, which converts to vitamin A, as and when required by the body. 1 cup of carrot juice, 2 sweet potatoes, 16 dried apricots and 4 cups of red cherries will each provide 25 mgs. Don't eat them all at once - people have been known to turn a little orange! A great juice to make yourself involves greens, sweetened by carrots and apples (for quercitin) and beetroot (for anthocyanins) with a helping of calming raw ginger. A real cancer fighting drink! Carotenoids are also found in natural food sources such as chlorella. Raw carrots are also high in pectins - your helpful gut bacteria will love you for eating pectins and give you more in return. A red pepper is the top source of vitamin C in the UK - even better than oranges.

3. **Ginger**

   Fresh, raw ginger has a number of very important benefits in cancer. It is a terrific anti-inflammatory agent in the body and reduces the effects of COX-2. This produces benefits throughout the body and especially in the gut, reducing rates of cancer spread. It also lowers blood sugar levels, and gingerols have been shown to have effects against prostate, breast, leukaemia and other cancer cells. Grate 5 gms or more of ginger each day into your juices. It is also full of helpful vitamins and minerals and is anti-parasitic.

4. **Seeds**

   Seeds are full of good oils, whole vitamins in a natural form (like vitamin E) and fibre to strengthen your gut flora. People who consume the highest levels of natural fibre have higher immune systems. For example:

Sunflower Seeds

High in zinc and natural vitamin E. Zinc helps vitamin C do its work and accelerates healing time. It is important to a healthy prostate. You need 15 to 25 mgs per day. Five tablespoons of sunflower seeds give you 10 mgs. Sunflower seeds will also provide a little selenium.

Pumpkin Seeds

Can be mixed with the sunflower seeds in your morning muesli. 5 tablespoons will each provide 20 mgs of vitamin E, the ultimate cancer buster, which inhibits cancer cell growth and protects immune cells from free radicals. Vitamin E boosts your immune system's fighting abilities. The target is 300-600 mgs and is difficult to achieve without supplements.

Sesame Seeds

The unique lignans can reduce blood pressure and lipid levels. Research shows they can fight inflammation and also cancer! Gamma tocopherol vitamin E reduces inflammation around the body. Both sesame and flax lignans are converted to compounds that can arrest oestrogen cancers.

5. **Nuts**

   Six cracked brazil nuts will give you your daily selenium; 100 to 200 mcgs is the goal. Selenium is a very potent anti-cancer agent. Eight slices of whole meal bread, an organic egg, or a large chicken breast will also be enough.

   (Tuna, onions, broccoli and tomatoes contain selenium too.)

   Walnuts and almonds are a helpful additions to your diet because they contain good oils and high natural fibre. People who eat nuts every day live longer according to research in Cancer Watch.

6. **Mushrooms**

   There's an enormous body of research evidence now that shows how 'medicinal' mushrooms (Shiitake, Maiitake, cordyceps etc) boost the immune system and fight cancer. Even the button mushroom has cancer fighting ingredients. We have a great review on medicinal mushroom.

7. **Tomatoes**

   Seven to ten helpings per week, especially cooked.

According to Harvard research 7-10 helpings a week cuts prostate symptoms by 40% and has an influence on many cancers e.g.: lung; colon; cervix; breast. Lycopene is the prime active ingredient, and 25 - 40 mgs the desired daily dose.

It is also found in strawberries, peppers, carrots and peaches, but one tin of tomato soup has 65 mgs alone. Lycopene helps reduce 'bad´ fat levels in the blood stream and is a strong antioxidant.

8. **Green leafy vegetables**

Along with avocado, beans, carrots, apricots, pumpkins, and egg yolk green vegetables will give you folic acid if your gut bacteria are strong.

This will help your DNA to replicate properly and protect it during radiotherapy.

400 micrograms is a recommended amount. Folate, biotin, choline and inositol, niacin and vitamin B12 are all B vitamins that help in the cancer fight. Niacin has been shown to kill cancer cells. Egg yolk, greens and whole grains are the best sources.

It doesn´t just stop there. Green vegetables and sprouting seeds are a source of sulforaphanes which have strong epigenetic (cancer correcting) benefits and have been shown to aid survival from colorectal cancer.

A diet rich in greens will help alkalyse your body. A slightly alkaline body is important as it improves the performance of your immune system and research shows it stops new metastases.

9. **Broccoli**

Like other green cruciferous vegetables (e.g. cabbage, kale, Brussels sprouts), broccoli contains fibre which helps eliminate toxins

Moreover, the fibre is rich in galactose, which binds to damaging agents in the intestine, and is one of the favourite foods of good, helpful gut bacteria (as are carrots, apples, chicory and onions).

Broccoli also contains indoles, and especially indole 3carbinol which, along with its metabolite DIM, modifies and diminishes aggressive oestrogen action, can modify cellular oestrogen receptor sites, and aids in fighting oestrogen-driven cancers like some breast, prostate, brain and colorectal cancers.

I3C and DIM were also found to have action in non-oestrogen driven cancers as they can also affect the *p27* cancer pathway.

10. **Garlic**

It is a truly wonderful food. Active ingredients like allicin seem to act to stop the spread of cancer in a number of ways, for example by stopping blood supply formation for tumours.

Garlic also kills microbes and yeasts - after taking drugs and antibiotics the body is often susceptible to these. Garlic is also anti-inflamatory in the body. It has a number of active ingredients. It contains selenium, tryptophan and sulphur-based active agents that attack cancer cells.

Two or three raw cloves of garlic raw per day will ward off more than vampires.

11. **Beetroot**

And cherries, aubergines, plums, red grapes - indeed any purple coloured fruits and vegeatables. They contain anthocyanins (and sometimes also resveratrol). Anthocyanins have been shown to kill cancer cells; Resveratrrol has research supporting its role in fighting certain cancers like blood and brain cancers too.

12. **Pulses**

Lentils, chickpeas, beans, peas, kidney beans and even soya beans are a great source of plant protein. Most importantly they release their carbohydrate slowly because of their high fibre content. They reduce blood glucose.

Pulses also contain isoflavones called phytoestrogens. People get confused about plant oestrogen. The cells of your body have oestrogen receptor sites. When one form of human oestrogen (oestradiol) binds to them, the result is havoc inside your cells. About 40 times less potent is human oestrogen oestrone and about 40 to 50 times less potent still are plant oestrogens. Now which would you rather have sitting on your receptors? Pulses also provide fibre like lignans that can help neutralise free-radicals in the gut and blood stream.

Phytoestrogens bind more weakly than human oestrogen and wash through the body - so you need to eat them daily.

Instructions for Patients with Peptic Ulcer

1. Pick four meals a day.

2. Select your meals at periodic times.

3. Consume your meals gradually; masticate your food thoughtfully.

4. Turn aside haste and hustle before and after meals. Relax for a few minutes before and after feeding.

5. Observe that you gain adequate sleep at night.

6. Bear in mind that distress and apprehension can tipped digestion.

7. Escape large, burdensome meals, fried foods and any item of food which you find disagrees with you.

8. Cet away from foods which are mechanically annoying or chemically exhilarating (see list below) and severely hot or intensely cold foods.

9. Do not smoke or consume alcohol prior to meals, when the stomach is vacuous.

10. Consume only sparingly at meals for this will help to assure suitable consumption, but drink abundance of water between meals.

11. Check with your dentist at periodic intervals.

   - *The ensuing foods should lie avoided at the time the acute stage of ulcer and taken sparingly during intermissions by those prone to recurrent attacks of ulcer. For those who sustain from ulcer only infrequently, no special restrictions may be inevitable, by trial and error the patient can find out which of the commodity listed below should be avoided ;*

     1. Alcohol, strong tea and coffee, gravies and soups made from meat extracts.

     2. Raw vegetables, celery, cucumber, onions, radishes, watercress, tomatoes, mushrooms.

3. Raw unripe fruit and dried fruit (e.g. currants, raisins and figs), nuts, and the pips skins and pee! of all fruits, whether cooked or in puddings, cakes or jam.

4. Pickles, spices and condiments.

5. Twice-cooked, or highly seasoned meats, including sausages, bacon and pork.

6. Salted fish and some fatty fish such as herring, mackerel, salmon and sardines.

7. Rich and heavy puddings.

8. Fried foods.

9. New bread and scones, hot buttered toast, whole meal bread or biscuits, rye or wheat crisp brcad, coarse cereals, pastry, cakes containing dried fruit or peel.

10. Excess sugar and sweets.

11. Any food that the particular patient finds to be indigestible.

- *The succeeding foods are permitted :*
    1. Milky tea or milk drink, e.g. Ovaltine.
    2. Dairy products i.e., milk, cream, butter, cream cheese, eggs (not fried).
    3. Fish - white fish, steamed, baked or grilled.
    4. Meat - Chichen, lean ham, tender beef, mutton or lamb.
    5. Crisp toast (buttered cold), rusts and white bread (not new).
    6. Plain biscuits and cakes, e.g. sponge cake. Honey, golden syrup, jellies.
    7. Cereals - refined and well cooked, e.g. cornflour, semolina, ground rice and oat four porridge.
    8. Puddings - junket, jellies, custards, blancmange, souffle, mousse.
    9. Vegetables - potatoes, e.g. creamed or mashed, and green and yellow vegetables finely sieved and purced with butter.
    10. Fruits - stewed and preferably sieved, and served as purees or fools, raw ripe banana and fruit juices, diluted with water, or used in jellies.

Foods for Diabetics

Approximately: Protein 80g, Carbohydrate 180g, Fat 80g, Energy 1,800 kcal (7.5 MJ)

Breakfast

- ✓ 1 protein exchange.
- ✓ 4 carbohydrate exchanges.
- ✓ Butter and milk from allowance.
- ✓ Tea or coffee (no sugar).

Mid-morning

- ✓ 1 carbohydrate exchange.
- ✓ Butter and milk from allowance.
- ✓ Tea or coffee (no sugar).

Mid-day meal

- ✓ Clear soup if desired.
- ✓ 3 protein exchanges.
- ✓ 4 carbohydrate exchanges.
- ✓ Vegetables if desired.
- ✓ Butter and milk from allowance.

Mid-afternoon

- ✓ 1 carbohydrate exchange.
- ✓ Butter and milk from allowance.
- ✓ Tea (no sugar).
- ✓ *Evening meal*
- ✓ 2 protein exchanges.
- ✓ 4 carbohydrate exchanges.
- ✓ Vegetables if desired.
- ✓ Tea or coffee (no sugar).

Before bed

- ✓ 1 carbohydrate exchange.
- ✓ Remainder of butter and milk from allowance.
- ✓ 1 carbohydrate exchange   =   50 kcal
- ✓ Protein exchange   -   70 kcal

✓ Fat exchange   = 110 kcal

✓ one pint of milk   = 410 kcal

(a) *The following foods may be taken in any amount*

✓ Tea, coffee (milk from allowance, no sugar)

✓ Tomato juice,

✓ Lemon juice.

✓ Diabetic fruit, and Sweetex.

✓ Clear soup.

✓ Herbs, seasonings and spices.

✓ Cabbage, carrots, cauliflower, celery, cucumber, French beans, lettuce, mushrooms, mustard or cress, onions, spring onions, runner beans, spinach, tomatoes, watercress.

(b) *The following foods should be taken in consultation with doctor:*

✓ Spirits,

✓ dry wines.

(c) *The following foods are not allowed :*

✓ Sugar,

✓ glucose,

✓ sweets,

✓ chocolate,

✓ honey,

✓ syrup,,

✓ jam,

✓ marmalade,

✓ cakes,

✓ biscuits (except those specified),

✓ pies,

✓ fruit tinned in syrup,

✓ fruit squash,

✓ lemonade, or similar aerated drinks.

Foods for Patients with Cirrhosis of Liver

1. No salt to be used in cooking or at table

2. Avoid all cured meat and fish

3. Avoid all foods made with bicarbonate of soda or baking powder

4. To increase the calories of the foods the following may be added: sugar, fruit, jam, marmalade etc.

5. High protein foods (120 gm) must be provided.

6. Low sodium diet should be allowed usually about 3-6 weeks. By that time if there is no clinical improvement persistence is useless and other therapeutic measures must be tried.

Instruction for patients suffering from arthritis

1. Regular exercise: Both the regulated active type in which muscles will operate the joints' and the passive type, in which the joints are moved by some other force. For active exercise, walking, hiking, swimming, bicycling etc. are approved. Weight lifting, deep knee bends and hard contact sports such as football are avoided. Passive exercise is a way of "Cheating : the muscles against antagonist system to keep the joint active despite painful arthritis. For instance, patient can passively work a shoulder that has been stiffened by bursitis (a form of arthritis) by bending at the waist and swinging the arms like a pendulum.

2. Heat techniques for arthritis patients comprise taking a warm bath or long hot shower soaking hands and   feet in warm water.

3. Any exercise in water (hydrotherapy) is also favored because the water supports 90 per cent of body weight, allowing greater freedom of movement and curtailing the risk of injury.

4. Movement should be slow and gentle. The patients should not exercise beyond the point of pain.

5. Patients should carry a handbag instead of handled purse, slide rather than lift heavy object.

6. Weight control is very significant for arthritis patients. Surplus weight puts extreme stress on weight bearing joints and interfere with smooth functioning of tendons, ligaments and muscles.

7. Refrain from excess carbohydrate, red meat, wine and smoking.

Take green vegetables, fish oil, soybean oil etc. adequately. These foods are rich in PUFF analogues.

Glossary of Botanical Names

A

Alangium amark 198

Acacia arab 43

Ananas saf 106

Abroma augusta 42, 101

Abrus precatorius 101

Acacia catechu 169

Acacia melanoxylon 42

Acacia modesta 43

Acacia nilotica 43

Acanthus ilicifolius 197

Achyranthes aspera 102

Aconitum ferox 43

Acorus Calamus 1-10

Actiniopteris radiata 102

Acunthus ebractectus 1-10

Adhatoda vasica 44, 103, 264

Adiantum capillus 44

Adiantum incisum 45

Aegle marmelos 45, 230

Aeschynomene indica 103

Agrimonia eupatoria 288

Alangium salvifolium 198

Albizia lebbeck 103

Albizia stipulata 46

Allium cepa 46, 104

Allium sativum 47, 104, 169, 198, 230, 283

Aloe barbadensis 48, 105, 264, 285

Aloe ferox 285

Aloe indica Royle 105

Aloe Vera 1-10

Alpina calcarata 199

Alpinia galanga 18, 49, 295

Alpinia officinarum 231

Althaea rosea 265

Ambroma augusta 101

Amoora rohituka 18

Anacardium occidentale 49, 199

Anagallis arvensis 106

Ananas comosus 106

Anaphalis contorta 231

Andrographis paniculata 2-10, 24, 169

Anemone obtusiloba 200

Angustifolia 283

Anisomeles malabarica 107

Anthemis cotula 200

Antirrhinum majus 265

Apiumg raveolens 282

Arctium lappa 49

Arctostaphylos uvaursh 288

Ardisia nerifolia 107

Areca catechu 50, 107

Aristoloca Indica-Iswarmul 2-10

Aristolochia bacteolata 231

Aristolochia indica 108

Arnebia hispidissima 200

Arnebia hispidissinia 4

Arnebia nobilis 232

Artabotrys odorautissimus 108

Artemisia annuta 2

Artemisia capillaries 170